Review and Resource Manual

Acute Care Nurse Practitioner

Volume 2

- CONTINUING EDUCATION RESOURCE
- NURSING CERTIFICATION REVIEW MANUAL
- CLINICAL PRACTICE RESOURCE

Pamela Smith, MSN, RN, ACNP-BC, CCRN
Tiffany Boysen, MSN, RN, ACNP-BC, CCRN
Julie Davey, MSN, RN, APRN-BC
Hope Moser, DNP, ANP, BC
Melanie Smith, MSN, RN, ACNP-BC

NURSING KNOWLEDGE CENTER

Library of Congress Cataloging-in-Publication Data

Acute care nurse practitioner : review and resource manual / by Pamela Smith ... [et al.].
    p. ; cm.
  Includes bibliographical references and index.
  ISBN 9781935213529 (pbk.)
  I. Smith, Pamela (Pamela Ann), 1955 May 11- II. American Nurses Credentialing Center.
  [DNLM: 1. Critical Care–methods–Outlines. 2. Nursing Care–Outlines. WY 18.2]

616.02'8–dc23
                          2011047808

The American Nurses Credentialing Center (ANCC), a subsidiary of the American Nurses Association (ANA), provides individuals and organizations throughout the nursing profession with the resources they need to achieve practice excellence. ANCC's internationally renowned credentialing programs certify nurses in specialty practice areas; recognize healthcare organizations for promoting safe, positive work environments through the Magnet Recognition Program® and the Pathway to Excellence® Program; and accredit providers of continuing nursing education. In addition, ANCC's Institute for Credentialing Innovation provides leading-edge information and education services and products to support its core credentialing programs.

ISBN 13: 9781935213529
© 2011 American Nurses Credentialing Center. 8515 Georgia Ave.,
Suite 400
Silver Spring, MD 20910
Reprinted under license from American Nurses Credentialing Center.
All rights reserved.

Acute Care Nurse Practitioner Review and Resource Manual

JANUARY 2012

Please direct your comments and/or queries to: revmanuals@ana.org

The healthcare services delivery system is a volatile marketplace demanding superior knowledge, clinical skills, and competencies from all registered nurses. Nursing autonomy of practice and nurse career marketability and mobility in the new century hinge on affirming the profession's formative philosophy, which places a priority on a lifelong commitment to the principles of education and professional development. The knowledge base of nursing theory and practice is expanding, and while care has been taken to ensure the accuracy and timeliness of the information presented in the **Acute Care Nurse Practitioner Review and Resource Manual**, clinicians are advised to always verify the most current national guidelines and recommendations and to practice in accordance with professional standards of care used with regard to the unique circumstances that apply in each practice situation. In addition, every effort has been made in this text to ensure accuracy and, in particular, to confirm that drug selections and dosages are in accordance with current recommendations and practice, including the ongoing research, changes to government regulations, and the developments in product information provided by pharmaceutical manufacturers. However, it is the responsibility of each nurse practitioner to verify drug product information and to practice in accordance with professional standards of care. In addition, the editors wish to note that provision of information in this text does not imply an endorsement of any particular products, procedures or services.

Therefore, the authors, editors, American Nurses Association (ANA), American Nurses Association's Publishing (ANP), American Nurses Credentialing Center (ANCC), and the Institute for Credentialing Innovation cannot accept responsibility for errors or omissions, or for any consequences or liability, injury, and/or damages to persons or property from application of the information in this manual and make no warranty, express or implied, with respect to the contents of the **Acute Care Nurse Practitioner Review and Resource Manual**. Completion of this manual does not guarantee that the reader will pass the certification exam. The practice examination questions are not a requirement to take a certification examination. The practice examination questions cannot be used as an indicator of results on the actual certification.

Published by:
American Nurses Credentialing Center
The Institute for Credentialing Innovation
8515 Georgia Avenue, Suite 400
Silver Spring, MD 20910-3402
www.nursecredentialing.org

Introduction to the Continuing Education (CE) Contact Hour Application Process for *Acute Care Nurse Practitioner Review and Resource Manual*

The Institute for Credentialing Innovation now offers the continuing education contact hours for this manual online at www.NursingWorld.org, the American Nurses Association's Web site. This process involves answering approximately 25–30 questions that test knowledge of the information contained within this manual. The continuing education contact hours can be completed at any time and a certificate can be printed from the Web site immediately upon successful completion of the test.

After studying the manual and given an online multiple-choice test, the exam candidate will be able to:

1. Pass the posttest with at least 75% of the answers correct.
2. Select responses to test questions based on key principles, standards of practice, and theoretical basis of nursing practice.
3. Choose accepted therapeutic interventions in answering questions related to quality nursing practice.
4. Utilize direct and indirect professional role responsibilities and applications regarding nursing practice in answering test questions.

Upon completion of this manual *and* the online CE test, a nurse can receive a total of 47 continuing education contact hours at a price of $90, only $2 per CE. (ANA members receive a discount on CEs.) **The entire process—online test and evaluation form—must be completed by December 31, 2013 in order to receive credit.** To begin the process, please e-mail **revmanuals@ana.org**. Your patience with this process is greatly appreciated.

Inquiries or Comments
If you have any questions about the CE contact hours, please e-mail The Institute at revmanuals@ana.org. You may also mail any comments to Editor/Project Manager, at the address listed below.

Duplicate CE Certificates
Once you have successfully passed the CE test, you may go back and re-print your certificate as often as you wish.

Conflicts of Interest
A conflict of interest occurs when an individual has an opportunity to affect educational content about health-care products or services of a commercial company with which she/he has a financial relationship.

The planners and presenters of this CNE activity have disclosed no relevant financial relationships with any commercial companies pertaining to this activity.

The Institute for Credentialing Innovation
American Nurses Credentialing Center
Attn: Editor/Project Manager
8515 Georgia Avenue, Suite 400
Silver Spring, MD 20910-3492
Fax: (301) 628-5342

A maximum of 47 contact hours may be earned by learners who successfully complete this continuing nursing education activity.

The American Nurses Association Center for Continuing Education and Professional Development is accredited as a provider of continuing nursing education by the American Nurses Credentialing Center's Commission on Accreditation.

ANCC Provider Number 0023

ANA is approved by the California Board of Registered Nursing, Provider Number 6178.

The ANA Center for Continuing Education and Professional Development includes ANCC's Institute for Credentialing Innovation.

Acknowledgements

The authors would like to gratefully acknowledge the foundational work provided by the authors of these review manuals:

Elizabeth Blunt, PhD, MSN, FNP-BC
    Editor of *Family Nurse Practitioner Review and Resource Manual, 3rd Edition*
Sally Miller, PhD, ACNP-BC, GNP-BC, ANP-BC
    Author of *Adult Nurse Practitioner Review and Resource Manual, 3rd Edition*

The authors would also like to acknowledge the following contributors for their work on this manual:

Shirlee Drayton-Brooks, PhD, FNP-BC
Deborah Gilbert-Palmer, MSN, RN, CS, FNP
Elizabeth Petit de Mange, PhD, MSN, NP-C, RN

Contents

V	**Introduction to the Continuing Education (CE) Contact Hour Application Process**
VII	**Acknowledgements**
1	**Chapter 1. Taking the Certification Examination** General Suggestions for Preparing for the Exam About the Certification Exams
11	**Chapter 2. Professional Responsibility** *Pamela Smith, MSN, RN, ACNP-BC, CCRN, and Melanie Smith, MSN, RN, ACNP-BC* Acute Care Nurse Practitioner (ACNP)–Patient Relationship ACNP Scope of Practice Ethical and Legal Principles Evidence-Based Practice Healthcare Delivery-Coordinating Patient Focused Care
39	**Chapter 3. General Assessment and Management** *Pamela Smith, MSN, RN, ACNP-BC, CCRN; Julie Davey, MSN, RN, APRN-BC; and Melanie Smith, MSN, RN, ACNP-BC* Assessment of the At-Risk Patient Evaluating the Plan of Care
53	**Chapter 4. Cardiovascular** *Julie Davey, MSN, RN, APRN-BC* Acute Coronary Syndromes and Coronary Artery Disease Contraindications to Thrombolytic Therapy Dyslipidemia Hypertension Heart Failure (HF) Valvular Disease Mitral Regurgitation (MR) Mitral Stenosis (MS) Mitral Valve Prolapse (MVP) Aortic Stenosis (AS) Aortic Regurgitation (AR) Peripheral Vascular Disease (PVD) Deep Vein Thrombosis Pulmonary Hypertension Cardiac Rhythm Disturbances Narrow Complex Supraventricular Tachycardia Ventricular Tachycardia Ventricular Fibrillation Asystole Complete Heart Block (3rd- Degree Atrioventricular Block) Pericarditis Cardiac Tamponade Cardiomyopathy Dilated Cardiomyopathy Hypertrophic Cardiomyopathy Restrictive Cardiomyopathy Anuerysm Endocarditis

111   Chapter 5. Pulmonary Disorders
Julie Davey, MSN, RN, APRN-BC
Chronic Obstructive Pulmonary Disease (COPD: Emphysema and Chronic Bronchitis)
Asthma
Bronchitis (Acute Bronchitis)
Respiratory Infections

147   Chapter 6. Endocrine Disorders
Tiffany Boysen, MSN, RN, ACNP-BC, CCRN; Shirlee Drayton-Brooks, PhD, FNP-BC; and Melanie Smith, RN, MSN, ACNP-BC
General Approach
Red Flags
Diabetes Mellitus
Diabetes Mellitus (Type 1)
Diabetes Mellitus (Type 2)
Diabetes Ketoacidosis (DKA)
Hyperosmolar Hyperglycemic Nonketosis (HHNK)
Hypoglycemia
Thyroid Disorders
Adrenal Disorders

193   Chapter 7. Neurologic Disorders
Tiffany Boysen, MSN, RN, ACNP-BC, CCRN, and Deborah Gilbert-Palmer MSN, RN, CS, FNP
General Approach
Red Flags
Stroke and Transient Ischemic Attack
Incidence and Demographics
Myasthenia Gravis
Guillan Barré Syndrome
Parkinson's Disease
Multiple Sclerosis (MS)
Head Trauma
Spinal Cord Trauma
Meningitis
Seizures and Epilepsy
Alzheimer's Disease (AD)/Multi-Infarct Dementia (MID)
Delirium
Case Studies

251   Chapter 8. Renal and Urologic Disorders
Pamela Smith, MSN, RN, ACNP-BC, CCRN
General Approach
Red Flags
Urologic Disorders
Renal Disorders

311 Chapter 9. Gastrointestinal Disorders
Pamela Smith, MSN, RN, ACNP-BC, CCRN
General Approach
Red Flags
Appendicitis
Acute Cholecystitis
Cirrhosis/Chronic Liver Disease
Crohn's Disease
Diverticulitis/Diverticulosis
Gastrointestinal Bleeding (GIB)
Acute Hepatic Failure
Acute Viral Hepatitis
Large Bowel Obstruction (LBO)
Mesenteric Ischemia
Acute Pancreatitis
Peptic Ulcer Disease (PUD)
Peritonitis
Small Bowel Obstruction (SBO)
Ulcerative Colitis (UC)

397 Chapter 10. Hematologic Disorders
Pamela Smith, MSN, RN, ACNP-BC, CCRN;
Tiffany Boysen, MSN, RN, ACNP-BC, CCRN, and
Elizabeth Petit de Mange, PhD, MSN, NP-C, RN
General Approach
Red Flags
Normocytic Anemias
Hypochromic Anemias
Megaloblastic Anemias
Coagulation Disorders
Oncology
Lymphoid Cancers
Lymphoma
Case Studies

505 Chapter 11. Immunologic Disorders
Pamela Smith, MSN, RN, ACNP-BC, CCRN
General Approach
Red Flags
Acquired Immunodeficiency Syndrome (AIDS) and Human Immunodeficiency Virus Infection (HIV)
Acute Allergic Reactions
Amyloidosis
Sarcoidosis
Scleroderma (Systemic Sclerosis)
Systemic Lupus Erythematosus (SLE)
Immunosuppression

553 Chapter 12. Muscoloskeletal Disorders
Julie Davey, MSN, RN, APRN-BC
Trauma
Degenerative Joint Diseases

575   **Chapter 13. Psychosocial Health Issues**
Julie Davey, MSN, RN, APRN-BC
Violence
Depression
Substance Abuse
Anxiety Disorders
Grief and Bereavement
Sexuality
Powerlessness
Altered Mental Status

603   **Chapter 14. Sexually Transmitted Infections**
Pamela Smith, MSN, RN, ACNP-BC, CCRN
General Approach
Red Flags
Chlamydia
Gonorrhea (GC)
Syphilis
Genital Herpes Simplex Virus (HSV) Infection
Human Papillomavirus Infection (HPV)

633   **Chapter 15. Palliative Care/End-of-Life Care**
Hope Moser, DNP, ANP, BC
Description
Palliative Care
Pain

647   **Chapter 16. Health Promotion**
Julie Davey, MSN, RN, APRN-BC
Diet and Nutrition
Disease Prevention
Recommended Adult Screening Practices
Recommended Adult Immunizations
Additional Risk Assessment Principles
General Influences on Health Care and Treatment Considerations

663   **Chapter 17. Nutritional Imbalances**
Pamela Smith, MSN, RN, ACNP-BC, CCRN
Description
Etiology
Incidence and Demographics
Risk Factors
Prevention and Screening
Assessment
Differential Diagnosis
Management
Special Considerations
When to Consult, Refer, or Hospitalize
Follow-Up

691 **Chapter 18. Transplants**
Melanie Smith, MSN, RN, ACNP-BC
Liver Transplantation
Lung Transplantation
Heart Transplant
Kidney (Renal) Transplant
Pancreas Transplantation
Transplant Terminology
Immunosuppressive Agents

719 **Chapter 19. Fever and Shock**
Pamela Smith, MSN, RN, ACNP-BC, CCRN
General Approach
Red Flags
Fever
Shock

737 **Chapter 20. Fluid, Electrolyte, and Acid–Base Balance**
Pamela Smith, MSN, RN, ACNP-BC, CCRN
Hyponatremia
Hyponatremia
Hypokalemia
Hyperkalemia
Hypocalcemia
Hypercalcemia
Hypomagnesemia
Hypermagnesemia
Hypophosphatemia
Hyperphosphatemia
Acid–Base Disorders
Metabolic Acidosis
Respiratory Acidosis
Respiratory Alkalosis

807 **Chapter 21. Poisoning and Drug Toxicities**
Pamela Smith, MSN, RN, ACNP-BC, CCRN
Specific Poisonings/Toxicities
Antiarrythmic Drug Overdose
Anticholinergic Agents
Anticonvulsant Agents
Antidepressant Toxicity
Antipsychotic Drug Toxicity
Carbon Monoxide Poisoning
Cardiac Glycoside Poisoning
Cholinergic Toxicity
Lithium Toxicity
Opioid Toxicity
Pesticide Poisoning
Salicyclate Toxicity
Sedative-Hypnotic Drug Toxicity
Stimulant Toxicity
Theophylline Toxicity

867   **Chapter 22. Infections**
Pamela Smith, MSN, RN, ACNP-BC, CCRN
Nosocomial Infections
Miscellaneous Nosocomial Infections
Community-Acquired Infections

905   **Appendix A. Immobility**
Pamela Smith, MSN, RN, ACNP-BC, CCRN

911   **Appendix B. Intravenous Fluid Management**
Pamela Smith, MSN, RN, ACNP-BC, CCRN
General Principles
Intravenous Fluid Administration

919   **Appendix C. Bites and Stings**
Pamela Smith, MSN, RN, ACNP-BC, CCRN
Snake Bites
Spider Bites and Scorpion Stings

925   **Appendix D. Wound Care**
Pamela Smith, MSN, RN, ACNP-BC, CCRN

933   **Appendix E. Review Questions**

941   **Appendix F. Answers to the Review Questions**

947   **Index**

963   **About the Authors**

ACUTE CARE NURSE PRACTITIONER REVIEW AND RESOURCE MANUAL

Note About This Two-Volume Set
Thank you for purchasing the Acute Care Nurse Practitioner Review Manual. Please note that this book is printed in two volumes; one volume alone does not contain information covering the entire test content outline for this exam. You will need to purchase both volumes in order to be eligible to obtain the continuing education for this manual.

Please visit www.nursingknowledgecenter.org for complete information on NKC review manuals. You can contact revmanuals@ana.org with any questions.

Immunologic Disorders

Pamela Smith, MSN, RN, ACNP-BC, CCRN

GENERAL APPROACH

- The treatment of patients with immunological disorders requires close monitoring over the patient's lifetime.
- These patients must be educated to obtain yearly influenza vaccinations, recommended cancer screenings, and pnemoccocal vaccine every 5 years, and have at a minimum yearly physical examination.
- Many serology markers overlap among diseases and the diagnosis is based on clinical manifestions, history, and laboratory correlations.

RED FLAGS

- The presence of infection in the immunocompromised patient
- Rapidly progressing multi-organ failure indicates a poor prognosis.
- HIV-positive individuals should be tested for coexisting sexually transmitted infections and treated accordingly.
- Patients presenting with signs and symptoms suspicious for HIV need to be educated regarding the need for testing because 1 in 5 affected people are not aware they are infected.

ACQUIRED IMMUNODEFICIENCY SYNDROME (AIDS) AND HUMAN IMMUNODEFICIENCY VIRUS INFECTION (HIV)

Description

- AIDS is a disease of the human immune system that is caused by HIV.
- It is a progressive disease that eventually disables the immune system and leaves the patient vulnerable to opportunistic infections and tumors.
- HIV infects cells that express the CD4 receptor.
  - Macrophages
  - CD4+ T lymphocytes
  - Monocytes
  - B-lymphocytes
  - Dendritic cells
  - Langerhans' cells of the skin
  - Central nervous system
    - Microglia of the nervous system
    - Astrocytes
    - Oligodendrocytes
    - Neurons—indirectly
- Transmission is through direct contact with a mucous membrane or body fluids such as blood, semen, vaginal fluid, preseminal fluid, and breast milk.
- Transmission may occur during sexual contact (vaginal, anal, oral sex); blood transfusion; the sharing of needles in IV drug users; mother to baby during pregnancy, childbirth, and breastfeeding; or exposure to the previously mentioned bodily fluids.
- HIV originated in west-central Africa during the late 19th or early 20th century.
- AIDS was first recognized in the United States by the Centers for Disease Control (CDC) in 1981, and HIV was identified in the early 1980s.

Etiology

- HIV
- Belongs to the family of human retrovirusis (*Retroviridae*) and the subfamily of lentiviruses

Incidence and Demographics

- CDC estimates there are more than 1 million people living with HIV in the United States.
  - 1 in 5 of these are unaware they are infected.
- The annual new numbers of HIV infections has remained stable.
  - 56,300 new HIV infections each year
    - Estimated rate of new AIDS cases in the United States per 100,000 adults/adolescents is 59.2 Blacks, 20.4 Latinos, 8.6 Native American/Alaskans, 6.1 Whites, 4.3 Asians, and 22.3 Pacific Islanders.

- There are an estimated 468,478 persons in the United States living with AIDS.
  - 76% are men, of whom 60% were exposed through male-to-male sexual contact, 18% were exposed through IV drug use, 11% were exposed through heterosexual contact, and 8% were exposured through both male-to-male sexual contact and IV drug use.
  - Women account for 23% of those with AIDS; 66% were exposed through heterosexual contact and 32% through IV drug use.
  - Children account for < 1% of living persons with AIDS
  - Approximately 18,000 patients die from AIDS each year.
- Worldwide there are an estimated 33.4 million persons infected with HIV.

Risk Factors

- Men who have sex with men
- IV drug use
- Women infected with HIV who are pregnant (transmission to infant)
- Unprotected sex
- High-risk sexual behavior
- Healthcare worker
  - Needlestick injury
  - Blood splatter
  - Dental procedures
- Presence of STIs
- Exposure to bodily fluids
- Uncircumcised male

Prevention and Screening

- Avoid unprotected sex
  - Use of male or female condoms
- Avoid multiple sex partners
- Avoid sharing needles during IV drug use
- To prevent mother-to-infant transmission
  - Azidothymidine (AZT)
  - Antiviral agents
  - Nevirapine
  - Avoid breastfeeding if other nutritional means are available.
- Use of personal protective equipment for healthcare workers
  - Proper and safe disposal of used needles, scalpels, and glass
- Health education and access to services through schools and community
- For all HIV-infected patients
  - CD4 counts every 3 to 6 months
  - Viral load tests every 3 to 6 months and 1 month after change in therapy

- PPD
- INH for positive PPD and normal chest x-ray
- RPR/VDRL
- Toxoplasma IgG serology
- Hepatitis serologies
- Pneumoccocal vaccine
- Hepatitis A vaccine for those without immunity
- Hepatitis B vaccine for those without immunity
- Tetanus and diphtheria vaccine
- HPV for women infected with HIV who are 26 years of age or younger
- *Haemophilus influenzae* type b vaccination
- Pap smear every 6 months for women
- Consider anal swabs for cytologic evaluation
- Patients who are infected with HIV with CD4 < 200 cells/mcL
  - *Pneumocystis jiroveci* prophylaxis
- HIV-infected patients with CD4 < 75 cells/mcL
  - *Mycobacterium avium* complex prophylaxis
- HIV-infected individuals with DC4 < 50 cells/mcL
  - Consider CMV prophylaxis (McPhee & Papadakis, 2011)

Assessment

History
- HIV infection
  - Document risk factors
  - Many individuals remain asymptomatic for years.
  - Fever
  - Chills
  - Fatigue
  - Night sweats
  - Weight loss
  - Diffuse erythematous rash
- AIDS
  - Anorexia
  - Nausea
  - Vomiting
  - Malabsorption
  - Diarrhea
  - Increased metabolic rate

Physical Examination
- Initially may be unremarkable except for unintended weight loss
- Symptomatic disease
  - Fever
  - Lymphadenopathy
  - Headache

- Infections normally kept in check by an intact immune system
  - Herpes zoster
  - Thrush
    - Oral
    - Mucocutaneous
    - Vaginal
- Pulmonary
  - Pneumocystis pneumonia
  - Bacterial, mycobacterial, viral pneumonia
  - Noninfectious
    - Kaposi sarcoma
    - Non-Hodgkin's lymphoma
    - Interstitial pneumonitis
- Sinusitis
  - Chronic
- Central nervous system (CNS)
  - Toxoplasmosis
  - CNS lymphoma
  - AIDS dementia complex
  - Cryptococcal meningitis
  - HIV myelopathy
  - Progressive multifocal leukoencephalopathy (PML)
- Peripheral nervous system
  - Inflammatory polyneruopathies
  - Peripheral neuropathies
    - May be drug-induced
- Rheumatology
  - Arthritis—single or multiple joints
  - Reiter's syndrome
  - Psoriatic arthritis
  - Sicca syndrome
  - Systemic lupus erythematosus
- Myopathy
  - Infrequent with the advent of antirectroviral therapy
- Retinitis
  - Complaints of visual changes must be evaluated immediately
  - CMV retinitis
  - Cotton wool spots common but benign
- Oral lesions
  - Oral candidiasis
  - Hairy leukoplakia because of Epstein-Barr virus
  - Angular cheilitis
  - Gingivial disease
  - Aphthous ulcers

- Gastrointestinal
  - Candidial esophagitis
  - Hepatic disease
    - Infectious
      - Hepatitis B, C
    - Drug-induced
  - Bililary disease
    - Cholecystitis
  - Enterocolitis
  - Gastropathy
  - Malabsorption
- Renal
  - HIV-associated nephropathy
  - Proteinuria
- Endocrine
  - Hypogonadism
  - Abnormal thyroid function tests
- Skin
  - Herpes simplex
  - Herpes zoster
  - Molluscum contagiosum due to a pox virus
  - *Staphylococcus*
    - Folliculitis
    - Furuncles
    - Bullous impetigo
    - Bacillary angiomatosis
    - Fungal rashes
    - Seborrheic dermatitis
- HIV-related malignancies
  - Kaposi sarcoma
  - Non-Hodgkin's lymphoma
  - Anal dysplasia and squamous cell carcinoma
  - Cervical dysplasia and neoplasm
- Gynecology
  - Vaginal candidiasis
  - Cervical dysplasia
  - PID
  - Neoplasia
- Coronary artery disease
  - Higher risk than age and gender counterparts
  - Changes in lipid metabolism from antiretroviral therapy
    - Stavudine
    - Most of the protease inhibitors
- Inflammatory reactions
  - Because of recovery of immune system indicated by rapid increase in CD4 count
  - Diagnosis of exclusion
  - Fever
  - Sweats
  - Malaise

- Vitreitis
- M. avium
  - Focal lymphadenitis or granulomatous masses
- Tuberculosis may worsen if present
- PML and cryptococcal meningitis may progress atypically

Diagnostic Studies
- CBC
  - Anemia
  - Neutropenia
  - Thrombocytopenia
- Serum chemistry with liver function studies
  - Elevated transaminase levels
- Hepatitis screening
- Fasting lipid profile
- Pap smear
- Chest radiograph
- Tuberculin skin test
- Screen for STIs
- Cytomegalovirus serology
- Varicella antibody testing
- HIV enzyme-linked immunosorbent assay (ELISA)
  - Screening test for HIV infection
  - Sensitivity 99%
  - 50% are positive in 22 days after infection.
  - 95% positive within 6 weeks.
- Western blot
  - Confirmatory test for HIV
  - Specificity with ELISA > 99.9%
- HIV rapid antibody
  - Screening test—if positive, confirmed with ELISA and Western blot
  - Five approved by FDA
    - Oraquick Advance
    - Uni-Gold Recombigen
    - Clearview Stat-Pak and Complete
    - Reveal G-3
    - Multispot
  - Are used in about 40% of hospitals
- Absolute CD4 lymphocyte count
  - Use as predictor of HIV progression
  - Risk of opportunistic infection or malignancy is high with CD4 < 200 cells/mcL in the absence of treatment
    - CD4 lymphocyte percentage
    - Risk of opportunistic infection or malignancy is high with < 14% in the absence of treatment

- HIV viral load tests
  - HIV RNA
  - Measures the amount of actively replicating HIV virus
  - Treatment indicated for viral loads > 100,000/mcL
  - May represent false positive with low-level viremia < 500 copies/ml

Differential Diagnosis

- Candidiasis
- Cytomegalovirus
- Idiopathic thrombocytopenia purpura
- Influenza
- Meningitis
- Mononucleosis
- Pharyngitis
- Syphilis
- Viral hepatitis
- Enterocolitis
- Inflammatory bowel disease
- Antibiotic-associated colitis

Management

Nonpharmacologic Treatment
- Education regarding safe sexual practices, avoidance of breastfeeding with HIV infection
- Only latex condoms should be used
- Healthcare maintenance—see Prevention and Screening

Pharmacologic Treatment
- Combination therapy will maintain maximal viral suppression
- Continual drug therapy is essential
- Treatment started when:
  - CD4 count < 500 cells/mcL or rapidly dropping
  - Viral load > 100,000/mcL
  - Dual infection with hepatitis B or C
  - Risk factors for cardiac disease
  - Risk factors for non–AIDS-related cancers
  - When patient is willing to commit to therapy
- Types of medications
  - Nucleoside reverse transcriptase inhibitors
    - Zidovudine
    - Didanosine
    - Zalcitabine
    - Lamivudine
    - Stavudine
    - Abacavir
    - Emtricitabine

- Nucleotide reverse transcriptase inhibitors
  - Tenovir
- Protease inhibitors
  - Saquinavir
  - Ritonavir
  - Indinavir
  - Nelfinavir
  - Lopinavir/ritonavir
  - Tipranavir/ritonavir
  - Darunavir/ritonavir
  - Atazanavir
- Nonnucleoside reverse transcriptase inhibitors
  - Nevirapine
  - Delavirdine
  - Efavirenz
  - Etravirine
- Entry inhibitors
  - Enfuviritide
  - Maraviroc
- Integrase inhibitor
  - Raltegravir
- The current standard is to use at least three agents from at least two classes concurrently.
- To avoid drug resistance, patient must comply with an effective drug regimen.

Special Considerations

- In the hospital setting, when there is suspicion of infection, screening should take place with the patient's knowledge.
- Positive results may require the assistance of the social worker, the chaplain, or both, if the diagnosis was not expected.
- HIV-1 drug resistance limits the ability to fully control HIV replication and is the leading cause for treatment failure.
  - Resistance has been documented for all currently available antiretrovirals, including the new class of fusion inhibitor.
  - Resistance testing is recommended as a part of standard baseline testing.

When to Consult, Refer, or Hospitalize

- Refer to infectious disease for expert management
- Hospitalize patients with opportunistic infections who are acutely ill, require IV medications, or both.
  - Febrile
  - Change in mental status
  - Respiratory distress

Follow-up

Expected Outcomes
- CD4+ cell count and HIV viral load should be evaluated at 1 month and then every 3 to 6 months.
  - CD4+ cell count should rise 100 to 150/mL in the first month of therapy.
  - HIV RNA levels should decrease tenfold to < 50 copies/mL.
  - Failure to achieve these endpoints indicates a need for adjustment of medication.
- AIDS develops within 10 years in about 50% of untreated seropositive patients
- Denmark study found that HIV-infected patients at age 25 years without hepatitis C had a life expectancy of 39 additional years
- For those patients who deteriorate despite therapy, referral to palliative care is appropriate.

Complications
- *Pneumocystis jiroveci* infection
- *Mycobacterium avium* complex infection
- Toxoplasmosis
- Lymphoma
- Cryptococcal meningitis
- Cytomegalovirus infection
- Esophageal candidiasis or recurrent vaginal candidiasis
- Herpes simplex infection
- Herpes zoster
- Kaposi's sarcoma
  - Limited cutaneous disease
  - Extensive or aggressive cutaneous disease
  - Visceral disease

ACUTE ALLERGIC REACTIONS

Description

- Allergic disorders may be local or systemic
- The immune system typically prevents a person from contracting disease, but it can cause detrimental reactions, which are known as *hypersensitivity reactions*.
- These reactions are manifested by tissue inflammation and organ dysfunction.
- Hypersensitivity reactions are classified as follows:
  - Type I
    - IgE-mediated (immediate) hypersensitivity
    - Release of histamine and other mediators from mast cells and basophils

- Atopy
  - Applied to a group of diseases that occur in individuals with an inherited tendency to develop antigen-specific IgE reactions to environmental allergens or food antigens
    - Allergic rhinitis
    - Allergic asthma
    - Atopic dermatitis
    - Urticaria or angioedema
    - Allergic gastroenteropathy
- Anaphylaxis—life-threatening
  - Certain allergens, such as medications, insect venoms, latex, or food, may produce an IgE antibody response, causing a generalized release of mediators from mast cells and resulting in systemic anaphylaxis.
- Type II
  - Cytotoxic
  - Involve immunoglobulin G or immunoglobulin M antibodies bound to cell surface antigens with complement fixation
- Type III
  - Immune complex reactions
  - Involve circulating antigen–antibody immune complexes that deposit in postcapillary venules, with subsequent complement fixation
- Type IV
  - Delayed hypersensitivity reaction
  - Cell-mediated immunity
  - Mediated by T-cells rather than antibodies

Etiology

- Genetic predisposition to form IgE antibodies in response to allergen exposure
- Environmental exposure

Incidence and Demographics

- Allergic rhinitis affects approximately 17% to 22% of the population.
- Asthma affects approximately 22.2 million people in the United States.
- Atopic dermatitis affects approximately 10% of the population.
  - Common allergens
    - Nickel
    - Formaldehyde
    - Potassium dichromate
    - Thiurams
    - Parabens
- The prevalence of anaphylaxis is about 1% to 3% in industrialized countries.
- Allergic rhinitis tends to decrease with age.

- Food allergies may resolve from childhood to adulthood; however, some food allergies last a lifetime.
  - Common food allergies
    - Peanuts
    - Tree nuts
    - Finned fish
    - Shellfish
    - Eggs
    - Soy
    - Wheat

Risk Factors

- Genetic predisposition
- Environmental exposure

Prevention and Screening

- Avoidence of the allergen
- Allergy testing and desensitization
- Educating the allergic patient to keep rescue medication available if desensitization is not possible

Assessment

History
- Anaphylaxis
  - Skin itching
    - Localized or diffuse
  - Dizziness
  - Faintness
  - Diaphoresis
  - Difficulty breathing
    - Angioedema of pharyngeal tissue
  - Nausea
  - Vomiting
  - Diarrhea
  - Abdominal cramping
  - Symptoms begin within minutes of exposure to allergens.
  - Patient may not be able to identify allergen.
  - Ask about new or recently changed medication.

- Allergic rhinoconjunctivitis
  - Sneezing
  - Congestion
  - Injected sclera
  - Itching of the palate or inner ear
  - Tearing, itching of the eyes
  - Chronic nasal congestion
- Allergic asthma
  - Cough
  - Shortness of breath
  - Wheezing
- Urticaria and angioedema
  - Diffuse hives or wheals
  - Localized tissue swelling
  - Exposure may be to unknown allergen, which may never be discovered
  - Angioedema of the pharynx can cause airway obstruction.
    - Stridor
    - Hoarseness
- Atopic dermatitis
  - Eczematous cutaneous eruption
  - Significant pruritus
  - Superinfection with staphylococcal organisms can occur
- GI allergies
  - Nausea
  - Vomiting
  - Abdominal cramping
  - Diarrhea
  - Eosinophilic esophagitis
  - Gastritis

Physical Examination
- Anaphylaxis
  - May exhibit circulatory or respiratory collapse
  - Urticaria
  - Angioedema
  - Wheezing because of bronchial constriction
  - Confusion
  - Altered mental status
- Allergic rhinoconjunctivitis
  - Frequent throat clearing because of postnasal drip
  - Injected sclera
  - Dark circles under the eyes
  - Pharynx may have cobblestone appearance
  - Frontal or maxillary sinus tenderness
- Allergic asthma
  - Cough
  - Dyspnea
  - Wheezing
  - Shallow breathing with prolonged expiratory phase
  - Cyanosis of lips, fingers, or toes because of hypoxemia

- Urticaria and angioedema
  - Wheals with surrounding erythema
  - Angioedema
- Atopic dermatitis
  - Mild cases
    - Normal, dry, or with erythematous papules
  - Severe cases
    - Extremely dry, lichenified, cracked, and crusted lesions

Diagnostic Studies
- Serum tryptase level
  - Elevated
- Eosinophil count
  - Elevated
- IgE levels
  - May be elevated in patients who are atopic, but the level does not always correlate with clinical symptoms
- Radioallergosorbent test (RAST)
  - Measures antigen-specific IgE
- Skin testing for allergens
- Spirometry and pulmonary function tests
  - Objective means of evaluating asthma
- Nasal smear tests
  - Elevated eosinophil can be indicative of allergic rhinitis
- Induced sputum
  - Evaluated for eosinophils—a measure of the inflammation seen in asthma
- Patch testing for atopic dermatitis

Differential Diagnosis

- Bronchitis
- Carcinoid lung tumors
- Cardiogenic shock
- Chronic obstructive pulmonary disease
- Congestive heart failure
- Irritable bowel syndrome
- Pulmonary embolism
- Syncope
- Upper respiratory tract infection
- Nonallergic rhinitis

Management

Nonpharmacologic Treatment
- Anaphylaxis
  - Withdraw offending agent
  - Secure the airway
  - Medic Alert bracelet
- Allergic rhinitis
  - Avoid known allergen
- Asthma
  - Avoid offending agent
- Urticaria and angioedema
  - Avoid offending agent
  - Atopic dermatitis
  - Hydrate
  - Avoid offending agent

Pharmacologic Treatment
- Anaphylaxis
  - Epinephrine
  - Vasopressors
    - Norepinephrine
    - Epinephrine
    - Dopamine
    - Diphenhydramine
    - Ranitidine
    - Cimetidine
    - Albuterol nebulizer
    - Corticosteroid
- Allergic rhinitis
  - H1-receptor blocker
    - Diphenhydramine
    - Azelastine
    - Cetirizine
  - H2-receptor blocker
    - Ranitidine
    - Cimetidine
  - Intranasal glucocorticosteroid
    - Fluticasone
    - Budesonide
  - Antigen-injection immunotherapy
    - Based on test results
- Asthma
  - Albuterol metered dose inhaler
  - Inhaled glucocorticosteriod
    - Budesonide
  - Leukotriene inhibitor
    - Montelukast

- Systemic corticosteroid
  - Prednisone
  - Hydrocortisone
  - Solumedrol
- Urticaria and angiodema
  - H1-receptor blocker
  - H2-receptor blocker
- Atopic dermatitis
  - Topical glucocorticosteroids
    - Hydrocortisone
    - Triamcinolone
  - Topical immunomodulators
    - Tacrolimus

Special Considerations

- In anaphylaxis, late-phase reactions can occur 4 to 6 hours after the initial episode and can be as severe as or worse than the original event; therefore, observation of the patient is important.
- Patients with a history of anaphylaxis should be prescribed two doses of autoinjectable epinephrine and instructed in their use.
- Patients with latex allergies should avoid all products with latex—gloves, balloons, elastic, condoms, etc.
- During pregnancy patients may experience improvement, worsening, or no change in the severity of their symptoms.
  - Chlorpheniramine and dihenhydramine are category B in pregnancy.
  - Some of the nonsedating antihistamines are category C.
  - Cetirizine, loratadine, and montelukast are category B.
- In older adults, first-generation antihistamines may have adverse anticholinergic effects—use with caution.
  - Second-generation antihistamines may have fewer side effects.
  - First generation
    - Brompherniramine
    - Chlorpheniramine
    - Diphenhydramine
    - Doxylamine
  - Second generation
    - Cetirizine
    - Fexofenadine
    - Desloratadine
    - Loratadine
- Corticosteroid side effects may prove problematic for older adults because they have a greater risk for osteroporosis, cataracts, and gastrointestinal ulcers.

When to Consult, Refer, or Hospitalize

- Consultation with an allergist or immunologist, a pulmonologist, a critical care specialist, or a combination of these may be needed, depending in the severity of the allergic reaction.
- Hospitalize patients with anaphylactic reactions for close monitoring of airway, circulatory status. and latent reaction.

Follow-up

Expected Outcomes
- Resolution of the allergic reaction with removal of offending agent and appropriate medications
- Avoidance of future episodes through patient education and medication

Complications
- Airway compromise
- Circulatory collapse
- Chronic rhinitis
- Sinusitis
- Skin
  - Fissuring
  - Lichenification
  - Dyspigmentation

AMYLOIDOSIS

Description

- An uncommon condition manifested by abnormal protein deposits in tissue that results in organ dysfunction as the protein builds up and leads to premature death
- Amyloid is classified according to the type of amyloid deposited
  - Primary
    - Immunoglobin light chain (AL)
    - Organs affected
      - Tongue
      - Intestines
      - Skeletal and smooth muscles
      - Nerves
      - Skin
      - Ligaments
      - Heart
      - Liver
      - Spleen
      - Kidneys

- Secondary
  - Serum protein A, produced in inflammatory conditions (AA)
  - Is the most common form of systemic amyloidosis worldwide
- Hereditary
  - Transthyretin (TTR) senile amyloid (atrial natriuretic peptide)
- Renal failure type
  - β-microglobulin, not filtered by dialysis membranes
- It is further classified as localized or systemic.

Etiology

- Primary: AL
  - Cause unknown
- Secondary: AA amyloid
  - Chronic infectious diseases
    - Tuberculosis
    - Leprosy
    - Bronchiectasis
    - Chronic osteomyelitis
    - Chronic pyelonephritis
  - Chronic noninfectious inflammatory diseases
    - Inflammatory bowel disease
    - Rheumatoid arthritis
    - Behçet's syndrome
    - Ankylosing spondylitis
    - Psoriatic arthritis
- Hereditary
  - Inherited autosomal dominant disorder
- Renal failure type
  - The result of long-term dialysis treatment

Incidence and Demographics

- Primary: AL
  - Estimates are 4.5 per 100,000, but numbers may be higher
  - Usually occurs after age 40
  - Occurs in about 15% of myelomas
- Secondary: AA
  - Absolute prevalence is unknown
- Hereditary
  - Incidence is unknown
- Renal failure type
  - Relatively common in older patients on dialysis more than 5 years
  - Hemodialysis membrane cannot completely remove the complex β-2 microglobulin and it builds up in the blood.

Risk Factors

- Primary
  - No known risk factors
- AA
  - Presence of chronic infectious and noninfectious disease—see Etiology
- Hereditary
  - Genetic predisposition
- Renal failure
  - Hemodialysis

Prevention and Screening

- Primary
  - No known preventative measures
- Secondary
  - Treatment and control of infectious and noninfectious inflammatory conditions
- Hereditary
  - Genetic counseling
- Renal failure
  - Delay onset of hemodialysis for as long as feasible

Assessment

History
- Primary
  - Fatigue
  - Numbness of hands and feet
  - Swallowing difficulties
  - Weight loss
  - Diarrhea
  - Joint pain
- Secondary
  - Weakness
  - Weight loss
  - Appearance of renal disease in a patient with chronic infectious or noninfectious diseases
- Hereditary
  - Renal disease
  - Diarrhea
  - GI obstruction
  - Numbness in extremities
  - Dizziness
  - Malnutrition
  - Abdominal pain
  - Weakness in the extremities

- Renal failure
  - Carpal tunnel syndrome
  - Arthralgias
  - Joint stiffness

Physical Examination
- AL
  - Macroglossia
  - Irregular heart rhythm
  - Peripheral edema
  - Clay-colored stool
  - Hoarseness
  - Carpal tunnel syndrome
  - Nephrotic syndrome
- AA
  - Hypertension
  - Peripheral edema
  - Deforming arthritis
  - Hepatosplenomegaly
- Hereditary
  - Macroglossia
  - Renal disease
- Renal failure
  - Bone cysts
  - Fractures
  - Ligament or tendon tears

Diagnostic Studies
Diagnosis involves identifying the fibrillar deposits in tissues and typing of amyloid
- AL
  - Abdominal ultrasound
    - Enlarged liver and spleen
  - Abdominal fat pad biopsy
  - Rectal mucosa biopsy
  - Bone marrow biopsy
  - Electrocardiogram
  - Echocardiogram
  - Nerve conduction velocity
  - Urinalysis
    - Proteinuria
    - Casts
    - Fat bodies
  - Serum chemistry
    - Elevated BUN and creatinine

- AA
  - Urinalysis
    - Proteinuria
    - Nephrotic syndrome
  - Avoid IV pyelography
    - Contrast exposure is linked to more frequent renal failure
  - Serum immunoglobulins
    - Elevated levels
  - Ultrasound
  - CT scan
    - Occasionally technetium binds to amyloid soft tissue deposits
  - 10% of cases have cardiac involvement
    - Echocardiogram
    - Electrocardiogram
    - Cardiac catheterization with endomyocardial biopsy
- Hereditary
  - Rectal mucosa biopsy
  - Abdominal fat pad aspiration
- Renal failure
  - Plain film radiography of affected bone and joints

Differential Diagnosis

- Membranous glomerulonephritis
- Renal vein thrombosis
- Congestive heart failure
- Coronary artery disease
- Hypertensive renal disease
- Trauma
- Liver disease
- Multiple myeloma
- Malignant lymphoproliferative syndromes
- Monoclonal gammopathy of undetermined significance

Management

Nonpharmacologic Treatment
- Supportive care
- Treatment of underlying disease process in all forms amyloidosis
- Renal transplant option for AA, hereditary amyloidosis with renal involvement, and dialysis-related amyloidosis
- TPN for hereditary amyloidosis with end-stage GI involvement and malnutrition
- Biomedical research currently developing dialysis membranes that can remove larger proteins

Pharmacologic Treatment
- AL
  - Chemotherapy directed at abnormal plasma cells
  - Stem cell transplantation
- AA
- Tumor necrosis factor-α inhibitors and interleukin-1 inhibitors
- Hereditary
  - Antiarrhythmics for cardiac involvement
- Renal failure
  - No medication option

Special Considerations

- The clinical syndromes of the amyloidoses have relatively nonspecific alterations in laboratory tests.
- Blood counts are usually normal, but sedimentation rate may be elevated.
- Patients with renal involvement can have as much as 30 g/day of protein in the urine, which produces hypoalbuminemia of < 1 g/dL.
- Patients with cardiac involvement often have elevated brain naturietic peptide (BNP), pro-BNP, and troponins.
- Patients with liver involvement usually develop cholestasis with an elevated alkaline phosphatase but minimal elevation of transaminases and preservation of liver function.
- In AL amyloid, patient may exhibit hypothyroidism, hypoadrenalism, or even hypopituitarism, but they are not specific to amyloidosis.
- Maintain nutrition and fluid balance.
- Analgesics to relieve pain
- Provide meticulous oral care when tongue is involved.
- Assess airway for patency and prevent respiratory compromise with enlarged tongue.

When to Consult, Refer, or Hospitalize

- All patients with amyloidosis should be referred to an oncologist or hematologist.
- Renal and cardiology consults when kidneys and heart are involved
- Gastroenterology consult for GI involvement
- Hospitalize to treat exacerbations of end-organ failure, to undergo autologous hematopoietic stem cell transplantation, and to treat infections.

Follow-up

Expected Outcomes
- AL
  - Severity of the disease depends on the organs involved
  - Cardiac and renal involvement lead to organ failure and death.
  - Systemic involvement is associated with death in 1 to 3 years.
- AA
  - Management of underlying disorder
  - Prognosis dependent on level of renal involvement
    - Poorer prognosis with serum creatinine > 2 mg/dL or a serum albumin level < 2.5 g/dL
  - Mean survival time is 2 to 3 years.
- Hereditary
  - Many patients survive until the seventh decade and often 10 years after initial diagnosis.
- Renal failure
  - Prognosis depends on the possibility of transplantation and patient's management of the ESKD.

Complications
- AL
  - Congestive heart failure
  - Endocrine dysfunction
  - Renal failure
  - Respiratory failure
  - Death
- AA
  - Renal failure
- Hereditary
  - Renal failure
- Renal
  - See Physical examination

SARCOIDOSIS

Description

- Sarcoidosis is a disease that is manifested by the presence of noncaseating granulomas.
- The condition commonly involves multiple organs and must have involvement of two or more organs to confirm a diagnosis.
- The disease can affect any organ in the body, but the lung is affected in about 90% of cases.

Etiology

- Unknown
- Infectious and noninfectious environmental triggers have been proposed.
    - *Propionibacter acnes* has been found in the lymph nodes of patients with sarcoidosis.
        - *P. acnes* can cause granulomatous response in mice.
    - Recent studies have identified *Mycobacterium tuberculosis* catalase-peroxidase (mKat) in the granulomas of some sarcoid patients
        - This protein is very resistant to degradation.
    - Environmental triggers
        - Insecticides
        - Mold
        - Healthcare workers have an increased risk.
    - Possible genetic predisposition

Incidence and Demographics

- The disease is reportedly higher in Blacks than in Whites in the United States.
- Women are slightly more susceptible than men.
- Higher rates occur in Ireland and Nordic countries.
- Often occurs in otherwise healthy young adults, with a second peak incidence in the 60s
- Uncommon under age 18
- In a study of > 700 new cases in the United States, half the patients were ≥ 40 years old at the time.

Risk Factors

- Healthcare workers
- Possible genetic component
    - African American, Northern European descent
- Exposure to potential triggers

Prevention and Screening

- No screening or known preventative measures
- Annual electrocardiogram in diagnosed patients

Assessment

History
- About 5% of cases are asymptomatic.
- In about 45% of cases:
  - Fever
  - Anorexia
  - Arthralgias
- With pulmonary involvement, these symptoms present in about 50% of cases:
  - Dyspnea on exertion
  - Cough
  - Chest pain
  - Hemoptysis—rare
- Löfgren's syndrome (uncommon in Black and Japanese patients)
  - Fever
  - Bilateral hilar lymphadenopathy (BHL)
  - Polyarthralgias

Physical Examination
- Pulmonary
  - Breath sounds are usually normal, but crackles may be present.
  - Exertional oxygen desaturation
  - Chest x-ray staging system for sarcoidosis
    - Stage 0: normal
    - Stage 1: BHL
    - Stage 2: BHL and infiltrates
    - Stage 3: infiltrates only
    - Stage 4: fibrosis
- Skin
  - Erythema nodosum
    - More common in women
  - Lupus pernio is the most specific skin lesion
    - A specific complex, involving the bridge of the nose, the area beneath the eyes, and the cheeks—diagnostic for a chronic form of sarcoidosis
  - Hyper- or hypopigmentation
  - Violaceous rash on cheeks or nose
  - Maculopapular plaques
    - Most common chronic form of the disease
- Ocular
  - Anterior or posterior granulomatous uveitis is most common
  - Conjunctival lesions and sclera plaques
  - Photophobia
  - Blurred vision
  - Dry eyes
  - If untreated, may progress to blindness
- Cardiac
  - Rarely heart failure
  - Heart block, sudden death
  - < 5% of patients have clinical cardiac disease at autopsy

- Neurological
  - Cranial nerve palsy
  - Hypothalamic or pituitary dysfunction
  - Lymphocytic meningitis is common
- Liver
  - Based on liver function tests, about 20% to 30% of patients have liver involvement
  - In about 5% of patients:
    - Hepatomegaly
    - Cholestasis leading to portal hypertension
- Renal
- < 5% of patients have renal involvement.
- Hypercalcemia
- < 1% to 2% have acute renal failure.

Diagnostic Studies
- CBC
  - Leukopenia
- Erythrocyte sedimentation rate (5%)
  - Elevated
- Serum chemistry with liver function studies
  - Hypercalcemia (5%)
- Urinary electrolytes
  - Hypercalceuria
- Angiotensin-converting enzyme (ACE)
  - Elevated levels (40% to 80%)
- Chest radiograph (see staging p. 529)
- High-resolution CT scan of the chest
  - Identifies active alveolitis versus fibrosis
- Pulmonary function testing
  - Used in evaluation and follow-up
  - Decrease in carbon monoxide diffusion capacity
  - Restrictive pattern in advance disease
  - 15% to 20% of patients have obstruction
- Cardiopulmonary exercise testing
  - Identifies and quantifies the extent of pulmonary involvement
- Annual electrocardiogram
  - Recommended by the American Thoracic Society
- Transbronchial biopsy (TBB)
- May be positive even with normal chest x-ray
- Tissue confirmation is essential prior to therapy

Differential Diagnosis

- Eosinophilic granuloma
- Non–small cell lung cancer
- Small (oat) cell lung cancer

- Lymphoma
- Tuberculosis
- Fungal infection
- Hypersensitivity pneumonitis

Management

Nonpharmacologic Treatment
- Monitor for disease progression
- Lung transplant for advanced disease that does not respond to treatment

Pharmacologic Treatment
- More than 75% of patients require only symptomatic therapy with nonsteroidal antiinflammatory medications.
- Corticosteroid therapy is the mainstay of therapy.
- About 10% of patients need treatment for extrapulmonary disease.
- Acute disease
  - No therapy may be indicated for patients with no or mild symptoms
  - Single organ disease—skin, eye, cough
    - Topical steroids for eye, skin disease
    - NSAIDS
  - Multiorgan disease or disease too extensive for topical therapy
    - Prednisone 20 to 40 mg/day—initial dose
    - Taper to 5 to 10 mg/day
    - If steroids not tolerated or ineffective
      - Methotrexate
      - Hydroxychloroquine
      - Cyclophosphamide
      - Azathioprine
      - Infliximab
      - Tetracyclines
        - Cutaneous sarcoidosis

Special Considerations

- The diagnosis of sarcoidosis requires both compatible clinical features and pathological findings.
- Because the etiology is not known, the diagnosis cannot be made with 100% certainty but rather with a reasonable likelihood based on history, physical examination, and laboratory and biopsy findings.
- Long-term therapy, once started, is required for months to years
- Serum ACE levels usually fall with treatment.

When to Consult, Refer, or Hospitalize

- Hospitalize for deteriorating pulmonary or cardiac status not responsive to therapy.
- Consult pulmonary, rheumatology, and transplant services as patient condition requires.

Follow-up

Expected Outcomes
- The prognosis is best for patients with hilar adenopathy alone.
- Radiographic evidence of lung involvement is associated with a worse prognosis.
- About 20% of patients with lung involvement develop irreversible lung damage manifested by progressive fibrosis, bronchiectasis, and cavitation.
- Patients require long-term follow-up
  - Yearly physical examination
  - Pulmonary function tests
  - Chemistry panel
  - Ophthalmologic examination
  - Chest x-ray
  - Electrocardiogram
- Death from pulmonary insufficiency occurs in about 5% of patients.

Complications
- Pneumothorax
- Hemoptysis
- Mycetoma formation in lung cavities
- Respiratory failure
- Cardiac dysrhythmias
- Restrictive cardiomyopathy
- Renal failure
- Blindness
- Death

SCLERODERMA (SYSTEMIC SCLEROSIS)

Description

- Scleroderma is a rare chronic disorder manifested by diffuse fibrosis of the skin and internal organs.
- The disease involves multiple organs, most commonly the lungs, GI tract, heart, and kidneys.
- Early stages of the disease are associated with inflammatory features and are then followed by the development of functional and structural dysfunction in multiple vascular beds and visceral organs because of fibrosis.

- American College of Rheumatology criteria for the classification of scleroderma:
  - For diagnosis patient must have one major or two minor criteria
    - Major
      - Symmetric thickening, tightening, and induration of the skin of the fingers and the skin that is proximal to the metacarpophalangeal or metatarsophalangeal joints
      - These changes may affect the entire face, neck and trunk (thorax and abdomen)
    - Minor
      - Sclerodactyly—thickening, induration and tightening of the skin limited to the fingers
      - Digital pitting scars or a loss of substance from the finger pad because of ischemia; depressed areas of the fingertips or a loss of digital pad tissue occurs
      - Bibasilar pulmonary fibrosis—has the appearance of diffuse mottling or a honeycomb lung that is the result of primary lung disease
- Limited disease (80% of cases)
  - Raynaud's phenomenon seen in 90% of patients with scleroderma
    - Defined as episodic vasoconstriction in the fingers and toes
    - May also affect the tip of the nose and earlobes
    - Attacks are triggered by exposure to cold, decrease in temperature, emotional stress, and vibration
    - Typical attacks begin with pallor, then cyanosis of variable duration
    - Erythema develops spontaneously or with rewarming of digit
    - Underlying pathology
      - Vasocontriction
      - Ischemia
      - Reperfusion
  - Skin induration limited to the fingers, distal extremities, and face; trunk not affected
  - A subset of patients have calcinosis cutis, Raynaud's phenomenon, esophageal dysmotility, sclerodactyly, and telangiectasia known as the CREST syndrome (these features may also be seen in diffuse disease).
- Diffuse disease (20% of cases)
  - Progessive skin induration, starting from the fingers and ascending from distal to proximal extremities, the face, and the trunk
  - These patients are at risk for pulmonary fibrosis and acute renal involvement.

Etiology

- Unknown
- These pathological changes are always present:
  - Endothelial injury
  - Fibroblast activation
  - Cellular and humoral immunologic derangement
- Environmental factors
  - Silica exposure
  - Solvent exposure—vinyl chloride, trichloroethylene, epoxy resins, benzene, or carbon tetrachloride
  - Radiation exposure or radiotherapy

Incidence and Demographics

- The incidence of systemic sclerosis is 19 cases per million people, and the prevalence is about 240 cases per million people.
- The prevalence has increased because of earlier detection and increased survival rate
- Limited cutaneous disease has a 10-year survival rate of 71%.
- Diffuse cutaneous diseae has 10-year survival rate of 21%.
- The risk of developing the disease is slightly higher in Blacks than in Whites; the risk in young Black women is 10 times higher.
- Oklahoma Choctaw Indians have an incidence of 472 per million people.
- Cluster cases of scleroderma exist in male patients who live in Coffee, Tennessee; Northhampton, North Carolina; and South Boston, Massachusetts.
- The risk is 4 to 9 times higher in women than in men.
- Peak age for development of the disease is 30 to 50 years of age.

Risk Factors

- Age
- Female gender
- Family history
- Geography—see Incidence and Demographics

Prevention and Screening

- Avoid cigarette smoking
- Protect feet and hands from injury and infection
- Moisturize the skin
- Avoid cold temperatures
- Physical therapy and exercise to keep joints flexible

Assessment

History
- Diffuse disease
  - Skin
    - Pruritis
  - Vascular system
    - Raynaud's phenomenon
    - The interval between appearance of Raynaud's phenomenon and other manifestations is usually weeks to months
  - Gastrointestinal system
    - Reflux
    - Dyspepsia
    - Bloating
    - Early satiety
    - Constipation alternating with diarrhea

- Respiratory system
  - Dyspnea
  - Chest pain
  - Cough
- Musculoskeletal system
  - Arthralgias
  - Myalgias
  - Muscle weakness
- Cardiovascular system
  - Dyspnea
  - Palpitations
  - Syncope
- Genitourinay system
  - Erectile dysfunction
  - Dyspareunia
- Ears, nose, throat
  - Poor dentition
  - Sicca syndrome
  - Hoarseness
- Endocrine
  - Hypothryroidism
- Renal
  - Chronic kidney diseaes
- Neurologic
  - Facial pain and decreased sensation
  - Hand paresthesias and weakness
  - Headache
  - Stroke
- Constitutional
  - Fatigue
  - Weight loss
- Limited
  - Vascular
    - Raynaud's phenomenon
    - The interval between the appearance of Raynaud's phenomenon and symptoms of the disease is usually several years.
    - More severe in limited disease
- History similar to diffuse with progression of the disease

Physical Examination
- Diffuse
  - Skin
    - Tightness and induration
    - Hypo- or hyperpigmentation
    - Shiny
    - Loss of hair
    - Skin thickening
    - Edematous or swollen skin on the hands
      - This precedes the induration sclerotic stage.
    - Calcinosis
  - Vascular
    - Healed pitting ulcers on the fingertips
    - Cutaneous and mucosal telengiectasis
    - Infarction, dry gangrene of the fingers
    - Nail fold capillary microscopy reveals fewer capillaries than normal and numerous dilated capillary loops
  - Respiratory
    - Dry crackles
    - Accentuated second heart sound
    - Right ventricular heave
    - Pulmonary vascular fibrosis
    - Pulmonary hypertension
  - Ears, nose, throat
    - Salivary production decreased
    - Xerostomia
    - Xerophthalmia
    - Oropharyngeal and esophageal cancers are more common with diffuse disease.
  - Musculoskeletal
    - Tendon friction rubs
    - Myositis
    - Dissolution of the distal end of the phalanx
    - Flexion contractures
  - GI
    - Esophagitis
    - Esophageal strictures
    - Gastric vascular ectasia
    - Diverticula
    - Anal sphincter incompetence
  - Renal
    - Renal crisis
      - Accelerated hypertension
      - Oliguria
      - Headache
      - Dyspnea
      - Edema
      - Rapidly rising serum creatinine levels

- Cardiovascular system
  - Pericardial effusion
  - Cor pulmonale
  - Conduction abnormalities
  - Infiltrative cardiomyopathy
- Neurological
  - Carpal tunnel syndrome
- Gynecology and obstretrics
  - Vaginal dryness
  - Menstrual irregularities
  - Symptoms may increase during pregnancy

- Limited
  - Manifestations of CREST syndrome

Diagnostic Studies
- Antinuclear antibodies are present in 90% to 95% of affected patients.
- Topoisomerase I antibodies Scl-70 are present in about 30% of patients with diffuse disease and 20% with limited disease
- Anticentromere antibodies are present in about 50% of patients with limited disease and are present in patients with diffuse disease
- ANA is positive in 80% to 90% of patients in both diffuse and limited disease.
- Rheumatoid factor is positive in about 30% of patients in both diffuse and limited disease.
- CBC
  - Mild anemia
- Peripheral smear
  - Microangiopathic hemolytica anemia with renal crisis
- Proteinuria and cylindruria with renal involvement
- High-resolution CT scan of the chest to evaluate pulmonary involvement
  - Ground glass appearance—lung fibrosis
  - Honeycombing—bronchiolectasis
- Chest x-ray
  - Only able to detect late findings of pulmonary fibrosis
    - Increased interstitial markings
- Echocardiography
  - Evaluates pulmonary artery pressure
  - Assesses septal fibrosis and pericardial effusions
- Right heart catheterization
  - Standard for evaluating pulmonary hypertension
  - Performed after an elevated pulmonary artery pressure is found on echocardiogram
- Pulmonary function testing every 6 months
- Serum pro-BNP
  - Elevated levels may correlate with early pulmonary hypertension

- 24-hour Holter monitoring to detect dysrhythmias and conduction defects
- Esophagogastroduodenoscopy, esophageal manometry, and pH monitoring studies to evaluate upper GI system
- Bronchoscopy with bronchoalveolar lavage
  - Assesses for active lung inflammation

Differential Diagnosis

- Eosinophilic fasciitis
- Graft-versus-host disease
- Nephrogenic systemic fibrosis
- Primary pulmonary hypertension
- Mycosis fungoides
- Reflex sympathetic dystrophy

Management

Nonpharmacologic Treatment
- Treatment is symptomatic, supportive, and focused on the organ system involved.
- Patients with delayed gastric emptying should eat small, frequent meals, and remain upright for 2 hours after eating.
- Esophageal reflux and the risk of scarring can be reduced by avoiding late night meals.

Pharmacologic Treatment
- Raynaud's syndrome may respond to calcium channel blockers
  - Long-acting nifedipine 30 to 120 mg/day p.o. *or*
  - Losartan 50 mg/day p.o. *or*
  - Sildenafil 50 mg p.o. 2 times daily
- PPI: Omeprazole 20 to 40 mg/day p.o.
- Long-term octreotide 0.1 mg subq 2 times daily helps with bacterial overgrowth and pseudo-obstruction
  - Bacterial overgrowth may respond to antibiotic—tetracycline 500 mg 4 times daily
- Hypertensive crisis must be treated early in the hospital with ACE-I.
- Prednisone has a role only if the patient has myositis.
- Cyclophosphamide improves dyspnea and pulmonary function tests.
- Bosentan—endothelin receptor antagonist—improves exercise capacity and cardiopulmonary hemodynamics in patients with pulmonary hypertension.
  - Also prevents digital ulceration
- Sildenafil or prostaglandins delivered by continuous infusion or intermittent inhalation may be used to treat pulmonary hypertension.

Special Considerations

- Overlap of scleroderma with other autoimmune syndromes, such as sicca syndrome, polyarthritis, cutaneous vasculitis, and biliary cirrhosis, occurs primarily in those with the limited form of the disease
- Breast and lung cancer may be more common in the scleroderma patient.

When to Consult, Refer, or Hospitalize

- Consult rheumatologist
- Severity of organ involvement determines referral to other subspecialists such as a pulmonologist or gastroenterologist
- Hospitalization for renal crisis, severe hypertension, and worsening pulmonary and cardiovascular status

Follow-up

Expected Outcomes
- The 9-year survival rate in scleroderma averages approximately 40%.
- Prognosis is worse in those with diffuse scleroderma, in Blacks, in males, and in the elderly
- Lung disease is the number one cause of mortality.
- If severe internal organ involvement does not occur in the first 3 years, then survival rate increases to 72% at 9 years

Complications
- Pulmonary hypertension
- Pulmonary fibrosis
- Digital infarctions
- Renal failure
- Wound infections

SYSTEMIC LUPUS ERYTHEMATOSUS (SLE)

Description

- SLE is an autoimmune inflammatory disorder manifested by autoantibodies to nuclear antigens.
- The disease may affect multiple organ systems with spontaneous remissions and relapses.
- Most of the clinical findings are the result of the trapping of antigen-antibody complexes in the capillaries of visceral structures or from autoantibody-mediated destruction of host cells.
- Severity ranges from a mild episodic condition to a fulminant life-threatening illness.
- Criteria for the classfication of SLE
  - A patient is classified as having SLE if any four of the following criteria are met:

- Malar rash
- Discoid rash
- Photosensitivity
- Oral ulcers
- Arthritis
- Serositis
- Kidney disease
    - > 0.5 g/d proteinuria *or*
    - > 3⁺ dipstick proteinuria *or*
    - Cellular casts
  - Neurologic disease
    - Seizures
    - Psychosis—without other cause
  - Hematologic disorders
    - Hemolytic anemia
    - Leukopenia: < 4,000/mcL
    - Lymphopenia: < 1500/mcL
    - Thrombocytopenia: < 100,000/mcL
  - Immunologic abnormalities
    - Positive LE cell preparation *or*
    - Antibody to native DNA
    - Antibody to Sm
    - False-positive serologic test for syphilis
  - Positive ANA (McPhee & Papadakis, 2011)
- Drug-induced lupus
  - Four features separate it from SLE
    - Sex ratio is nearly equal
    - Nephritis and central nervous system features are not usually present.
    - Hypocomplementemia and antibodies to native DNA are absent.
    - The clinical features and most laboratory abnormalities usually return to normal when the offending drug is removed.

Etiology

- Multiple immune disturbances may predispose an individual to SLE.
  - Inate susceptibility
    - HLA type DR3/2
    - Immunoregulatory genes
    - Complement levels
    - Hormonal levels
  - Environmental stimuli
    - UV exposure
    - Microbial response
    - Medications

- Autoimmune proliferation
  - Hyperactive B-cell or T-cell activation
  - High ratio of CD4:CD8 T-cells
  - Defective immune complex clearance
- Autoantibody production
  - Apoptosis and self-exposure
  - Self-recognition
  - Foreing-Ab cross reaction

Incidence and Demographics

- Approximately 85% of patients are women.
- Most cases develop after menarche and before menopause.
- About 250,000 persons have SLE in the United States.
- Higher rates are reported in the Black, Asian, and Hispanic populations.
- Among older adults, the gender distribution is about equal.
- There is a familial occurrence.
  - The disorder is concordant in 25% to 70% of identical twins.
  - If a mother has SLE, her daughter's risk is 1:40 and the son's risk is 1:250.
  - Positive antinuclear antibody is seen in asymptomatic family members.

Risk Factors

- Familial predisposition
- Exposure to environmental triggers—see above
- Female gender
- Black, Hispanic, or Asian descent
- Presence of other autoimmune disorders
- Smoking

Prevention and Screening

- Avoidance of environmental triggers
- Smoking cessation
- No routine screening
- Yearly influenza vaccine
- Pneumococcal vaccine every 5 years

Assessment

History
- Fever
- Anorexia
- Malaise
- Weight loss
- Arthritis
- Synovitis
- Blurred vision
- Photosensitivity
- Pleurisy
- Abdominal pain
- Psychosis
- Cognitive impairment
- Peripheral and cranial neuropathies
- Transverse myelitis
- Stokes
- Depression

Physical Examination
- Characteristic "butterfly" malar rash is seen in 50% of patients
- Discoid lupus
- Fingertip lesions
- Periungual erythema
- Nail fold infarcts
- Splinter hemorrhages
- Alopecia
- Raynaud's phenomenon—20% of patients
- Conjunctivitis
- Photophobia
- Transient or permanent monocular blindness
- Cotton wool spots on the retina (cytoid bodies) represent degeneration of nerve fibers because of occlusion of retinal blood vessels
- Pleural effusion
- Bronchopneumonia
- Pneumonitis
- Alveolar hemorrhage—rare but life-threatening
- Myocarditis
- Hypertension
- Cardiac dysrhythmias
- Atypical verrucous Libman-Sacks endocarditis
- Mesenteric vasculitis
- Ileus
- Peritonitis or perforation
- Glomerulonephritis
  - Mesangial
  - Focal proliferative
  - Diffuse proliferative
  - Membranous

Diagnostic Studies
- Antinuclear antibody tests are sensitive but not specific for SLE
  - They are present in all SLE patients, but they are also present in several other disorders.
- Antibodies to double-stranded DNA and to Sm are specific to SLE but not sensitive.
  - They are present in only 60% to 70% of patients.
  - Anti–double-stranded DNA levels correlate with disease activity; Sm levels do not
- Depressed serum complement is suggestive of disease activity and usually returns to normal during remissions.
- Serum chemistry panel with liver function studies
  - Liver enzymes may be elevated in drug-induced SLE.
- Creatine kinase
  - May be elevated in myositis
- Laboratory abnormalities in SLE
  - Anemia: 60%
  - Leukopenia: 45%
  - Thrombocytopenia: 30%
  - Biologic false-positive tests for syphilis: 25%
  - Antiphospholipid antibodies
    - Lupus anticoagulant: 7%
    - Anti-cardiolipin antibody: 25%
    - Direct Coomb's test, positive: 30%
  - Proteinuria: 30%
  - Hematuria: 30%
  - Hypocomplementemia: 60%
  - ANA: 95% to 100%
  - Anti–native-DNA: 50%
  - Anti-Sm: 20% (McPhee & Papadakis, 2011)
- With renal lesions: urinary sediment, red blood cells, with or without casts, and proteinuria—usually resolve with remission
- Chest radiograph to monitor interstitial lung disease
- Brain MRI/MRA to evaluate for CNS lupus white matter changes, vasculitis, or stroke
- Echocardiography
  - Pericardial effusion
  - Pulmonary hypertension
  - Verrucous Libman-Sacks endocarditis
- Lumbar puncture to exclude other disease
- Renal biopsy
  - To identify type of glomerulonephritis
- Skin biopsy
  - To aid in diagnosis

Differential Diagnosis

- Anti-phospholipid syndrome
- Fibromyalgia
- Hepatitis C
- Infectious mononucleosis
- Infective endocarditis
- Lyme disease
- Lymphoma B-cell
- Rheumatic fever
- Rheumatoid arthritis
- Thrombotic thrombocytopenic purpura (TTP)
- Undifferentiated connective-tissue disease
- Mixed connective-tissue disease

Management

Nonpharmacologic Treatment
- Patient education and emotional support
- Joint rest
- Patients with photosensitivity should avoid sun exposure and use high-block sunscreen

Pharmacologic Treatment
- Minor joint symptoms
  - NSAIDS
- Lupus rash or joint symptoms
  - Hydroxchloroquine 200 or 400 mg/d p.o., not > 6.5 mg/kg/d
    - Annual monitoring for retinal changes
- Thrombocytopenia not responsive to steroids
  - Dehydroepiandrosterone (DHEA)
- Glomerulonephritis, hemolytic anemia, pericarditis or myocarditis, alveolar hemorrhage, CNS involvement, and TTP
  - Prednisone 40 to 60 mg initially, then the dose is tailored to keep symptoms at a minimun
- If resistant to corticosteroids:
  - Cyclophosphamide
  - Mycopenolate mofetil
  - Azathioprine
- Treatment of severe lupus nephritis
  - Cyclophosphamide
  - Mycophenolate mofetil
- Antiphospholipid syndrome
  - Anticoagulation
  - Warfarin to keep INR 2.0 to 3.0

Special Considerations

- Pregnant patients with recurrent fetal loss should be treated with low–molecular-weight heparin plus aspirin
- When cyclophosphamide is needed, gonadotropin-releasing hormone analogs can be administered to prevent premature ovarian failure

When to Consult, Refer, or Hospitalize

- SLE requires management by a rheumatologist.
- Consults to other subspecialites are determined by the course of the disease.
- Hospitalize for rapidly progressing glomerulonephritis, pulmonary hemorrhage, transverse myelitis, or other life-threatening organ failure.
- Admit for treatment of infections, especially if the patient is immunosuppressed, for close monitoring.

Follow-up

Expected Outcomes
- 10-year survival rates are exceeding 85%.
- However, some patients have a virulent course that leads to serious dysfunction of the heart, lung, brain, and kidneys.
  - Multi-organ involvement can lead to death.
- In the early years after diagnosis, infections are the leading cause of death.
- In the later years, accelerated atherosclerosis from chronic inflammation is a major cause of death.
  - Myocardial infarction is five times higher in those with SLE.

IMMUNOSUPPRESSION

Description

- Immunodeficiency disorders are a reduced or absent response from the body's immune system.
- The immune system is composed of bone marrow, lymph nodes, thymus, tonsils, parts of the spleen, and GI tract.
- The immune system is divided into humoral and cellular components.
  - Humoral
    - Antibodies
    - Complement system

- Cellular
  - T cells
  - Natural killer cells
  - Macrophages
  - Neutrophils
- Patients with humoral deficiencies have recurrent infections
  - Encapsulated bacteria
  - Occasionally enteric viruses
- Patients with cellular deficiencies have recurrent infections with *Pneumocystis carinii*, fungi, viruses, and mycobacteria predominantly.
- Primary immunodeficiencies are classified according to mode of inheritance and whether the genetic defect affects T cells, B cells, or both.

Etiology

- Immunodeficiency syndromes may be congenital, spontaneously acquired, or iatrogenic.
- Defects in the humoral response may occur from lack of production, inadequate production or dysfunction of antibodies, and antibody consumption.
- Immune system dysfunction can result from altered activity of any type of cell types (T cell, macrophage, neutrophil, or NK)
- Congenital immunodeficiency
  - Often X-linked—only males affected
    - 60% of people with congenital immunodeficiency disorders are male.
  - Both B and T cells may be affected singly or in combination.
  - Phagocytes
  - Complement proteins
  - About one-half of these disorders involve B cells.
  - Common disorders
    - B cells
      - Common variable immunodeficiency
      - Deficiency of a specific antibody (immunoglobulin)
      - X-linked agammagloblinemia
    - T cells
      - Chronic mucocutaneous candidiasis
      - DiGeorge syndrome
      - X-linked lymphoproliferative syndrome
    - B and T cells
      - Ataxia-telangiectasia
      - Hyperimmunoglobulinemia E syndrome
      - Severe combined immunodeficiency
      - Wiskott-Aldrich syndrome
    - Dysfunction of phagocytes
      - Chédiak-Higashi syndrome (rare)
      - Chronic granulomatous disease
      - Leukocyte adhesion defects
    - Dysfunction of complement proteins
      - Complement component 1 (C1) inhibitor deficiency (hereditary angioedema)
      - C3 deficiency

- C6 deficiency
- C7 deficiency
- C8 deficiency
- Acquired immunodeficiency disorders
  - Most commonly result from medications
    - Primarily immunosuppresants
    - Corticosteroids
    - Chemotherapy
    - Radiation therapy
    - Common causes of acquired immunodeficiency disorders
      - Medications
        - Anticonvulsants
          - Carbamazepine
            - Phenytoin
            - Valproate
        - Immunosuppresants
          - Azathioprine
          - Mycophenolate mofetil
          - Cyclosporine
          - Sirolimus
          - Tacrolimus
        - Corticosteroids
          - Methylprednisolone
          - Prednisone
        - Chemotherapy
          - Alemtuzumab
          - Busulfan
          - Cyclophosphamide
          - Melphalan
        - Monoclonal antibodies
          - Muromonab (OKT3)
      - Disorders
        - Aplastic anemia
        - Leukemia
        - Myelofibrosis
        - Sickle cell disease
        - Cancer
        - Down syndrome
        - Cytomegalovirus
        - Epstein-Barr virus
        - HIV infection
        - Measles
        - Varicella
        - Diabetes
        - Uremia
        - Nephrotic syndrome
        - Hepatitis
        - Rheumatoid arthritis

- SLE
- Splenectomy
- Alcoholism
- Burns
- Malnutrition

Incidence and Demographics

- Primary immunodeficiency disorders are relatively common.
- IgA deficiency (the most frequent) occurs in approximately 1 in 600 persons in the United States.
- Common variable immunodeficiency is the next most common disorder.
- These disorders become clinically evident as young adults.
- The more severe forms of primary immunodeficiency are somewhat rare, have onset in early life, and often result in death in childhood.
- Patients with congenital hypogammaglobulinemia may live relatively healthy lives with adequate antibody-replacement therapy.

Risk Factors

- See Etiology
- Genetic predisposition
- Medications—corticosteroids
- History of splenectomy
- Diabetes
- Increasing age
- HIV/AIDS
- Malignancy or chemotherapy
- Transplant recipient
- Malnutrition

Prevention and Screening

- Genetic testing
- HIV: safe sex practices, avoidance of sharing needles
- Malignancy: return of immune system function usually occurs after successful treatment
- Diabetes: maintaining control of blood sugars will promote more effective cellular immune response
- Immunodeficiency disorders resulting from a deficiency of antibodies may be treated with immune globulin.
  - Avoid undercooked food
  - Obtain routine dental care
  - Consume only bottled water
  - Avoid individuals who have an infection

Assessment

History
- Weight loss
- Recurrent infections
  - Ear
  - Skin
    - Sore throats
    - Frequent colds
    - Chronic diarrhea
    - Chronic sinusitis
    - Assessment of risk factors—see above

Physical Examination
- Rashes
- Pyoderma
- Petechiae
- Alopecia
- Chronic cough
- Hepato- and/or splenomegaly
- Lymphadenopathy
  - Cervical lymph nodes and tonsillar or adenoid tissue, or both, may be small in X-linked and T cell disorders
  - In chronic granulomatous disease, lymph nodes of the head and neck may be enlarged.
- Tympanic membranes may be scarred or perforated.
- Nostrils may be crusted.
  - Purulent nasal discharge
- Crackles on pulmonary examination
- Muscle mass and fat deposits of the buttocks are decreased.

Diagnostic Studies
- Complete blood count with differential
  - Neutropenia
- Peripheral blood smear
  - Howell-Jolly bodies
- Quantitative Ig measurements
- Antibody titer measurements
- Skin testing for delayed hypersensitivity
- If tests are positive then further testing is warranted, oriented toward the suspected disorder.

Differential Diagnosis

- Cystic fibrosis
- Primary ciliary dyskinesia

Management

Nonpharmacologic and Pharmacologic Treatment
- Severe combined immunodeficiency
  - Bone marrow transplant
  - Exogenous ADA if bone marrow match not available
  - Hematopoietic stem cell gene therapy
  - These patients must be recognized and treated early.
  - Live viral vaccines or blood transfusions must be avoided because they may cause fatal infections and graft-versus-host disease.
- Primary T cell immunodeficiency
  - Symptomatic treatment
  - Live vaccines and blood transfusions should be avoided.
  - Exposure to x-radiation should also be avoided.
  - Epithelial thymic transplant can repair T cell deficiency in patients with nude syndrome where T cells are absent.
  - Bone marrow transplant
  - Immunoglobulin infusions
- Immunoglobulin deficiency syndromes
  - Replacement therapy with human immunoglobulin
  - Maintain IgG > 6.0 g/l

Special Considerations

- Medication-induced immunosuppression is often reversible after discontinuation of the offending medication.
- Patients receiving chemotherapy or corticosteroids should be instructed to seek medical care for a fever > 100.5° F or if they develop a cough and shortness of breath, thrush, or headache with a stiff neck.

When to Consult, Refer, or Hospitalize

- When diagnosis made, referral to an immunologist should be made.
- Hospitalize for complications, therapeutic interventions, or both.
- Patient made need referral to tertiary care center for treatment.

Follow-up

Expected Outcomes
- Patients with primary immunodeficiency disorders require lifelong surveillance and specialized treatment.
- Secondary immunodeficiency prognosis depends on the underlying etiology.

Complications
- Progression of disease
- Persistent infections, opportunistic infections, or both
- Death

REFERENCES

Anand, M., & Routes, J. (2010). *Hypersensitivity reactions, immediate.* Retrieved from www.emedicine.com/article/136217

Azar, E. (2007). Evaluation of the adult with suspected immunodeficiency. *American Journal of Medicine, 120,* 764–768.

Barkley, T., & Myers, C. (2008). *Practice guidelines for acute care nurse practitioners.* (2nd ed.). St. Louis, MO: Elsevier.

Beers, M., Porter, R., Jones, T., Kaplan, J., & Berkwitz, M. (2007). *The Merck manual of diagnosis and therapy.* Whitehouse Station, NJ: Merck Research Laboratories.

Chifflot, H., Fautral, B., Sordet, C., Chatelus, E., & Sibilia, J. (2008). Incidence and prevalence of systemic sclerosis: A systematic literature review. *Seminars in Arthritis and Rheumatism, 37*(4), 223–235.

Fauci, A., Braunwald, E., Hauser, S., Jameson, J., Kasper, D., Longo, D., & Loscalzo, J. (2008). *Harrison's principles of internal medicine* (17th ed.). New York: McGraw Hill.

Goldman, L., & Ausiello, D. (Eds.). (2007). *Cecil medicine.* Philadelphia: Saunders Elsevier.

Kamanger, N., & Schorr, A. (2009). *Sarcoidosis.* Retrieved from www.emedicine.com/article/301914

McPhee, S., & Papadakis, M. (Eds.) (2011). *Current medical diagnosis and treatment.* New York: McGraw Hill

Morimoto, Y. (2008). Immunodeficiency overview. *Primary Care, 35,* 159–173.

Obici, L., Perfetti, V., Palladini, G., Moratti, R. (2005). Clinical aspects of systemic amyloid diseases. *Biochemica et biophysica acta, 1753*(1), 11–22.

Tran, M., & Nettleman, M. (2010). *HIV/AIDS overview.* Retrieved from www.emedicinehealth.com

12

Musculoskeletal Disorders
Julie Davey, MSN, RN, ANP-BC, ACNP-BC

TRAUMA

SHOULDER PAIN

Description

- Acute or chronic pain in the shoulder girdle as the result of a variety of arthritic, inflammatory, or traumatic causes

Etiology, Incidence, and Demographics

- Acute injury more common in younger adults
- Chronic, inflammatory injury more common in older adults

Trauma
- Fracture of proximal humerus, greater tuberosity, clavicle, scapula
- Rotator cuff strain, tear
- Dislocation
- Acromioclavicular separation
- Sternoclavicular injury

Inflammatory Conditions
- Bursitis
- Rotator cuff tendonitis
- Rheumatoid arthritis
- Impingement syndrome

Degenerative Conditions
- Osteoarthritis

Miscellaneous
- Chronic instability
- Adhesive capsulitis

Risk Factors

- Repetitive overhead activity (occupational, recreational)
- Rheumatoid arthritis or osteoarthritis
- Previous shoulder injury

Assessment

Diagnostic Studies

Plain film x-rays
- Assess for fracture
- Deformity of acromioclavicular (AC) separation
- Arthritic changes
- Osteophytes
- Calcified tendinitis

Magnetic resonance imaging
- Tendinitis
- Rotator cuff tear
- Cartilage injury

Fracture
- Fall directly onto shoulder or outstretched arm
- Localized pain, edema
- Decreased range of motion (ROM)
- No bruising evident for first few days after injury
- Patient holds arm close to body
- Point tenderness
- Varying degree of deformity dependent upon bone fractured
- Decreased ROM

Rotator cuff tear
- Age usually > 50 years
- Pain may radiate into deltoid area.
- May have felt "pop" or "something give" in shoulder
- Inability to raise arm overhead
- Weakness or inability to externally rotate arm
- Inability to sleep on affected side
- Weakness or inability to externally rotate shoulder
- Limited abduction, forward flexion of shoulder
- Inability to maintain resisted abduction at 90°

Dislocation
- Direct blow to shoulder or trying to avoid fall by grabbing onto a brace; shoulder in abducted, externally rotated position
- Sensation of shoulder slipping out of joint
- "Popping" or clicking of joint
- May be edematous
- Positive apprehension test—shoulder abducted to 90° and elbow flexed to 90°; shoulder then passively externally rotated; resistance by patient constitutes a positive test
- Palpable clicking with ROM
- Deformity may be visible

Separated shoulder
- Typically, history of direct blow or fall onto top of shoulder
- Pain with adduction of arm
- Edema
- Deformity depends upon severity of injury
- Tenderness over acromioclavicular (AC) joint
- Ecchymosis

Inflammatory conditions
- Progressive pain with certain activities (usually overhead)—may progress to constant pain
- Pain often worse with lifting, pushing objects away
- Difficulty lying on affected side
- Tenderness over inflamed tendons
- Weak abduction
- Painful arc (pain at 70° to 120° of abduction)

Adhesive capsulitis
- Middle-aged women more likely to be afflicted
- May be history of trauma
- Progressive loss of motion
- Pain varies from minimal to severe
- Marked restriction in active and passive ROM
- Pain over anterior joint, rotator cuff

Differential Diagnosis

- Septic joint
- Gout
- Chondroclavicular disease
- Acromegaly

Management

Nonpharmacologic and Pharmacologic Treatment
- Treat arthritic or inflammatory conditions as indicated.

Rotator cuff injury/tear
- NSAIDs and/or moist heat
- Rest or immobilization for short period (< 14 days)
- Passive, active, resistive exercises
- For those unresponsive to conservative therapy
  - Intra-articular corticosteroid preparation injection
  - Physical therapy
- Surgical intervention for those unresponsive to several months of therapy or with complete tears

Adhesive capsulitis
- Manipulation of joint

ACUTE KNEE INJURY

Description

- Damage to the knee or its supporting structures, typically caused by trauma. Medial meniscus tears are most common.

Etiology, Incidence, and Demographics

- Direct or indirect force against the knee—direction and intensity of force determines specific type of injury
- Occurs most commonly during sports that require rapid changes in direction, acceleration–deceleration, or both

Risk Factors

- Participation in contact, running sports
- Osteoarthritis
- Steroid use
- Osteoporosis
- Poor conditioning
- Poorly fitting footwear
- Falls

Assessment

Diagnostic Studies
- Plain film radiograph: assess for fractures, osteoarthritis
- Magnetic resonance imaging: differentiate among ligamentous, cartilaginous injuries
- Joint aspiration: has both diagnostic and therapeutic utility

Fracture
- Trauma
- Sudden edema, pain, warmth
- Effusion (hemarthrosis)
- Tenderness or pain to palpation
- Decreased ROM
- Difficulty bearing weight

Meniscus tear
- Pain with twisting of the knee (getting in or out of automobile)
- Sense of knee "locking" or "giving way"
- More difficult going downstairs than climbing up
- Edema
- Tenderness over medial or lateral tibial joint line
- Positive McMurray test

Medial collateral ligament (MCL) injury
- Sudden valgus stress to knee
- May report "pop" sensation
- Medial knee pain
- Localized edema over 1 to 4 hours
- Tenderness to palpation over medial aspect

Lateral collateral ligament (LCL) injury
- Direct blow to medial aspect of knee
- Similar to MCL injury but lateral
- Tenderness to palpation over lateral aspect
- Varying degree of joint laxity

Anterior cruciate ligament (ACL) injury
- Pain and almost immediate edema following sudden deceleration, jumping
- Weight-bearing difficult because of sense of knee instability
- Effusion
- Hemarthrosis
- Pain or tenderness in posterolateral joint
- Positive anterior drawer test
- Positive Lachman test

Posterior cruciate ligament (PCL) injury
- Forced hyperextension of knee
- Direct blow to anterior proximal knee while knee is flexed and foot planted
- Mild to moderate effusion
- Positive posterior drawer test
- Positive Godfrey's test

Differential Diagnosis

- Progressive osteoarthritis
- Septic joint
- Gout
- Tumor

Management

- NSAIDs for acute pain relief
- Narcotic analgesia when indicated for severe pain
- Physical therapy for strength and ROM improvement
- Immobilization as appropriate (fractures)
- Non–weight-bearing as appropriate
- Surgical repair sometimes necessary

Table 12-1. Clinically Relevant Tests of the Knee

Test Name	How to Perform
Valgus stress (tests MCL)	With patient's knee in 20° to 30° of flexion, the examiner stabilizes the leg with one hand while applying inward-directed pressure to the joint. Test is repeated with knee in full extension.
Varus stress (tests LCL)	As above, but stress at joint is directed from medial to lateral direction
Anterior drawer (tests ACL)	With patient supine, his or her knee is flexed to 90° while examiner stabilizes patient's tibia (usually by sitting on it). Examiner grasps proximal posterior tibia, pulling it forward. Anterior movement (translation) of tibia greater than uninvolved side is positive test.
Posterior drawer (tests PCL)	Patient and examiner in same position as for anterior drawer, but examiner pushes tibia posteriorly.
Lachman test (more accurate than anterior drawer)	With patient supine, his or her knee is flexed to 30°. Using one hand, examiner stabilizes patient's distal femur while using the other hand to pull proximal tibia anteriorly.
McMurray test (for meniscus injury)	Patient's knee maximally flexed then internally rotated; as leg is passively extended, examiner simultaneously externally rotates leg while palpating tibial joint line. Repeat with leg externally rotated, internally rotating while extending. Positive test is palpable click or tibial joint line pain.

Adapted from "Arthritis and musculoskeletal diseases" by D. B. Hellman & J. H. Stone, 2007, in Tierney, L. M., McPhee, S. J. Jr., & Papadakis, M. A. (Eds.), *Current medical diagnosis and treatment* (pp. 826–886), New York, NY: Lange Medical Books/McGraw-Hill.

ANKLE SPRAIN

Description

- Stretching, tearing, or both of the ligaments around the ankle, typically involving the lateral ligament complex. Ankle sprain is the most common sports injury.

Etiology, Incidence, and Demographics

- Usually a forced inversion (affects lateral ankle) or eversion injury (affects medial ankle)
- Most common musculoskeletal injury
- Occurs in 1 in 10,000 persons per day
- Males more often affected

Risk Factors

- Sports events requiring sudden turns
- Jumping

Assessment

Diagnostic Studies
- Radiograph indicated according to Ottawa Ankle Rule
  - There is pain near the malleoli *and*
  - Bone tenderness is present at the posterior edge of the distal 6 cm or the tip of either malleolus *or*
  - The patient is unable to bear weight for at least four steps at the time of injury and evaluation
  - Otherwise, diagnostic studies not indicated

Grade I
- Stretching but no tearing of ligament; no joint instability
- Local tenderness
- Minimal edema
- Ecchymosis typically insignificant or absent
- Full range of motion remains although may be uncomfortable
- Patient retains weight-bearing ability.

Grade II
- Partial (incomplete) tearing of ligament; some joint instability but definite endpoint to laxity
- Pain immediately upon injury
- Localized edema and ecchymosis
- Significant pain with weight-bearing
- Range of motion is limited.

Grade III
- Complete ligamentous tearing; joint unstable with no definite end point to ligamentous stressing
- Severe pain immediately upon injury
- Significant edema along foot and ankle
- Profound ecchymosis due to hemorrhage—worsens over several days
- Patient cannot bear weight.
- No range of motion to ankle

Differential Diagnosis

- Fracture
- Tendonitis

Management

Nonpharmacologic and Pharmacologic Treatment
- All grades, including III (unless severe grade III) respond well to RICE
  - **R**est: weight-bearing should be avoided for the first several days
  - **I**ce: should be applied on top of the compression dressing as quickly as possible following injury, 30 minutes on and off alternately
  - **C**ompression: immediately securing compression will minimize edema and support stability of the ankle
  - **E**levation: for several days following injury reduces pain and edema and promotes recovery
- NSAIDs for pharmacologic pain relief

FRACTURES

Description

- A complete or incomplete break in bone, typically as a result of trauma but can occur pathologically as a result of a variety of disorders.

Etiology, Incidence, and Demographics

- Trauma to otherwise healthy bone
- Pathologic occurrence in bone weakened as a result of:
  - Osteoporosis
  - Osteomalacia
  - Osteomyelitis
- Most common demographic is White women

Risk Factors

- Trauma
- Falls
- Neoplasms
- Osteoporosis
- Osteomyelitis
- Smoking
- Chronic corticosteroid use

Assessment

History
- Immediate pain in affected area
- Significant, rapid onset edema

Physical Examination
- Pain intensifies with movement or palpation of affected bone.
- Obvious deformity or asymmetry may be present.

Diagnostic Studies
- Plain x-ray typically most useful study
- Bone scan for stress or occult fracture
- CT scan for compression fracture

Differential Diagnosis

- Severe sprain
- Hematoma
- Tumor

Management

Nonpharmacologic and Pharmacologic Treatment
- Immobilization by splinting or casting
- Narcotic analgesia typically indicated
- NSAID analgesia to augment narcotic—may be primary pain drug after first 48 to 72 hours
- Maintain neurovascular integrity

When to Consult, Refer, Hospitalize (refers to all musculoskeletal injuries)

- Admission may be required for fractures or trauma, depending upon the severity and presence of additional complications. Otherwise, immobilization with splinting or casting and discharge home is appropriate.
- Consult orthopedics to determine the treatment plan and need for possible surgical intervention.

Follow-up (for all musculoskeletal injuries)

- Avoid high-risk behavior that may lead to injury.
- Discuss importance of rest and immobilization when appropriate.
- Explain procedure in detail as indicated (e.g., cast, surgical procedures).

DEGENERATIVE JOINT DISEASES

RHEUMATOID ARTHRITIS

Description

- Chronic, inflammatory, systemic disease with its most pronounced symptoms from progressive destruction of synovial joints with loss of cartilage and bone. It is also characterized by
  - Damaged ligaments and tendons
  - Loss of physical function and quality of life with disability and underemployment
  - Life expectancy reduced by 5 to 15 years
  - Extra-articular manifestations later in disease
    - Cardiovascular disease presents 10 years earlier.
    - Increased incidence of gastrointestinal bleeding
    - Increased incidence of pulmonary disease
    - Twice the incidence of cancer as in the general population
    - 6 to 9 times the rate of serious infection as compared to the general population

Etiology, Incidence, and Demographics

- Believed to be autoimmune
- Susceptibility genetically determined; most patients have human leukocyte antigen (HLA) class 2
- Onset commonly at ages 40 to 60
- Female to male ratio 3:1
- Occurs in 1% to 2% of the population

Risk Factors

- HLA-2
- Family history
- Personal history of other autoimmune disease

Prevention and Screening

- None

Assessment

- Highly variable
- Prodromal symptoms of malaise, weight loss
- Infrequently, onset may be triggered by physical or emotional stress.
- Characteristic symmetric joint edema with stiffness, warmth, tenderness, and pain
- Stiffness prominent in the morning and subsides during the day
- Duration of stiffness an indicator of disease activity
- May develop permanent deformity
- May have vasculitis and other systemic inflammation
- Any joint may be affected; interphalangeal joints, wrists, knees, ankles, and toes most common
- Palmar errythema
- Subcutaneous nodules over bony prominences
- Extra-articular manifestations
  - Dryness of mucous membranes
  - Ocular manifestations
  - Aortitis
  - Skin or muscle atrophy
  - Splenomegaly
  - Lymphadenopathy

Diagnostic Studies
- Acute phase reactants
- Elevated erythrocyte sedimentation rate (ESR)
- Elevated C-reactive protein (CRP)
- Rheumatoid factor
  - Less than 20% of patients positive within the first 6 months
  - Only 85% ever positive
  - Not specific to RA
  - Higher titers correlate to worse prognosis
  - Once positive, does not need to be repeated
- Anti–cyclic citrullinated peptide (CCP) antibodies
  - Higher specificity for rheumatoid arthritis (RA) than rheumatoid factor (RF)
  - Similar or higher sensitivity for RA than RF
    - Found in up to 40% of patients who are RF negative
    - But, not all RA patients will be CCP-positive
      - May be seen earlier than RF
      - High positive predictive value for RA
      - Predictive of prognosis (erosive disease and joint damage)
- Antinuclear antibody in 20% patients
- Hypochromic,of normocytic anemia is common
- Platelet and leukocyte count may be elevated

- Joint fluid shows inflammatory changes
  - > 3.5 cc
  - Translucent to opaque
  - Yellow to opalescent
  - 3,000 to 50,000 white blood count (WBC)
  - > 50% polymorphonuclear neutrophilic leukocyte (PMN)
  - Culture negative
  - Glucose present but lower than serum
- X-ray shows soft-tissue edema and juxta-articular demineralization
- Later x-ray changes include joint space narrowing and erosion

Differential Diagnosis

- Systemic lupus erythematosus
- Psoriatic arthritis
- Osteoarthritis
- Gout
- Lyme disease

Management

- Early intervention is of paramount importance

Nonpharmacologic Treatment
- Physical therapy
- Rest as indicated—complete bed rest may be necessary during acute exacerbation
- Passive range of motion and active joint exercise as tolerated
- Splinting
- Heat or cold application for comfort
- Assistive devices as indicated

Pharmacologic Treatment (see Table 12–2)

Table 12–2. Pharmacologic Treatment for Rheumatoid Arthritis

NSAIDs	Methotrexate	Tumor Necrosis Factor (TNF) Inhibitors	Hydroxychlorquine
First-line agent for those with high risk of gastrointestinal bleeding	Treatment of choice for those not responding to NSAIDs	Produce marked improvement in the majority of patients	Another alternative for those unresponsive to NSAIDs
COX-2 inhibitors *or*	Contraindicated in patients with any form of chronic hepatitis	TNF important in physiologic response to infection	Useful primarily for mild disease
COX-1 *with*	Common adverse effects include stomatitis and gastric irritation	TNF inhibitors should be discontinued in the patient with evidence of systemic infection (e.g., fever)	Low incidence of toxicity
Concomitant misoprostol (Cytotec) *or*	Rare but life-threatening interstitial pneumonitis may occur	Very expensive	May produce visual loss—ophthalmic exam every 6 to 12 months
Concomitant proton-pump inhibitors	Co-administer with folic acid supplementation		Neuropathies and myopathies may occur

Adapted from "Arthritis and musculoskeletal diseases", by D. B. Hellman & J. H. Stone, 2007, in Tierney, L. M., McPhee, S. J. Jr., & Papadakis, M. A. (Eds.), *Current medical diagnosis and treatment* (pp. 826–886). New York, NY: Lange Medical Books/McGraw-Hill.

Corticosteroids	Gold Salts	Minocycline (Minocin)	Leflunomide (Arava)
Produce dramatic relief	Used for patients not responsive to methotrexate	Mechanism of action unclear	Food and Drug Administration (FDA)–approved for rheumatoid arthritis treatment
Should be reserved for short-term use in severe exacerbation or in severe disease not responsive to other therapies	Less common now with newer options	Used in mild disease	Monitor liver function tests
			May produce alopecia, diarrhea
			Carcinogenic; should not be used by men or women trying to conceive

When to Consult, Refer, or Hospitalize

- Refer to rheumatology for detailed testing to ensure accurate diagnosis and determine treatment course
- Hospital admission may be required for complications of rheumatoid arthritis such as cardiovascular manifestations or disease

Patient Education

- Educate patients on the disease process and goals of treatment.
- Educate patients on medications and side effects as appropriate.
- Discuss the use of assistive devices such as splints and application of heat or cold.
- Inform patients of self-help programs and classes.

OSTEOARTHRITIS

Description

- Degenerative disorder of the movable joints characterized by degeneration of cartilage and bone hypertrophy, and formation of osteophytes and subchondral cysts. There is no systemic involvement.

Etiology, Incidence, and Demographics

- Articular cartilage roughens, is worn away
  - May occur as a result of injury (secondary osteoarthritis)
    - Fracture—acute injury
    - Overuse, metabolic disease—chronic injury
  - Cause not always identifiable (primary osteoarthritis)
- Synovial membrane thickens
- Enzymatic destruction increases cartilage degradation.
- Proteoglycans and collagen synthesis are decreased.
- Changes in the proteoglycans render cartilage less resistant to compressive forces.
- Decreased strength of cartilage is compounded by adverse alterations of the collagen.
- Elevated levels of collagen degradation place excessive stresses on the remaining fibers, leading to mechanical failure.
- The diminished elastic return, reduced contact area of the cartilage, and cyclic nature of joint loading causes the situation to worsen over time.
- Affects 20 million people in the United States
- Greatest prevalence in Native Americans
- Age of symptom onset typically 55 to 65 years old
- 80% to 90% of persons > 65 years of age are affected.

Risk Factors

- Advancing age
- Repetitive joint use
- Trauma
- Obesity
- Heredity

Prevention and Screening

- None

Assessment

History
- Initially articular stiffness, developing into pain with motion
- Pain relieved by rest—at best upon awakening, worsens throughout the day

Physical Examination
- Heberden's nodes—nodes in the proximal interphalangeal joints
- Bouchard's nodes—nodes in the distal interphalangeal joints
- Coarse crepitus in the joint
- Decreased range of motion (ROM) of the affected joint
- No gross deformity but interphalangeal joint enlargement may be prominent
- Joint enlargement is hard and cold.
- Limited range of motion

Diagnostic Studies
- Markers of systemic inflammation and autoimmune disease are within normal limits.
  - Erythrocyte sedimentation rate
  - Serum antinuclear antibody
  - Rheumatoid factor
- Classic radiographic findings
  - Unequal narrowing of joint space on x-ray
  - Thick, dense subchondral bone
  - Bone cysts
  - Osteophytes
  - Sharpened articular margins

Differential Diagnosis

- Rheumatic disease
- Fibromyalgia
- Gout

- Osteoporosis
- Multiple myeloma
- Acute injury

Management

Nonpharmacologic Treatment
- Weight loss if indicated
- Physical activity—supervised walking
- Ambulation aids
- Physical therapy

Pharmacologic Treatment
- Acetaminophen
- Acetylsalicylic acid (ASA) or other nonsteroidal anti-inflammatory drugs (NSAIDs) for failure to respond to acetaminophen—high doses as used for rheumatoid arthritis unnecessary
- Cyclooxygenase (COX)-2 inhibitors only for those with high risk for gastrointestinal bleeding
- Knee with effusion—intra-articular triamcinolone no more than two to three times yearly
  - Intra-articular hyaluronic acid (Hyalgan, Synvisc)
- Pain unresponsive to conservative measures may require joint surgery or replacement

When to Consult, Refer, Hospitalize

- Rarely do patients require hospital admission unless complications occur such as fracture or acute injury.
- Consult orthopedic surgery for patients with severe pain, functional impairment, or both; surgical intervention may be indicated.

Follow-up

- Educate patients on the disease process and goals of treatment.
- Educate patients on medications and side effects as appropriate.
- Inform patients of self-help programs and classes.
- Discuss the benefits of a daily exercise regimen.
- Discuss the use of assistive devices when appropriate (e.g., cane, walker).
- Educate the patient and family regarding surgical procedures when appropriate.

GOUT

Description

- A group of metabolic diseases arising from deposition of uric acid or monosodium urate crystals in supersaturated extracellular fluids (particularly in and around joints and tendons), resulting in recurring acute arthritis that later deteriorates to chronic, deforming, tophaceous arthritis. Gout is the most common cause of monoarticular joint inflammation

Etiology, Incidence, and Demographics

- Hyperuricemia secondary to overproduction or underexcretion
- Hyperuricemia as a result of chronic medication use
  - ASA
  - Thiazide diuretics
  - Niacin
- Chronic ethanol (ETOH) ingestion
- More common in persons of Asian descent
- 90% of patients are male
- Age of onset: > 30 men, postmenopause for women

Risk Factors

- Heredity
- Obesity
- Overproduction of urate
  - High intake of purine-rich foods (e.g., organ meats, shellfish, peas, lentils, beans)
  - Hemolytic diseases
  - Psoriasis
  - Glycogen-storage diseases
- Underexcretion of uric acid
  - Reduced renal function
  - Lactic acidosis
  - Ketoacidosis
  - Diuretics
  - Dehydration
  - Certain drugs (ethambutol, cyclosporine)

Prevention and Screening

- Avoid ETOH abuse.

Assessment

- Frequently no apparent cause
- Sudden onset of red, hot, edematous, exquisitely tender joint
- First metatarsophalangeal (MTP) joint is most susceptible—known as podagra
- Foot, ankle, knee are most common sites; wrist, elbow, finger also may be affected
- Fever, chills, malaise may accompany acute attack
- Desquamation and pruritus during resolution of acute attack
- Tophi (sodium urate crystals deposited in soft tissue) present in chronic tophaceous gout; usually 2 to 10 years after onset of acute intermittent gout
- Joint edema, restricted movement in late and chronic stages because of arthritis

Diagnostic Studies
- Serial uric acid measurements > 7.5 mg/dL in 95% patients
- Elevated erythrocyte sedimentation rate
- Elevated leukocyte count
- Joint fluid aspiration
  - Sodium urate crystals
  - Negatively birefringent crystals on polarized light microscopy
- Radiographic changes
  - None in early disease
  - "Punched-out" erosions in later disease
  - Soft tissue tophi

Differential Diagnosis

- Septic joint
- Acute rheumatic fever
- Cellulitis
- Pyogenic arthritis

Management

Acute Attack
- NSAIDs drug of choice—indomethacin most frequently used but others just as efficacious
- COX-2 inhibitor for those at high risk of gastrointestinal bleeding
- Colchicine effective but less frequently used because of gastrointestinal effects—should be given within the first few hours of symptom onset
- Corticosteroids—for those who cannot take NSAIDs
- Bed rest through 24 hours after acute attack

Chronic Management
- Weight loss
- Decrease purines in diet
- Moderate alcohol use
- Increase fluids; maintain > 2L urine output daily
- Colchicine may reduce number of acute attacks
- Pharmacologic blockade of renal reabsorption of uric acid
  - Allopurinol (Zyloprim)
  - Probenecid (Benemid)
  - Require maintenance of high urine output

When to Consult, Refer, or Hospitalize

- Rarely requires hospital admission
- Consult rheumatology for recurrent acute gouty attacks.

Follow-up

- Educate patients on the underlying disease process and treatment goals.
- Discuss medication side effects as necessary.
- Discuss the importance of weight reduction if appropriate.
- Educate patients on the importance of rest during acute attacks.
- Discuss elimination of ETOH.
- Instruct patients to try application of cold compress during acute attacks.

REFERENCES

Barkley, T. W., & Myers, C. (2008). *Practice guidelines for acute care nurse practitioners.* Philadelphia: W. B. Saunders.

Beers, M., Porter, R., Jones, T., Kaplan, J., & Berkwits, M. (Eds.). (2006). *The Merck manual of diagnosis and therapy.* Whitehouse Station, NJ: Merck Research Laboratories.

Buttaro, T., Trybulski, J., Bailey, P., & Sandberg-Cook, J. (2008). *Primary care* (3rd ed.). St. Louis, MO: Mosby.

Fauci, A. S., Braunwalk, E., Kasper, D. L., Hauser, S. L., Longo, D. L., Jameson, J. L., et al. (2008). *Harrison's principles of internal medicine* (17th ed.). Philadelphia: McGraw Hill.

Fiebach, N. H., Barker, L. R., Burton, J. R., & Zieves, P. D. (2007). *Principles of ambulatory medicine* (7th ed.). Philadelphia: Lippincott Williams and Wilkinson.

McPhee, S. J., Tierney, L. M., & Papadakis, M. A. (2007). *Current medical diagnosis & treatment* (46th ed.). New York: McGraw-Hill.

McPhee, S., & Papadakis, M. (2010). *Current medical diagnosis and treatment* (49th ed.). New York: Lange/McGraw-Hill Publishers.

Parrillo, J., & Dellinger, R. (Eds.). (2008). *Critical care medicine: Principles of diagnosis and management in the adult* (3rd ed.). St. Louis, MO: Mosby.

Psychosocial Health Issues
Julie Davey, MSN, RN, ANP-BC, ACNP-BC

VIOLENCE

Description

- The act of aggression resulting in injury to others or destruction of property

Etiology, Incidence, and Demographics

- May be a genetic predisposition toward aggression
- Personality disorders
  - Antisocial
  - Narcissistic
  - Borderline
- Environmental stressors
- Low self-esteem
- Exposure to violence at an early developmental age

- Comorbid medical disease may include
  - Depression
  - Schizophrenia
  - Mania
  - Temporal lobe dysfunction

Risk Factors

- Poverty, lack of education, lack of vocational skills
- Psychiatric diagnosis
- Alcohol or substance abuse
- Physical or emotional disabilities
- Family or personal history of physical or sexual abuse
- Long-term exposure to violence
- Social isolation, lack of support systems
- Environmental factors such as unemployment, financial difficulty, housing problems, overcrowding

Prevention and Screening

- Avoid stressful situations and environmental stressors

Assessment

Abuser
- Trouble expressing anger
- Verbal threatening
- Impulsivity
- Increased muscle tension
- Agitation
- Substance abuse
- Depression, anxiety

Abused Person
- Withdrawn, fearful, evasive
- Poor personal hygiene, neglect
- Bruises, burns, fractures
- Injuries inconsistent with explanation offered
- Significant delay between time of injury and treatment
- Suicidal or homicidal ideation
- Somatization of symptoms
- Frequent pain complaints

Diagnostic Studies

Abuser
- Mental status exam
- Toxicology screening

Abused Person
- As indicated by presenting symptoms

Differential Diagnosis

Abuser
- See Etiology (personality disorders and comorbid disease)

Abused Person
- Hypochondriasis
- Accidental injuries
- Borderline personality disorder

Management

Abuser
- Allow the patient to ventilate
- Attempt verbal, chemical, physical restraint as deemed appropriate based on the situation
  - Speak in a soft, calm manner. Use a nonthreatening posture.
  - Anxiolytics (lorazepam, diazepam)
  - Neuroleptics (haloperidol)
  - Physical restraints if necessary
- Psychiatric consultation

Abused Person
- Establish safe, supportive environment
- Develop plan of action regarding safety and escape
- Provide community resources, shelters, and hotlines
- Cognitive–behavioral therapy
- Antidepressants or anxiolytics may be indicated, dependent upon specific situation
- Treatment as indicated for posttraumatic stress disorder

When to Consult, Refer, or Hospitalize

Abuser
- Hospitalize if chemical or physical restraint necessary
- Inpatient psychiatric consultation

Abused Person
- As deemed necessary based on injuries, emotional condition
- Counseling and support groups

Follow-up

- Provide information on outpatient treatment programs and support groups.

DEPRESSION

Definition

- A complex mood disorder resulting from a variety of genetic, environmental, and developmental influences. Four major types of depression are identified, with additional subtyping in two of the groups. The predominant feature of major depression is a disturbance in mood (the sustained internal emotional state of an individual) with duration of at least 2 weeks, accompanied by anhedonia (the loss of interest or pleasure) in nearly all activities, and guilt. Subtypes of depression include (1) adjustment disorder with depressed mood, (2) depressive disorders (major depressive disorder, dysthymia, premenstrual dysphoric disorder), (3) bipolar disorder (mania, cyclothymic disorder), and (4) mood disorders due to illness and drugs.

Etiology, Incidence, and Demographics

- Biological
  - Abnormalities in neurotransmitter concentration—serotonin, norepinephrine, dopamine, and gamma aminobuteryic acid (GABA)
  - Dysregulation of the hypopituitary axis
  - Structural changes in the brain, including specific changes in the prefrontal lobe and hippocampus that influence emotions
- Psychoanalytic—anger turned inward
- Developmental problems
  - Cognitive distortion
  - Childhood events
  - Personality disturbances
- Environmental—stressful life events
  - Divorce
  - Unemployment
  - Legal problems

- The World Health Organization (WHO) has identified major depression as a leading cause of disability worldwide and a greater source of morbidity for women than any other illness.
- Women have a 2 to 3 times greater risk of being depressed than men.
- 13% to 20% of the general population has experienced depressive symptoms.
- 5% of the total world population suffers from major depression.
- 15% of individuals diagnosed with severe major depression die of suicide.
- Depression is the most common mental illness seen in primary care practices.
- Lifetime rates of depression for the U.S. population are 7% for women and 3% for men.
- Major depression occurs more often in divorced or separated persons.
- Patients with depression have 2 to 3 times the normal death rate at any age (independent of suicide) and are more likely to incur long-term medical consequences such as premature osteoporosis, coronary artery disease, dysfunction of inflammatory mediators and the immune system, and increased insulin resistance.
- The prevalence of depression does not differ among races.
- Bipolar disorder occurs equally in men and women.
- Dysthymic disorder occurs up to seven times more often in women than in men.

Risk Factors

- History of depression
- Family history in a first-degree relative
- Alcohol and substance abuse
- Postpartum period
- Significant psychosocial stressors
- Periods of prolonged stress

Prevention and Screening

- Avoid ETOH and substance abuse
- Screen patients with depression for suicidal ideations

Assessment

- Major depressive disorder
  - Irritable mood or increased agitation
  - Psychomotor agitation or retardation
  - Changes in appetite or weight
  - Difficulty concentrating or making decisions
  - Change in sleep patterns (insomnia or hypersomnia)
  - Low self-esteem
  - Feelings of worthlessness or excessive, inappropriate guilt
  - Recurrent thoughts of death, morbid thoughts, or preoccupations
  - Suicidal ideation with or without a plan
  - Loss of enjoyment or pleasure in activities
  - Difficulty getting along with others
  - Increased social isolation and withdrawal with increased solitary behavior

- Decreased energy and increased fatigue
- Inattention to self-hygiene and appearance
- Feelings of sadness or hopelessness
- Increased oversensitivity to real or perceived rejections or failures
- Self-destructive behaviors
- Increased somatic complaints such as headache
- Substance abuse
- Impaired judgment
• Adjustment disorder
  - Symptoms occur within 3 months of identifiable stressor
  - Mild sadness
  - Inability to concentrate
  - Excess worry
  - Somatic complaints
• Bipolar disorders
  - Extreme swings in mood
  - Hyperactivity
  - Flight of ideas
  - Decreased need for sleep
  - Grandiosity
  - Impaired judgment
  - Depression
  - Aggressive behavior
  - Sexual acting out
  - Delusions or ideation

Diagnostic Studies
- As indicated to rule out all medical causes of symptoms
- Electrocardiogram (ECG) prior to initiation of tricyclic antidepressant
- Complete blood count (CBC), thyroid profile, sedimentation rate, electrolytes, chemistry profile, syphilis screening
- Electroencephalogram (EEG)—abnormalities seen in 90% of inpatients and 60% of outpatients
- Psychometric tests include Minnesota Multiphasic Personality Inventory (MMPI-2).
- Self-report scales commonly used are the Beck Depression Inventory, Hamilton Rating Scale for Depression, and Zung Self-Rating Depression Scale.

Differential Diagnosis

- Hypo- or hyperthyroid
- Substance abuse
- Cushing's syndrome
- Addison's disease
- Neurological disease
- Head trauma

- Electrolyte imbalance
- Parkinson's disease
- Grief
- Psychotic disorders
- Infection
- Seizure disorder
- Anxiety and panic disorders

Management

- A complete diagnostic evaluation is essential—assess suicide risk.

    ### Nonpharmacologic Treatment
    - Cognitive–behavioral therapy with a focus on cognitive distortions
    - Psychoanalysis or psychotherapy with a focus on intrapsychic phenomena
    - Electroconvulsive therapy for severely depressed or suicidal patients unresponsive to pharmacological agents

    ### Pharmacologic Treatment
- SSRIs are the first-line drug of choice for the treatment of major depression because of their effectiveness and safety record.
    - Mainstay of pharmacologic therapy
    - May produce central nervous system (CNS) activation
    - Sexual adverse effects include retrograde ejaculation, loss of libido, erectile dysfunction
    - Although generally regarded as noncardiotoxic, events of angina have been reported
    - Other adverse effects include tinnitus, insomnia, headache
- Serotonin-norepinepinephrine reuptake inhibitors (SNRIs) are the next choice for those refractory to SSRI treatment; may be used as initial choice for the patient with comorbid neuropathic pain or who presents with more severe depression
    - May produce adverse effects described for SSRI
    - In higher doses, venlafaxine may produce hypertensive episodes; blood pressure should be monitored.
- Tricyclic antidepressants (TCAs) are also effective in the treatment and management of major depression; however, they are associated with a greater incidence of side effects that may be dangerous (cardiotoxicity) and reduce patient compliance.
    - Produces typical anticholinergic effects—dry mouth, urinary retention, constipation, and sedation
- May be cardiotoxic; avoid in patient with preexisting cardiac disease
- Most TCAs produce sedation; may be useful in patients with comorbid insomnia
- Monoamine oxidase inhibitors (MAOs) used in the treatment of refractory or treatment-resistant depression—because of potentially serious and lethal side effects, patients in need of these types of medications should always be referred to a psychiatrist

When to Consult, Refer, or Hospitalize

- All patients who present with suicidal ideation, a prior attempt, or plan should immediately be referred to an emergency room or psychiatrist for further evaluation and treatment.
- Patients who are severely impaired by their symptomology or present with comorbid disorders, such as obsessive–compulsive disorder, substance abuse, eating disorder, or no social support, should be referred to a psychiatrist or other mental health specialist.
- Patients who represent a clear and present danger to themselves or others should be immediately hospitalized.

Follow-up

- Discuss depression as a medical condition and outline the treatment plan.
- Discuss expected treatment outcomes.
- Discuss medication side effects as appropriate.
- Discuss coping mechanisms such as meditation, relaxation techniques, and the like.

SUBSTANCE ABUSE

ALCOHOLISM

Description

- The physiological dependence on alcohol as indicated by evidence of tolerance, symptoms of withdrawal, and impairment of function in social, interpersonal, and occupational areas of one's personal life; typically coincident with depression and blackouts

Etiology, Incidence, and Demographics

- Genetic predisposition
- Social and cultural conditioning
- Male to female ratio for treatment is 4:1
- Alcoholism rates are highest in Black and Hispanic males.
- 50% of violent crimes occur under the influence of alcohol.

Risk Factors

- Underlying psychiatric disorder
- Abuse of other substances
- Cultural conditioning
- Domestic violence or abuse
- Presence of a psychiatric disorder
- College students
- Japanese ethnicity—40% of Japanese have aldehyde dehydrogenase deficiency, which increases susceptibility to alcoholism

Prevention and Screening

- High-risk patients should avoid alcohol use (see below)
- CAGE questionnaire for screening (see below)

Assessment

- Acute intoxication
  - Drowsiness
  - Psychomotor dysfunction
  - Disinhibition
  - Ataxia
  - Nystagmus
  - Delayed responses
- Overdosing
  - Respiratory depression
  - Stupor
  - Seizures
  - Coma
- Chronic indicators of alcoholism
  - Flushed face
  - Scleral injection
  - Frequent accidents
  - Unexplained work or school absences
  - Positive response to CAGE questionnaire (see below)

  ### Diagnostic Studies
  - CAGE questionnaire
    - **Cut down**—Do you feel the need to cut down on drinking?
    - **Annoyed**—Do you feel annoyed when people criticize you for drinking?
    - **Guilt**—Do you feel guilty about your drinking?
    - **Eye opener**—Do you need an "eye opener" in the morning?
  - Liver function tests may be elevated—isolated gamma glutamyltransferase (GGT) elevations is suggestive of alcoholism.
  - Aspartate aminotransferase (AST) > alanine aminotransferase (ALT) by a factor of 2

- Advanced alcoholic cirrhosis
  - Prolonged prothrombin time
  - Decreased albumin

Differential Diagnosis

- Polysubstance abuse
- Mood disorders
- Psychotic disorder
- Cushing's syndrome
- Hyperthyroidism

Management

- Should involve a substance abuse specialist

  ### Nonpharmacologic Treatment
  - Substance abuse counseling
  - Alcoholics Anonymous program
  - Substance abuse treatment programs and halfway houses
  - Cognitive-behavioral therapy
  - Psychoanalysis

  ### Pharmacologic Treatment
  - Acute detoxification—benzodiazepines for seizure prophylaxis (atenolol may be used as adjunctive therapy)
  - Clonidine (Catapres), carbamazepine (Tegretol) are other alternatives when benzodiazepines are undesirable
  - Management of comorbid medical and psychiatric illness
  - Disulfiram (Antabuse) as aversive therapy in select situations—mixed results
  - Thiamine, folic acid, and vitamin B complex supplements

OTHER SUBSTANCE ABUSE

Description

- A maladaptive pattern of the use of intoxicating substances manifested by recurrent, significant adverse medical, psychosocial, and legal consequences related to the repeated use of the substance. Drug dependence clinically manifests as substance-seeking behaviors and physical dependence is accompanied by the presence of tolerance and withdrawal.

Etiology, Incidence, and Demographics

- Genetic predisposition
- Neurotransmitter abnormalities
- Environmental stressors
- Psychodynamic factors
    - Impaired developmental stages
    - Unstable childhood
    - Personality disorders
- Social and cultural
    - Increased availability and prevalence
    - Cultural acceptance and peer pressure
    - Impaired primary relations
    - Psychosocial stressors
- Abuse and dependence more common in men
- Marijuana is the most commonly used substance, excluding alcohol.
- Highest prevalence of abuse occurs from ages 18 to 25
- 1.9 million admissions to publicly funded treatment centers occur annually.
- 70% of all admissions to treatment programs are men.
- The economic costs of substance abuse are estimated to be $97.7 billion annually.

Risk Factors

- Genetic vulnerability
- Personal or family history
- Social, cultural, peer acceptance, and frequent use
- Psychiatric diagnosis
- Chronic pain

Prevention and Screening

- Avoid use of illicit drugs.
- Avoid abuse of prescription medications.
- Urine or blood drug screening if suspicious

Assessment

- Personal, family history of abuse
- Patterns of use, substance of choice
- History of accident, trauma, overdose
- Legal problems
- Stimulants

- Anxiety, agitation, panic, restlessness, irritability, aggression
- Mood swings, grandiosity, elated mood, hallucinations
- Tachycardia, arrhythmias, chest pain, hypertension
- Hypothermia, hyperthermia
- Abdominal pain, nausea, vomiting
- Insomnia
- Impotence
- Mydriasis
- Frequent urination
* Depressants
  - Dysphoria, depressed affect, apathy
  - Psychomotor retardation
  - Slurred speech
  - Drowsiness
  - Diaphoresis
  - Hypotension
  - Miosis
  - Nausea, vomiting
  - Myalgia, muscle pain
  - Rhinorrhea, sneezing, headache
  - Ataxia, tremors, impaired coordination
  - Mood swings, aggression, combativeness, lack of impulse control, disinhibition
  - Impaired attention, memory, and judgment; hallucinations; paranoia
* Hallucinogens
  - Dilated pupils, nystagmus
  - Tachycardia
  - Hypertension
  - Ataxia
  - Severe anxiety, panic
  - Mood swings, aggression
  - Hallucinations, paranoia, flashbacks
  - Tremors
  - Impaired concentration, memory, judgment, ability to make decisions
* Cannabis
  - Paranoia, confusion, distortion of time, hallucinations
* Inhalants and solvents
  - Odor on breath
  - Ataxia
  - Slurred speech
  - Euphoria
  - Tachycardia, arrhythmias
  - Agitation
  - Delirium, confusion, stupor, hallucinations
  - Organic brain damage

Diagnostic Studies
- Urine and serum toxicology screening
- Liver and renal profiles
- As indicated to rule out medical differential diagnoses

Differential Diagnosis

- Polysubstance abuse
- Psychiatric disorders
- Thyroid disease
- Head trauma
- Seizure disorder
- Delirium

Management

Nonpharmacologic Treatment
- Acknowledgement of problem of paramount importance—minimization and denial are significant barriers to treatment
- Inpatient detoxification indicated for some substances
- Behavioral therapy
- Narcotics Anonymous
- Residential treatment programs

Pharmacologic Treatment
- Buprenorphine (Buprenex)
- Methadone
- Clonidine (Catapres)
- Stimulant abuse
  - Diazepam (Valium) for cocaine toxicity
  - Monitor cardiac rate and rhythm
- Depressant abuse
  - Phenobarbital for withdrawal
  - Centrally acting antiadrenergic agonists
- Prognosis and recovery are highly dependent on personal motivation and social support.
- Residential treatment must exceed 90 days to be effective.
- Role of the primary provider is diagnosis, referral, and management of medical consequences.

When to Consult, Refer, or Hospitalize (refers to all substance abuse disorders)

- Admit for detoxification.
- Admit for suicidal ideation.
- Admit for hemodynamic instability.
- Consult psychiatry to assist in management.

Follow-up (for all substance abuse disorders)

- Discuss ways to eliminate one's exposure to prescription or illicit drugs, ETOH, or both in the future to avoid relapse.
- Discuss and refer patient to community self-help, support groups

ANXIETY DISORDERS

Description

- A group of disorders characterized by both psychological and somatic symptoms in response to an irrational, pervasive fear. The anxiety may be seemingly without cause or may appear disproportionate to everyday stressors. Types of anxiety disorders include generalized anxiety disorder (GAD), substance-induced anxiety disorder, panic disorder, obsessive–compulsive disorder (OCD), posttraumatic stress disorder (PTSD), and a variety of social and specific phobias.

Etiology, Incidence, and Demographics

- A variety of theories are postulated; the most widely accepted is that a variety of biopsychosocial factors interact with stressors to produce the disorder.
- Norepinephrine and serotonin are the primary neurotransmitter mediators.
- The autonomic nervous system mediates peripheral symptoms.
- One of the most common mental illnesses in the United States
- 19 million people are affected each year.
- Onset typically age 25 to 30
- Women account for 60% of cases diagnosed and treated.
- Lifetime prevalence of up to 5% of the general population; varies according to specific disorder
- Anxiety is a common concomitant disorder in patients with a history of early traumatic experiences such as abuse, separation, or loss of a parent.

Risk Factors

- Family history
- Exposure to traumatic events
- Genetic predisposition

Prevention and Screening

- Avoid stressful situations that may promote anxiety or a panic attack
- No specific screening

Assessment

- Excessive fear of "losing one's mind" or of death
- Difficulty concentrating
- Tension
- Irritable, agitated mood
- Feelings of impending doom or dread
- Feelings of depersonalization
- Motor restlessness
- Tachycardia
- Hyperventilation
- Palpitations
- Diaphoresis
- Chills or hot flashes
- Paresthesias
- Tremor
- Nausea
- Diarrhea
- Sleep disturbances

Diagnostic Studies
- As indicated to assess for organic disease
- Generalized anxiety disorder is characterized by excessive worry accompanied by at least three of the following:
  - Restlessness
  - Easy fatigue
  - Difficulty concentrating
  - Irritability
  - Muscle tension
  - Sleep disturbance
  - Anxiety scales
    - State and Trait Anxiety Scale
    - Hamilton Anxiety Scale

Differential Diagnosis

- Hyperthyroidism
- Substance abuse or withdrawal
- Adverse medication effects
- Dysrhythmia
- Seizure disorder

Management

Nonpharmacologic Treatment
- Cognitive–behavioral therapy
- Stress management
- Community support
- Behavioral conditioning

Pharmacologic Treatment
- Selective serotonin-reuptake inhibitors (SSRIs) are the treatment of choice for chronic anxiety syndromes.
- Tricyclic antidepressants (TCAs) or antiepileptic drugs in select patients
- Benzodiazepines as short-term adjunct or for PRN management of acute anxiety and panic situations

When to Consult, Refer, or Hospitalize

- Rarely require inpatient admission unless additional factors or disease processes involved
- Consult psychiatry for patients with severe anxiety and those that are difficult to manage despite medical therapy.

Follow-up

- Discuss, prepare in advance, and guide patients through procedures and illness.
- Discuss deep breathing exercises as a relaxation technique.

GRIEF AND BEREAVEMENT

Description

- The emotional and physiological reaction to significant loss, such as the death or loss of a loved one. A normal reaction that may present as depressed mood that is situational and time-limited—should be evaluated for mood disorder when duration exceeds 2 months.

Etiology, Incidence, and Demographics

- Recent history of significant loss as identified in the definition
- Occurs in all populations

Risk Factors

- All persons are at risk for uncomplicated grief
- Risk for extension to complicated mood disorder
  - Poor coping skills
  - Lack of support person
  - History of mood disorder
  - Alcohol or substance abuse

Prevention and Screening

- No prevention because grief is a normal process
- Screen for mood disorder when duration exceeds 2 months.

Assessment

- Feelings of sadness and profound loss
- Crying spells
- Insomnia
- Loss of appetite and weight loss
- Survivor guilt
- Should demonstrate significant improvement by 8 weeks

Diagnostic Studies
- None for grief and bereavement
- Depression screening as indicated if symptoms progress beyond 8 weeks, are accompanied by functional impairment, or both

Differential Diagnosis

- Major depressive illness
- Mood disorder

Management

Nonpharmacologic Treatment
- Encourage expression of grief and mourning.
- Reassure the patient that grief is a normal, nonpathologic, self-limited reaction to loss.
- Encourage participation in support groups.
- Provide emotional support.

Pharmacologic Treatment
- Mild antianxiety agents in lowest effective dose—use is controversial

When to Consult, Refer, or Hospitalize

- Refer to community resources
- Consider mental health referral if:
  - The patient is elderly.
  - The patient has limited social support.
  - Suicidal ideation is verbalized.
  - The patient has a history of suicidal ideation or a mental health disorder.
  - Symptoms last longer than 8 weeks.
  - There is significant functional impairment.

Follow-up

- Discuss with the patient and family that grief is a normal reaction to loss.

SEXUALITY

Description

- Expression of person's identification, feelings, and identity as a human being
- The acute care nurse practitioner should ensure safe, comfortable environment in which to discuss sexuality in nonjudgmental fashion

Assessment

- Discuss any concerns about sexual function with the patient.
- Assess patient's comfort with sexual orientation.
- Assess for unprotected sexual encounters and multiple sexual partners.
- Assess for symptom of sexually transmitted infactions (STIs).

Diagnostic Studies

- STI and HIV testing if high-risk behavior or symptoms are present

Management and Patient Education

- Provide empathy and support to facilitate a safe environment for patients to express feelings and concerns.
- Discuss safe-sex practice and contraception (if appropriate)
- Refer to appropriate medical professional if sexual dysfunction is an issue.

POWERLESSNESS

Description

- Subjective sense of inability to control one's environment or situation. This develops because of the sudden nature of a critical illness without sufficient time to adapt.

Etiology, Incidence, and Demographics

- Etiology
  - Healthcare environmental factors
  - Interpersonal interactions
  - Individual beliefs (often cultural and religious beliefs)
- Common occurrence among critically ill patients

Risk Factors

- Hospitalization, specifically in the ICU

Prevention and Screening

- Involve patient in care and daily decision-making.

Assessment

- Feelings of anxiety
- Delayed decision making
- Expression of self-doubt
- Expressions of the sense of lost control or influence over the situation
- Unwillingness to participate in care when opportunities are provided

Diagnostic Studies
- None

Differential Diagnosis

- Anxiety
- Hopelessness
- Depression

Management

- Encourage the patient to express feelings.
- Provide emotional support, including acknowledgement of the normalcy of the patient's feelings of powerlessness.
- Facilitate patients' sense of power by actively involving them in decisions about their health care, including seemingly "small" decision such as diet choices and timing of treatments.
- Incorporate family and friends as much as possible, based on the patient's wishes.

When to Consult, Refer, or Hospitalize

- Consult psychiatry if needed for extreme or prolonged cases in patients unresponsive to management outlined above.

Follow-up

- Educate patients and family on their medical condition and the ICU environment.
- Explain all procedures and treatments and allow patient to be an active participant in care when possible.

ALTERED MENTAL STATUS (DELIRIUM, DEMENTIA, PSYCHOSIS)

DELIRIUM

Description

- Acute disorder of attention with onset of hours to days. Confusion and disorientation fluctuate over the course of a day. "Sundowning" is mild to moderate delirium that occurs at night and is more common in hospitalized patients.

Etiology, Incidence, and Demographics

- Hypoxia or hypercapnia
- Severe organ dysfunction (renal, hepatic, cardiac)
- Polypharmacy
- Infections

- Metabolic and electrolyte disorders
- Vascular disease (cerebrovascular)
- Urinary retention
- Fecal impaction
- Dehydration
- Anesthesia
- Environmental change
- Incidence is approximately 20% to 50% among ICU patients.

Risk Factors

- History of dementia
- History of alcoholism
- Malnutrition states
- Diabetes mellitus
- Carcinomas

Prevention and Screening

- Monitor patients closely for signs of delirium in order to provide early treatment.
- Review medications and discontinue medications as appropriate to avoid polypharmacy.

Assessment

- Impaired judgment and memory
- Unorganized thinking
- Decreased ability to maintain attention to external stimuli
- Acute anxiety
- Disrupted speech
- Tachycardia or bradycardia
- Hypertension or hypotension
- Assessment may identify underlying etiology (e.g., cardiomegaly, carotid bruits, thyroid enlargement).

Diagnostic Studies
- Mini Mental Status Exam
- CBC with differential, electrolyte, thyroid function test, hepatic and renal function, test for specific STIs
- Toxicology screening
- Electrocardiogram
- Urinalysis
- Chest x-ray
- Additional tests as appropriate based on the differential diagnosis (e.g., CT scan, lumbar puncture).

Differential Diagnosis

- Dementia
- Acute agitation or ICU psychosis
- Other mental health disorders

Management

Nonpharmacologic Treatment
- Identify and treat the underlying medical condition
- Frequent orientation to person, place, time, and situation
- Modify the environment to promote less stimulation (e.g., dim lights, quiet music, combine nursing interventions to avoid frequent awakening).
- Close patient monitoring and supervision while acutely agitated

Pharmacologic Treatment
- Benzodiazepines (lorazepam)—often used; however, may worsen delirium, especially in the elderly
- Neuroleptics (haloperidol)

When to Consult, Refer, or Hospitalize

- Consult psychiatry for difficult-to-manage patients in order to determine the best pharmacologic regimen.
- Consult specialists as appropriate if underlying organic etiology is present.

Follow-up

- Frequent orientation
- Educate family on the temporary nature of the condition.
- Reassure the family that the patient is unaware of his or her actions and not responsible for aggressive or combative behavior.

DEMENTIA

Description

- Organic mental syndrome that is characterized by gradual decline in intellectual functioning. Progress occurs over months to years. May become sever enough to interfere with activities of daily living.

Etiology, Incidence, and Demographics

- Reversible causes
  - Nutritional deficiencies (B_{12}, folate, thiamin)
  - Infections
  - Polypharmacy
  - Metabolic disorders (hypothyroidism)
  - Cerebral trauma (subdural hematoma)
- Irreversible causes
  - Multi-infarct dementia
  - Alzheimer's dementia
  - Parkinson's disease
- Prevalence is approximately 30% to 50% at age 85.
- Females have a higher incidence.
- 2/3 of cases are the result of Alzheimer's dementia.

Risk Factors

Alzheimer's Dementia
- Older age
- Female gender
- Positive family history
- Low education level

Multi-Infarct Dementia
- Hypertension
- Hyperlipidemia
- Diabetes mellitus
- CVA

Prevention and Screening

- Screening for cognitive impairment (clock-drawing task, three-item word recall)
- Assess decision-making capacity.

Assessment

- Memory issues
- Personality changes
- Behavioral issues
- Hallucinations

Differential Diagnosis

- Mild cognitive impairment
- Delirium

Diagnostic Studies
- CBC
- Electrolytes
- Thyroid function tests
- Vitamin B_{12} levels
- Rapid plasma reagin (RPR)
- HIV testing
- CT without contrast or MRI to assess for other causes such as normal pressure hydrocephalous, subdural hematoma, previous CVA.

Management

Nonpharmacologic Treatment
- Modify the environment to protect patient from injury

Pharmacologic Treatment
- Cholinesterase inhibitors (donepazil)
- NMDA receptor antagonist

When to Consult, Refer, or Hospitalize

- Admission may be required for advanced disease with declining health status.
- Institutionalization at a long-term-care facility is often required as patients lose the ability to care for themselves.

Follow-up

- Educate family on the disease and its typical progression.
- Provide information to the family and patient on the Alzheimer's Association for detailed education, community resources, and caregiver support.
- Inform the family of local area support and respite care.

PSYCHOSIS

Description

- Acutely confused state that effects a person's orientation to person, time, and place and the ability to process incoming stimuli, follow direction, and maintain concentration. ICU psychosis may occur because of the stressful nature of the ICU environment.

Etiology, Incidence, and Demographics

- Occurs more frequently in individuals age 60 and older
- Sleep deprivation
- Sensory overload
- Immobilization
- Certain medications may contribute (e.g., digoxin, antibiotics, steroids, respiratory stimulants).

Risk Factors

- 60 years of age or older
- Chronic brain disorder (e.g., Alzheimer's)
- Sleep deprivation
- Increased arousal
- Social isolation
- Mechanical ventilation

Prevention and Screening

- Awareness of this condition will prompt early recognition and treatment.
- Assess patients daily for signs and symptoms.

Assessment

- Altered mental status or confusion
- Hallucinations
- Agitation
- Violence
- Tachycardia
- Diaphoresis

Diagnostic Studies
- Mental Status Exam
- Toxicology screening as appropriate
- Additional tests as appropriate according to the differential diagnosis (i.e., if specific underlying cause suspected)

Differential Diagnosis

- Delirium
- Dementia

Management

Nonpharmacologic Treatment
- Identify and treat the underlying medical condition.
- Provide frequent orientation to person, place, time, and situation.
- Modify the environment to promote less stimulation (e.g., dim lights, quiet music, combine nursing interventions to avoid frequent awakening).
- Close patient monitoring and supervision while acutely agitated

Pharmacologic Treatment
- Neuromuscular blocking agents may be needed for patients requiring mechanical ventilation to decrease agitation and thereby oxygen demand and consumption.
- Benzodiazepines (lorazepam)—often used; however, may worsen psychosis, especially in older persons
- Neuroleptics (haloperidol)

When to Consult, Refer, or Hospitalize

- Consult psychiatry for difficult-to-manage patients in order to determine the best pharmacologic regimen.
- Consult specialists as appropriate if underlying organic etiology is present.

Follow-up

- Frequent orientation
- Educate the family on the temporary nature of the condition.
- Reassure family that the patient is unaware of his or her actions and not responsible for aggressive or combative behavior.

REFERENCES

Beers, M., Porter, R., Jones, T., Kaplan, J., & Berkwits, M. (Eds.). (2006). *The Merck manual of diagnosis and therapy.* Whitehouse Station, NJ: Merck Research Laboratories.

Buttaro, T., Trybulski, J., Bailey, P., & Sandberg-Cook, J. (2008). *Primary care* (3rd ed.). St. Louis, MO: Mosby.

Fauci, A. S., Braunwalk, E., Kasper, D. L., Hauser, S. L., Longo, D. L., Jameson, J. L., et al. (2008). *Harrison's principles of internal medicine* (17th ed.). Philadelphia: McGraw Hill.

Fiebach, N. H., Barker, L. R., Burton, J. R., & Zieves, P. D. (2007). *Principles of ambulatory medicine* (7th ed.). Philadelphia: Lippincott Williams & Wilkins.

McPhee, S. J., Tierney, L. M., & Papadakis, M. A. (2007). *Current medical diagnosis and treatment* (46th ed.). New York: McGraw-Hill.

McPhee, S., & Papadakis, M. (2010). *Current medical diagnosis and treatment* (49th ed.). New York: Lange/McGraw Hill Publishers.

Parrillo, J., & Dellinger, R. (Eds.). (2008). *Critical care medicine: Principles of diagnosis and management in the adult* (3rd ed.). St. Louis, MO: Mosby.

14

Sexually Transmitted Infections
Pamela Smith, MSN, RN, ACNP-BC, CCRN

GENERAL APPROACH

- The most common sexually transmitted infections (STIs) are gonorrhea, syphilis, human papillomavirus (HPV)–associated condyloma acuminatum, chlamydial genital infections, herpes viral genital infections, trichomonas vaginitis, chancroid, granuloma inguinale, scabies, louse infection, and bacterial vaginosis (in women who are sexually active with other women). Other diseases that may be spread by sexual contact (oral-anal) include shigellosis; hepatitis A, B, and C; amebiasis; giardiasis; crytosporidiosis; salmonellosis; and campylobacteriosis.
- Use of the male latex condom is highly protective if condoms are used consistently.
- Use of female condoms and other barriers used for contraception may protect against some but not all STIs.
- Safe sex practices reduce the incidence of human immune deficiency virus (HIV) in high-risk groups.
- A quadrivalent vaccination against human papilloma virus (HPV) types 6, 11, 16, and 18 is recommended for females aged 9 to 26.
- Risk assessments and screening tests help to reduce the incidence of STIs and should be done on every sexually active adult and adolescent.
- Follow Centers for Disease Control and Prevention treatment guidelines for management of STIs.

RED FLAGS

- An infectious disease specialist should be consulted for pregnant women with hepatitis B virus (HBV), primary cytomegalovirus (CMV), primary genital herpes, or group B streptococcal infection, and women with syphilis who are allergic to penicillin.
- If patient reports a sexual assault, consult local law authorities regarding procedures for obtaining evidence.
  - Test for *Trichomonas vaginalis*, bacterial vaginosis, yeast, *Chlamydia*, gonorrhea, HIV, hepatitis B, and syphilis.
  - Empiric antibiotic therapy can be started for suspected *Chlamydia*, gonorrhea, *Trichomonas*, and bacterial vaginosis, as well as prophylactic treatment for hepatitis B, pregnancy testing, and emergency contraception if indicated.

CHLAMYDIA

Description

- Chlamydiaceae is a family of gram-negative obligate intracellular parasites that closely resemble gram-negative bacteria.
- In this family are two genera of human pathogens: *Chlamydia*, which includes *Chlamydia trachomatis*, and *Chlamydophila*.
- *C. trachomatis* can cause several different infections, which involve the eye (trachoma, inclusion conjunctivitis) and the genital tract (lymphogranuloma venereum, nongonococcal urethritis, cervicitis, salpingitis).
  - Lymphogranuloma venereum (LGV) is primary genital lesion
    - *C. trachomatis* types L1 to L3
    - Acquired during sexual intercourse through contact with contaminated exudate from active lesions
    - Incubation period is 5 to 21 days
    - After the genital lesion disappears, the infection spreads to lymph channels and nodes of the genital or rectal areas
    - Undiagnosed and latent diseases are not uncommon.
  - Nongonococcal urethritis, cervicitis, salpingitis
    - *C. trachomatis* immunotypes D to K
    - Isolated in 50% of nongonoccocal urethritis and cervicitis
    - Important cause of postgonococcal urethritis
    - Coinfection with gonococci and chlamydiae is common.
    - Postgonococcal (chlamydial) urethritis may persist after successful treatment of the gonorrhea.
- *Chlamydophila* genera include *Chlamydophila psittaci* and *Chlamydophila* pneumoniae, which can cause respiratory tract infections.

Etiology, Incidence, and Demographics

- Chlamydia is an infection caused by the bacterium *Chlamydia trachomatis*.
- Infected epithelial cells initially display neutrophilic infiltration, followed by the invasion of lymphocytes, macrophages, plasma cells, and esosinophils.
- Chlamydia have a biphasic life cycle that make them adaptable to both intracellular and extracellur environments.
- Chlamydia can be transmitted during vaginal, anal, or oral sex.
- Chlamydia can also be passed from an infected mother to her baby during vaginal childbirth in about 50% of cases.
- *Chlamydia trachomitis* infections are the most commonly reported infectious disease in the United States.
- In 2009, 1,244,180 chlamydial infections were reported to the Centers for Disease Control and Prevention (CDC) from 50 states and the District of Columbia, which was an increase of 2.8% from 2008.
- In 2009, the overall rate of reported cases was three times higher in females.
- Among women, the highest age-specific rates were from the ages of 15 to 19 and 20 to 24 years of age; for men, from the ages of 20 to 24 years.
- Blacks have a chlamydia infection rate eight times higher than Whites.
- Among adults, about 5% of the population is estimated to be infected; among sexually active adolescent females, about 10% are infected.

Risk Factors

- Sexual contact with multiple partners
- Non-White race
- Unprotected sex
- Young adults
- Vaginal, anal, oral sex
- Lower socioeconomic status
- Mother-to-infant transmission

Prevention and Screening

- Use of condoms
- Treatment of sexual partners
- Abstinence from sexual intercourse until treatment is complete
- Routine chlamydia screening in sexually active young women is recommended.
  - Women
    - Sexually active under the age of 24
    - Have new or multiple sexual partners
    - Have a history of sexually transmitted disease within the last year (no age limit)
    - Have partners who have had multiple partners within the last year (no age limit)
    - Test all pregnant women at least once, regardless of age, including those who plan to terminate the pregnancy.
    - Rescreen all women who test positive (especially adolescents) 3 to 4 months after treatment because of the high risk of reinfection.

- Men
  - Risk factors for sexually transmitted disease
  - HIV-positive men
  - Men who have sex with men

Assessment

History
- In women, 70% to 80% of cases do not exhibit symptoms.
- In men, 25% to 50% of cases do not exhibit symptoms.
- Women
  - Easily induced cervical bleeding
  - Dysuria
  - Abdominal pain
  - Fever
  - Intermenstrual bleeding
- Men
  - Dysuria
  - Urinary frequency, urgency, or both
  - Fever
  - Unilateral scrotal pain
  - Perineal fullness (related to prostatitis)

Physical Examination
- Women
  - Urethritis or cervicitis
    - Yellow, mucupurulent endocervical discharge (less painful, purulent and watery than gonorrhea)
    - Cervical motion tenderness
  - LGV
    - Early anorectal manifestations
    - Proctitis
    - Bloody purulent drainage
    - Late manifestations
      - Chronic scarring and inflammation of the rectal and perirectal tissue
    - These changes may lead to intractable constipation, rectal stricture, and rectovaginal and perianal fistulas
- Men
  - Urethritis
    - Urethral discharge—white or cloudy, watery
    - Unilateral scrotal tenderness, swelling, or both
  - LVG
    - Initial vesicular or ulcerative lesion on external genitalia may go unnoticed.
    - Inguinal swelling of the lymph nodes appears 1 to 4 weeks after exposure, usually bilateral and tending to fuse, then soften and break down to form draining sinuses with scarring.

Diagnostic Studies
- All patients with any STI should be evaluated for chlamydial infection.
- Urogenital infection
  - Cell culture
    - Incubation 40 to 72 hours
    - Specificity 50% to 90%, sensitivity 99%
    - Expensive
    - Many false negatives because of difficulty culturing organism
- Antigen detection and nucleic acid hybridization
  - Direct fluorescent antibody (DFA)
    - 50% to 80% sensitivity, 99% specificity
    - Labor-intensive
    - Used to confirm other assays
  - Enzyme-linked immunosorbent assay (ELISA)
    - 40% to 60% sensitivity, 99% specificity
    - Inexpensive
    - Most commonly used test in the emergency department and clinics
- DNA amplification testing (NAAT)
  - Detection of chlamydial DNA using specific probes
  - 80% to 92% sensitivity, 99% specificity
    - No difference in urine specimen vs. genital specimen for men
  - Expensive, but becoming more cost-effective
  - Serology
    - Complement testing
      - 15% of men with urethritis and 45% of women with endocervical infection have titers 1:16 or greater
  - Microimmunofluorescence test
    - More sensitive than complement fixation test
    - Results positive in 99% or more of women with cervicitis and 80% to 90% of men with urethritis
- LVG
  - Complement fixation testing
    - Titer > 1:64 coupled with appropriate clinical scenario is considered diagnostic
- NAATs
  - Urine specimen
  - Sensitivity 96% to 100%, specificity 99% to 100%

Differential Diagnosis

- Urethritis or cervicitis
  - Herpes simplex
  - Gonorrhea
  - *Trichomonas* infection
  - Periurethral abscess
  - *Myocplasma genitalium* infection
  - Prostatitis
  - Pelvic inflammatory disease
  - Orchitis
  - Urinary tract infection
  - Vaginitis
- LVG
  - Chanchroid
  - Colitis
  - Granuloma inguinale
  - Herpes simplex
  - HSV-2
  - Syphilis

Management

Nonpharmacologic Treatment
- Perform a pregnancy test
- Provide information and counseling regarding STIs and consider referral for HIV testing

Pharmacologic Treatment
- Urethritis
  - Azithromycin 1 gram p.o. x 1 dose (safe in pregnancy)
  - Doxycyline 100 mg p.o. daily for 7 days (contraindicated in pregnancy)
  - Levofloxacin 500 mg p.o. daily for 7 days (contraindicated in pregnancy)
  - Alternative regimens
    - 50 mg erythromycin base 4 times daily for 7 days
    - 800 mg erythromycin ethylsuccinate 4 times a day for 7 days
    - 300 mg ofloxacin 2 times a day for 7 days
- LVG
  - Doxycycline 100 mg p.o. 2 time daily for 21 days (contraindicated in pregnancy)
  - Erythromycin 500 mg 4 times daily for 21 days
  - Azithryomycin 1 gram p.o. x 1 dose or weekly for 3 weeks

Special Considerations

- Inform patients that a possible long-term complication from the infection is infertility.
- Treatment is also indicated for sexual partners of the index case if the time of the last sexual encounter was within 60 days of onset.

When to Consult, Refer, or Hospitalize

- Consult obstetrics/gynecology for any patient with severe pelvic inflammatory disease (PID) or any pregnant patient with chlamydia.
- Hospitalize for PID with any of the following:
  - Tubo-ovarian abscess
  - Pregnancy
  - Failure of outpatient treatment
  - Immunodeficiency
  - Severe abdominal pain
  - Inability to tolerate p.o. medications
  - Perihepatitis

Follow-up

Expected Outcomes
- 95% of patients are successfully treated with first-time therapy.
- Prognosis is excellent if treated early and the entire course of antibiotics is completed.
- All patients should receive follow-up care with a primary care provider to decrease risk of reinfection and for cervical cancer screening.

Complications
- Infertility
- Urethral scarring in men
- PID
- Chronic pelvic pain
- Perihepatitis
- Cervical cancer

GONORRHEA (GC)

Description

- A sexually transmitted disease caused by *Neisseria gonorrhoeae* that causes a purulent infection of mucous membrane surfaces and is highly infectious
- Inflammation is localized, causing urethritis, epididymitis, proctitis, cervicitis, bartholinitis, PID, and pharyngitis.
- Common sites of infection in women are the urethra, endocervix, upper genital tract, pharynx, and rectum.
- Common sites of infection in men are the urethra, epididymis, prostate, rectum, and pharynx.

Etiology

- *Neisseria gonorrhoeae* is a gram-negative diplococcus usually found inside polymorphonuclear cells.
- Transmission is through sexual contact and vaginal birth.
- Gonococcal bacteremia infection (GCI) leads to a disseminated systemic condition.
    - Intermittent fever
    - Arthralgias
    - Skin lesions
        - Maculopapular
        - Pustular
        - Hemorrhagic
    - Endocarditis
    - Meningitis

Incidence and Demographics

- 60% to 90% of women become infected after exposure.
- Greatest incidence is in sexually active persons aged 15 to 29.
- About 15% of infected women may develop PID with possible sterility if untreated.
- Men typically have symptoms that cause them to seek treatment.
- Infected women often do not have symptoms until complications are present.

Risk Factors

- History of STIs
- Presence of other STIs, including HIV
- Multiple sexual partners or new partner
- Drug use, partner who uses drugs, or both
- Homosexual or bisexual men and their partners
    - Homosexual males have a 10 times greater incidence.
- Lack of consistent use of barrier contraceptives

Prevention and Screening

- Emphasize the importance of screening because many STIs are asymptomatic.
- Counsel the adolescent or adult patient regarding sexual abstinence and monogamy.
- Consistent and correct use of barrier contraceptives
- Safe sex practices
- Screen sexually active men and women < 25 years of age if located in an area with a high incidence of GC. Screen all pregnant women at the initial prenatal visit and again early in the third trimester.
- Prophylactic treatment for contacts of infected patients
- Women and men at high risk should be encouraged to undergo HIV testing and receive the hepatitis B vaccine.

Assessment

History
- Short incubation
  - Urethritis in 2 to 5 days
  - Cervicitis in 5 to 10 days
- Women
  - Often asymptomatic
  - Dysuria
  - Urinary frequency
  - Pelvic pain
  - Fever
- Men
  - May be asymptomatic
  - Dysuria
  - Urinary frequency
  - Testicular pain
- Both may have conjunctivitis or pharyngitis as well
- Disseminated gonorrhea
- Fever

Physical Examination
- Women
  - Vaginal discharge
  - Spotting or abnormal menses
  - Purulent discharge from cervix
  - Inflammation of Bartholin's glands
  - Positive cervical motion tenderness (CMT)
  - If untreated, signs of PID
  - Proctitis
  - Lower abdominal tenderness
- Male
  - Copious purulent, blood-tinged penile discharge
  - Signs of prostatitis or epididymitis if left untreated
  - Periurethral inflammation or strictures (chronic infection)
  - Rectal symptoms
    - Erythematous
    - Discharge
    - Pain with defecation
- Both male and female may have conjunctivitis or pharyngitis.
- Disseminated gonorrhea infection (DGI)
  - Rash: maculopapular, pustular, hemorrhagic
  - Tenosynovitis
  - Arthritis

Diagnostic Studies
- Gram stain
  - Rapid and inexpensive test
  - Predictive value for urethral infection is high, but a negative value does not rule out infection in asymptomatic males
  - Sensitivity and specificity are lower for endocervical and rectal specimens.
  - Test is not useful in the diagnosis of pharyngeal infection.
- Culture
  - Swab from the site of infection is a standard for diagnosis at all potential sites of infection and can guide treatment with antibiotic sensitivity.
  - Empiric therapy is often needed because culture results are not ready for 24 to 48 hours.
  - Cultures are useful when the diagnosis is unclear, in treatment failure, when contact tracing is problematic, and if there are legal concerns.
- Nucleic acid amplification tests (NAAT)
  - Offer the most specimen sites because of the Food and Drug Administration's (FDA) approval for use with endocervical, vaginal, male urethral swabs, and female or male urine specimens
  - These tests are designed to amplify sequences of DNA unique to a specific pathogen.
- Suspected DGI
  - Blood and joint effusions should be sent for gram stain and culture.
  - Cerebrospinal fluid should be tested if there are signs or symptoms of meningitis.
- Ultrasound and abdominal CT scan
  - Pelvic ultrasound or CT scan may reveal thick, dilated fallopian tubes or abscess formation.
  - Used to rule out ectopic pregnancy when a patient has signs or symptoms of possible PID

Differential Diagnosis

- PID
- Nongonococcal cervicitis
- *Chlamydia*
- Urethritis
- Proctitis
- Nongonoccocal pharyngitis
- Ectopic pregnancy
- Testicular torsion
- Vaginitis
- Urinary tract infection
- Herpes simplex urethritis

Management

Nonpharmacologic Treatment
- Screening
- Limit sexual partners
- Obtain an accurate, detailed history from patients to determine their risk for STI.

Pharmacologic Treatment
- Infected persons with *N. gonorrhoeae* are often also infected with *C. trachomatis*. The recommendation for treatment is to use medications that are effective against both organisms. However, patients with a negative NAAT result at the time of treatment do not need to be treated simultaneously.
- Uncomplicated gonorrhea
  - Ceftriazone 125 mg intramuscularly (IM) in a single dose *or*
  - Cefixime 400 mg orally (p.o.) as a single dose
  - Other single-dose regimens
    - Ceftizoxime 500 mg IM *or*
    - Cefoxitin 2 gram IM administered with probenecid 1 gram orally *or*
    - Cefotaxime 500 mg IM
- Pharyngeal
  - Ceftriaxone 125 mg IM
  - For concomitant chlamydial infection (unless ruled out with a negative NAAT)
    - Doxycycline 100 mg p.o. twice daily for 7 days *or*
    - Azithromycin 1 gram p.o. as a single dose
    - Administer with ceftriaxone
- DGI
  - Ceftriaxone 1 gram intravenously (IV) daily until 48 hours after improvement begins; at that time therapy may be changed to cefixime 400 mg p.o. daily for at least once week
  - If organism is susceptible, oral fluoroquinolones for 7 days may also be may also be effective
    - Ciprofloxacin 500 mg p.o. twice daily
    - Levofloxacin 500 mg p.o. once daily
- Endocarditis
  - Ceftriaxone 2 gram IV every 24 hours for at least 3 weeks
- Postgonococcal urethritis or cervicitis: doses as above
  - Doxycycline
  - Azithromycine
- PID
  - Cefoxitin 2 grams IM/IV every 6 hours *or*
  - Cefotetan 2 grams IV every 12 hours
  - Also effective
    - Clindamycin 900 mg IV every 8 hours *plus* gentamycin IV as a 2 mg/kg loading dose followed by 1.5 mg/kg every 8 hours
      - Outpatient regimen
        - Cefoxitin 2 grams IM plus probenecid 1 gram p.o. as a single dose followed by a 14-day course of doxycycline 100 mg 2 times daily
  - Concurrent treatment for chlamydial infection is indicated.
- Gonococcal conjunctivitis
  - Ceftriaxone 1 gram IM in a single dose

Special Considerations

- Pregnant women should be treated with a cephalosporin.
- Pregnant or lactating women should not be treated with quinolones or tetracycline.

When to Consult, Refer, or Hospitalize

- Hospitalize for DIG.
- Hospitalize patients who are unresponsive to treatment.
- Hospitalize patients with PID in the presence of the following:
  - Tubo-ovarian abscess
  - Pregnancy
  - Pain, high fever, persistent nausea and vomiting
  - Immunodeficiency
  - Gonococcal conjunctivitis
  - Abdominal peritonitis or perihepatitis
- Consult a gynecologist for severe PID.
- Consult an ophthalmologist for every patient with gonococcal conjunctivitis because the disease may progress rapidly and cause permanent blindness.

Follow-up

Expected Outcomes
- Prompt response to therapy

Complications
- Urethral scarring in men; may lead to decreased fertility or bladder-outlet obstruction
- Scarring of the upper reproductive tract in women with PID; may lead to infertility, chronic pelvic pain, or ectopic pregnancy
- In pregnant women: possible pematurity, neonatal infection, or miscarriage
- Postpartum sepsis
- Possible corneal scarring and permanent vision impairment or blindness
- Possible permanent deficits from gonococcal meningitis
- Destruction of joint articular surfaces
- Destruction of cardiac valves
- Death from congestive heart failure or meningitis
- Epididymitis
- Prostatitis
- DGI

SYPHILIS

Description

- An infectious disease caused by *Treponema pallidum*—a spirochete that can infect nearly any organ or tissue in the body
- Divided into two clinical stages, which are separated by a symptom-free latent phase
- During the early part of the latent stage, infectious lesions may recur.
  - Early (infectious)
    - Primary lesions (chancre and regional lymphadenopathy) and secondary lesions (involving skin, mucous membranes, sometimes bone, central nervous system, and the liver)
    - These lesions have a large number of spirochetes with minimal tissue reaction.
  - Late
    - Benign (gummatous) lesions that involve the skin, bones, and viscera
    - May cause cardiovascular disease, primarily aortitis, and central nervous system and ocular syndromes
    - This form of syphilis is not contagious.
    - The lesions contain a small number of spirochetes, but tissue reactivity is severe and can cause vasculitis with necrosis.
- The primary and secondary lesions are self-limiting in nature (even without treatment) and will resolve without tissue damage.
- Late syphilis can be very damaging and lead to death.
- It is believed that the infection is almost never completely eliminated without treatment.
- Most infections remain latent without symptoms and only a small percentage advance to further disease.

Etiology

- *Treponema pallidum* spirochete
- Transmission occurs through sexual contact, and spirochetes enter the body by way of small genitali or extragenital skin or mucosal lesions.
- Once inside the body, spirochetes rapidly multiply and spread to regional lymph nodes.
- Congenital syphilis occurs from transplacental passage of the organism occurring any time during gestation and may result in spontaneous abortion (second trimester) or stillbirth.
- Occurs rarely through blood transfusions, nonsexual contact

Incidence and Demographics

- The risk of infection after an unprotected sexual encounter with an infected individual is 30% to 50%.
- With the introduction of penicillin during and after World War II, there was a reduction in the incidence of syphilis.
- There was a resurgence of the disease in the 1960s and 1970s.

- In the early 1980s, the incidence increased with a particularly high rate among homosexual men and other men who have sex with men (MSM).
- In the mid-1980s, there was a slight decrease because of the changes in sexual practices in response to the AIDS epidemic.
- Between 1985 and 1990, there was a large increase in cases—more than 50,000 cases of primary and secondary syphilis were reported in 1990.
  - Broad-based, affecting both men and women in inner-city, urban, and rural areas, especially in the southern regions of the United States
  - Adolescent and young Blacks were most affected, but other racial and ethnic groups were also affected, as well as those over 60 years of age.
    - Limited access to health care, decreases in health department clinical services, increased use of illicit drugs, the difficulty of contact tracing with multiple partners, and the exchange of money for sex were all contributing factors to the increased number of cases.
  - With the increase in sexually transmitted syphilis, there was also an increase in congenital syphilis.
- These high rates declined in the latter part of the 1990s, and in 1998 the United States Congress allocated funds for a syphilis elimination program.
  - Efforts were initially successful, achieving a decrease in cases in 2000 to 5,979 compared to 7,035 cases in 1998.
- In 2008, the number of cases was 13,470, the highest since 1995; contributing factors were
  - MSM
  - Internet sexual partners
  - Substance abuse
  - Decreased use of condoms
- Most cases in the United States occur in MSM.
- From 2007 to 2008, the number of cases of primary and secondary syphilis increased among White, Black, and Hispanic men and women.
  - The highest rates were in Black men, with 28 cases/100,000 people.
  - In 2008, half of the reported cases were in the southern region of the United States.

Risk Factors

- High-risk sexual activity
  - Unprotected sex
  - Multiple partners
  - Sexual activity while under the influence of alcohol or drugs
  - MSM
  - Exchange of money for sex
- Infection with HIV

Prevention and Screening

- Early diagnosis and treatment with partner notification and treatment
- Use of condoms protects covered areas only.
- Routine screening for those < 25 years of age in high-prevalence areas and those with other STIs

- MSM should be screened every 6 to 12 months.
- Patients must abstain from sexual activity for 7 to 10 days after treatment or until lesions have resolved.
- In pregnancy, screening at the first prenatal visit, then repeat for high-risk populations at 28 weeks and at delivery
- Patients with HIV infection or patients treated with a nonpenicillin regimen should be monitored for life.

Assessment

History
- Primary
  - This stage may be unrecognized.
  - Incubation is about 3 weeks and ranges from 10 to 90 days after the exposure.
  - Primary chancre is highly infectious and heals spontaneously after 1 to 5 weeks, and patient may not seek treatment.
- Secondary
  - May occur from 6 weeks to 6 months after primary stage; most contagious
  - Fever
  - Arthritis
  - Iritis
  - Serologic tests positive
  - Hepatitis
  - Meningitis
  - Osteitis
  - Arthralgias or myalgias and "flu-like" symptoms
- Latent
  - Often asymptomatic
  - Early
    - The first year after a primary infection
      - May relapse to secondary syphilis if undiagnosed or untreated
      - Relapse associated with rising titer in serologic testing
      - About 90% of relapses occur in the first year after infection.
      - If not treated, a small number of patients may progress to tertiary syphilis.
    - History of syphilis with subtherapeutic treatment
  - Late
    - This is the stage after the first year of latent syphilis.
    - Difficult to distinguish early latent from late latent stage if duration of symptoms is unknown
- Tertiary
  - Rarely seen because of treatment with antibiotics
  - May occur any time after secondary syphilis
  - Periostitis
  - Osteitis
  - Arthritis

- Myalgia and myositis
- Pain more severe at night
- Gastric involvement because of diffuse infiltration into the stomach wall or focal lesions that may resemble lymphoma or carcinoma
  - Epigastric pain
  - Early satiety
  - Regurgitation belching
  - Weight loss
- Gummatous infiltrates of larynx, trachea, and pulmonary parenchyma
  - Hoarseness
  - Respiratory distress
  - Wheezing
- Cardiovascular lesions may be progressive, disabling, and threaten existence.
  - Arteritis in the aorta and progress to one or more of the following:
    - Narrowing of the coronary arteries leading to angina or myocardial infarction
    - Scarring of the aortic valves
    - Weakness of the aortic wall with saccular aneurysm formation and occasional rupture
- Associated symptoms
  - Hoarseness
  - Brassy cough
  - Back pain
- Neurosyphilis
  - Can occur at any stage of the disease
  - Four clinical types
    - Asymptomatic
    - Meningovascular syphilis (meningeal involvement, changes in the vascular structures of the brain, or both)
      - Headache
      - Irritability
    - Tabes dorsalis (chronic progressive degeneration of the parenchyma of the posterior columns of the spinal cord and of the posterior sensory ganglia and nerve roots)
      - Impairment of proprioception and vibration sense
      - Paresthesias
      - Sharp recurrent pains in the muscles of the leg
      - Crises are common in tabes dorsalis—may begin suddenly, last for hours to days, and cease abruptly
      - Gastric crisis
        - Sharp abdominal pain with nausea and vomiting
      - Laryngeal crisis
        - Paroxysmal cough
        - Dyspnea
      - Neurogenic bladder
        - Overflow incontinence
      - Urethral crisis
        - Painful bladder spasm
      - Rectal crisis

- General paresis (generalized involvement of the cerebral cortex with insidious onset of symptoms)
  - Decrease in concentration
  - Memory loss
  - Dysarthria
  - Change in personality
    - Confusion
    - Irresponsibility
    - Psychosis

Physical Examination
- Primary
  - Painless, nonpurulent, indurated ulcer (chancre) appears at the site of inoculation 3 to 4 weeks after exposure
    - Usually the penis, labia, cervix, or anorectal region
    - Chancre sores may also appear on the lips, tongue, tonsils, breasts, or fingers.
    - About 30% of lesions fit this description.
    - Heals spontaneously after 1 to 5 weeks
  - Anorectal lesions are common in MSM.
  - 10 to 90 days postexposure, a small erosion quickly develops into a painless, superficial ulcer with a clean, firm base and indurated margins.
  - This is associated with enlargement of regional lymph nodes, which feel rubbery, discrete, and nontender.
  - If a bacterial infection is present, the chancre sore may be painful.
  - Multiple chancre sores may be present in patients infected with HIV.
- Secondary
  - Symptoms appear a few weeks to 6 months after the development of the chancre sore.
  - Most common manifestations appear in the skin and mucous membranes.
  - Generalized maculopapular rash
    - May be present on palms and soles
    - Rash lasts 2 to 6 weeks, then spontaneously heals
  - Mucous membrane lesions
    - Patches
    - Ulcers
  - Condylomas in moist skin areas
  - Generalized nontender lymphadenopathy
  - Many treponemes in mucous membrane scrapings or skin lesions as shown by immunofluorescence
- Latent
  - Early
    - No physical signs
    - Positive serologic tests
  - Late
    - Cerebrol spinal fluid (CSF) negative when evaluated for neurosyphilis
    - No signs of cardiovascular involvement
    - False-positive tests for syphilis have been ruled out
    - Latent phase may last months to a lifetime
    - Positive serologic tests

- Tertiary
  - Rarely seen because of the efficacy of antibiotics
  - Lesions, probably because of a delayed hypersensitivity, divided into two types:
    - A localized gummatous reaction with rapid onset and prompt response to therapy
    - Diffuse inflammatory onset that usually involves the central nervous system and large arteries
    - May be fatal if not treated
    - Gummas may involve any area or organ of the body but most often affect skin and bones.
    - Multiple nodular lesions that may ulcerate or resolve by forming atrophic, pigmented scars
    - Solitary gummas start as painless subcutaneous nodules, then enlarge and ulcerate.
    - Ocular lesions
      - Gummatous iritis
      - Chorioretinitis
      - Optic atrophy
      - Cranial nerve palsies
    - Gummas found in the liver form benign, asymptomatic hepar lobatum
      - Occasional symptoms similar to Laënnec's cirrhosis may be evident with liver involvement.
- Neurosyphilis
- Asymptomatic
  - Cerebral spinal fluid (CSF) abnormalities
    - Positive serology
    - Increased cell count
    - Occasionally increased protein
    - Controversy regarding significance of CSF fluid in the absence of neurological symptoms
- Meningovascular syphilis
  - Cranial nerve palsies
  - Unequal reflexes
  - Irregular pupils
  - CSF
    - Increased cells
    - Protein
    - Usually positive serology
- Tabes dorsalis
  - Muscular hypotonia
  - Hyporeflexia
  - CSF
    - Normal or increased cell count
    - Elevated protein
    - Variable results of serologic testing
- General paresis
  - Dysarthria
  - Tremor of the fingers and lips
    - Asymptomatic and meningovascular syphilis occur months to years after infection and, at times, manifest at the time of primary and secondary syphilis.
    - Tabes dorsalis and general paresis occur 2 to 50 years after infection.

Diagnostic Studies
- Microscopic examinations—early, infectious syphilis
- Darkfield microscopic examination
  - Skilled observer
  - Fresh exudates from lesions or material aspirated from regional lymph nodes
  - Usually only available in select sexually transmitted disease clinics
  - Not recommended for oral lesions
- Immunofluorescent staining technique
  - Dried smears of fluid taken from early syphilitic lesions
  - Not widely used
  - Simple, high specificity, convenient for clinicians
  - Has replaced darkfield microscopy in some centers
- Serologic testing
  - Used in primary, secondary, latent (early & late), tertiary, and neurosyphilis
  - Nontreponemal antigen tests
    - Veneral Disease Research Laboratory (VDRL)
    - Rapid plasma reagin (RPR)
    - Are usually positive 4 to 6 weeks after infection or 1 to 3 weeks after the appearance of a primary lesion
    - Nearly always positive in the secondary stage of syphilis with elevated titers (> 1:32)
    - In the late stage, titers are lower (< 1:4).
    - Not highly specific, may be positive with the following:
      - Non–sexually acquired treponematoses
      - Connective tissue disorders
      - Infectious mononucelosis
      - Malaria
      - Febrile states
      - Leprosy
      - Injection drug use
      - Infective endocarditis
      - Elderly
      - Hepatitis C
      - HIV-positive patients
      - Pregnancy
      - False positives usually have a low titer
      - Distinguished from true positives by specific treponemal antibody tests
      - False negatives occur when high antibody titers are present (prozone phenomenon)
        - If test is negative and syphilis is suspected, the specimen should be diluted to detect a positive reaction
    - Used to track the adequacy of treatment
    - When the VDRL or RPR becomes negative depends on the stage of the disease, the level of the initial titer, and whether the infection is an initial or repeat episode.
    - Patients with advanced disease, high initial titers, or repeat infections, or who are HIV-positive, have slower seroconversion rates.
    - It may take 6 months to see a fourfold decrease in a titer and 12 months to see an eightfold decrease.
    - With early latent syphilis, a four-fold drop may take 12–24 months.

- Treponemal antibody tests
  - Measure the antibodies capable of reacting with *T. pallidum* antigens.
  - *T. pallidum* hemagglutination (TPHA) test
  - *T. pallidum* particle agglutination (TPPA) test
  - These are used to confirm the diagnosis of syphilis after a positive nontreponemal antigen test or in patients with clinical evidence of syphilis and a negative nontreponemal antigen test.
  - May revert to negative with adequate therapy
  - False positives in the following:
    - Systemic lupus erythematosus (SLE)
    - Disorders associated with elevated gamma-globulins
    - Malaria
    - Leprosy
    - Other spirochetal infections
    - Lyme disease
- Polymerase chain reaction
  - Used for genital ulcer disease
  - Not widely available in the United States
- Neurosyphilis
  - Same serological testing as above
  - Lumbar puncture
    - Not recommended in early syphilis unless neurological signs or symptoms present
    - Recommended in later stages
    - Patients positive for HIV
    - Evidence of treatment failure
    - When neurological symptoms are present
  - Spinal fluid examination
    - Findings variable
    - Elevated protein
    - Lymphocytic pleocytosis and a positive VDRL
    - CSF fluid may be negative

Differential Diagnosis

- Chlamydia
- Endometriosis
- Ectopic pregnancy
- Genital ulcers
- Genital herpes
- Chancroid
- Neoplasm
- Lymphogranuloma venereum
- Mucupurulent cervicitis
- Testicular torsion
- Septic arthritis

- Sexual assault
- Superficial fungal infections
- Urinary tract infection
- Vaginitis

Management

Nonpharmacologic Treatment
- Abstainence from sexual activity until treatment complete
- Early infection—primary, secondary, early latent, and congenital syphilis are reportable to the local public health agency in all states.
- Contacts must be treated.
- Reinfection may occur; patients should be monitored at 3 to 6 months.

Pharmacologic Treatment
- Primary, secondary, early latent
  - Benzathine penicillin G 2.4 million units IM, single dose
  - Alternative
    - Doxycycline 100 mg orally twice daily for 14 to 28 days *or*
    - Tetracycline 500 mg orally 4 times daily for 28 days *or*
    - Ceftriaxone 1 gram IM daily for 8 to 10 days
- Late latent or unknown duration
  - Benzathine penicillin G 2.4 million units IM weekly for 3 weeks
  - Alternative
    - Docycycline 100 mg orally twice daily for 28 days *or*
    - Tetracycline 500 mg orally 4 times daily for 28 days
- Tertiary without neurosyphilis
  - Benzathine penicillin G 2.4 million units IM weekly for 3 weeks
  - Alternative
    - Doxycycline 100 mg orally 2 times daily for 28 days *or*
    - Tetracycline 500 mg orally 4 times daily for 28 days
    - CSF evaluation recommended
  - Neurosyphilis
    - Aqueous penicillin G 18 to 24 million units IV daily given in 3 to 4 million units every 3 to 4 hours or as a continuous infusion for 10 to 14 days
    - Patients who are allergic to penicillin should be desensitized.
  - Alternative
    - Procaine penicillin 2.4 million units IM daily with probenicid 500 mg orally 4 times a day for 10 to 14 days *or*
    - Ceftriaxone 2 grams IM daily for 10 to 14 days
  - Follow treatment with benzathine penicillin G 2.4 million units IM weekly for up to 3 weeks for slowly dividing organisms that may persist after the 10- to 14-day treatment.
- Pregnancy
  - The only acceptable treatment for syphilis in pregnancy is penicillin.
  - It prevents congenital syphilis in 90% of cases.
  - Those with a penicillin allergy must be desensitized.
  - Tetracycline, doxycycline, and erythromycin are contraindicated.

Special Considerations

- Syphilis and patients infected with HIV
  - Treatment and interpretation is the same as for patients who are negative for HIV.
  - Neurosyphilis must be considered in the differential
  - If serological testing is negative and syphilis is suspected, biopsy, darkfield examination, or direct fluorescent antibody staining should be done.
  - Patients who are penicillin-allergic must be desensitized.
  - Primary and secondary syphilis should have VDRL/RPR serology testing at 3, 6, 9, 12, and 24 months.
  - If titers increase fourfold, titers fail to decrease fourfold at 3 months, or symptoms persist, retreatment is indicated.
- Pregnancy
  - All pregnant women should have a nontreponemal serologic test for syphilis at the time of the first prenatal visit.
  - Seropositive women should be treated.
  - The infant should be evaluated immediately and at 6 to 8 weeks of age.
  - Women treated in the second trimester are at risk for premature labor, fetal distress, or both.
- Congenital syphilis
  - Transplacentally transmitted infection that occurs in infants of untreated or inadequately treated mothers
- CSF pleocytosis may occur in 10%–20% of patients with primary syphilis.
- All patients may experience Jarish-Herxheimer reaction.
  - Occurs because of lysis of treponemes and is not IgE-mediated
  - Most common in early syphilis
  - Fever, chills, headache, myalgias, rash
  - Treat with antipyretics and antihistamine.

When to Consult, Refer, or Hospitalize

- Refer to an infectious disease specialist: pregnant women, patients with congential syphilis, and patients who are HIV positive
  - Women in late pregnancy treated for early syphilis need close outpatient monitoring or inpatient admission because the Jarish-Herxheimer reaction may cause premature labor.
  - Hospitalize for IV treatment of neurosyphilis
  - Consultation with the public health department may be useful for treatment records and helpful in complicated cases.

Follow-up

Expected Outcomes
- Primary stage lasts 1 to 5 weeks, secondary stage 2 to 6 weeks
- Primary and secondary syphilis
  - Examine clinically and obtain serologic testing at 6 or 12 months
  - If serologic titer has not decreased fourfold 6 months after therapy, treatment failure must be considered.

- Latent syphilis
  - Serological testing at 6, 12, and 24 months
  - Evaluate for neurosyphilis and retreat for titers that increase fourfold, an initially high titer that fails to decline at least fourfold in 12 to 24 months, or if patient is symptomatic.

Complications
- Jarish-Herxheimer reaction
- Tertiary syphilis—see Physical examination section
  - Cardiovascular involvement
  - Gastric involvement
  - Respiratory involvement

GENITAL HERPES SIMPLEX VIRUS (HSV) INFECTION

Description

- Infection with herpes simplex type 2, which causes lesions similar in morphology to herpes simplex type I on the genitalia of both sexes

Etiology

- HSV-2 transmitted through sexual contact with direct contact of mucous membranes and secretions
- May occasionally be caused by HSV-1
- Many HSV-2-infected patients have not been diagnosed and are unaware of transmission.
- Herpes viruses establish lifelong latency in neural ganglia and may reactivate.

Incidence and Demographics

- About 25% of the U.S. population has serologic evidence of HSV-2 infection.
- In monogamous heterosexual couples where one partner has HSV-2 infection, seroconversion of the noninfected partner occurs in 10% over a 1-year time frame.
  - Up to 70% of such infections are transmitted during asymptomatic periods.
- Highest frequency occurs in the 15- to 29-year-old age group.
- Incidence of primary or recurrent herpes in about 10% of pregnant women

Risk Factors

- Same as for other STI transmission

Prevention and Screening

- Condoms may not block transmission from some lesions.
- Abstinence from sexual activity during outbreaks or if prodromal symptoms are present
- No routine screening

Assessment

History
- First episode symptoms
  - Hyperesthesias
  - Burning
  - Itching
  - Dysuria
  - Pain
  - Fever
  - Myalgia
  - Malaise
  - Healing of initial lesion—may be up 21 days, average 12 days
- Prodromal symptoms in recurrent episodes
  - Unusual sensation in the affected area before eruption
  - Usually recur in the same area
  - Length of shedding reduced—about 7 days
  - Healing in about 5 days

Physical Examination
- Tenderness in the genital area
- Genital lesions occur 2 to 14 days after exposure.
  - Painful papules followed by vesicles, ulceration, crusting, and healing
- Enlarged lymph nodes in inguinal areas

Diagnostic Studies
- Direct immunofluorescent antibody slide tests
- Viral culture
- Herpes serology is not used in the diagnosis of an acute genital ulcer.
- HSV-2 serology by Western blot assay or enzyme-linked immunosorbent assay (ELISA) can determine who is infected with HSV and possibly infectious.
  - Useful for couples in which only one partner reports a history of genital herpes

Differential Diagnosis

- Syphilis
- Chancroid
- Folliculits
- *Molluscum contagiosum*

Management

Nonpharmacologic Treatment
- Cool perianal compresses, sitz baths, loose-fitting clothes to alleviate pain
- Handwashing and hygiene to avoid inoculation of other areas of the body

Pharmacologic Treatment
- Three systemic agents available for treatment
  - Acyclovir
    - Available for IV administration
  - Valacyclovir
  - Famciclovir
- For first clinical episodes: treatment duration 7 to 10 days
  - Acyclovir 400 mg p.o. 5 times daily *or*
  - Acyclovir 800 mg p.o. 3 times daily *or*
  - Valacyclovir 1000 mg 2 times daily *or*
  - Famciclovir 250 mg 3 times daily
- Most cases of recurrent infections are mild and do not require therapy, but if therapy is needed:
  - The treatment must be started at first sign of recurrence
  - Valacyclovir 500 mg p.o. 2 times daily for 3 days *or*
  - Acyclovir 200 mg p.o. 5 times daily for 5 days *or*
  - Famciclovir 125 mg p.o. 2 times daily for 5 days
  - Alternate therapy
    - Valacyclovir 2 grams p.o. 2 times daily for one day *or*
    - Famciclovir 1 gram p.o. once or twice for one day
  - The addition of a topical corticosteroid three times daily can help reduce the duration, size, and pain of the lesions.

Special Considerations

- HIV positive or immunocompromised patients
  - Acyclovir 400 mg p.o. 3 times daily for 5 days *or*
  - Famciclovir 500 mg twice daily for 5 days
- First clinical episode in pregnancy may be treated with acyclovir
- Cesarean section recommended when active lesions are visible at the onset of labor

When to Consult, Refer, or Hospitalize

- Consult HIV specialist if resistance to therapy is suspected in a patient who is positive for HIV.
- Hospitalize for suspected encephalitis, pneumonitis, hepatits, or congenital infection

Follow-up

Expected Outcomes
- Most lesions heal promptly in about 12 days.
- No recurrent treatment unless there are severe recurrent episodes and resistance to therapy

Complications
- Pyoderma
- Eczema herpeticum
- Herpetic whitlow
- Herpes gladiatorum (epidemic herpes in wrestlers transmitted by contact)
- Proctitis
- Esophagitis
- Keratitis
- Encephalitis

HUMAN PAPILLOMAVIRUS INFECTON (HPV)

Description

- Infection with certain types of HPV or genital warts causing flat, papular, or pedunculated growth on the genital mucosa
    - HPV types 6, 11, 30, 42, 43, 44, 45, 51, 52, 54
- Visible warts are called *condyloma acuminate.*
- Sexually transmitted
- Pregnancy and immunosuppresion favor growth
- Vulvular lesions may be wartlike or diagnosed after application of 4% acetic acid and colposcopy, after which they appear whitish with prominent papillae.

Etiology

- Virus enters the body during sexual activity through an epithelial defect
- Infects the squamous epithelium of the lower genital tract
- HPV usually persists throughout the patient's life in a dormant state with intermittent recurrence.
- Usually benign
- Highly contagious—90% to 100% of male partners of infected women become infected
- HPV types 16, 18, and 31 are associated with cervical dysplasia.
- HPV implicated in epithelial cancers, especially anorectal carcinoma, and vulvar or penile cancer

Incidence and Demographics

- One of the most commonly transmitted STIs
- Number of patients has increased markedly over the past 20 years.
- Immunosuppressed and those with defects in cell-mediated immunity are especially susceptible to developing HPV infections.
- Anogenital warts or condylomata acuminate are the most commonly diagnosed viral STI in the United States.
- Annual incidence is between 500,000 and 1 million cases.
- The prevalence of HPV is 22% to 35% in women and 2% to 35% in men.
- The incidence is highest among college-aged women and men.

Risk Factors

- Early onset sexual intercourse
- Risk factors same as for other STIs
- Growth of warts may be stimulated by oral contraceptives, pregnancy, and/or immunosuppresion
- Folate deficiency
- Smoking

Prevention and Screening

- Quadrivalent HPV recombinant vaccine
  - Girls and women age 9 to 25: 0.5 ml for 3 doses—0, 2, and 6 months
  - If age 26 reached before vaccine series completed, may complete after age 26 years
  - Routine immunization should begin at about age 12 years
- First vaccine indicated to prevent cervical cancer, genital warts, and precancerous genital lesions
- Annual Papanicolaou (Pap) smear
- Condoms may not eliminate risk of transmission.

Assessment

History
- Usually asymptomatic
- May be unknown history of contact
- Incubation period can be weeks to a year or longer.

Physical Examination
- Small, flesh-colored, cauliflower-type lesions that are usually found near moist surfaces
- Genital warts may also be found on dry surfaces, such as the shaft of the penis.
- May be seen in the perianal area, vaginal introitus, vagina, labia, and vulva

Diagnostic Studies
- Cytologic testing
  - Pap smear is the standard screening test for cervical neoplasia
    - Detects koilocytosis indicative of HPV
- HPV DNA typing
  - Hybrid Capture II
  - Polymerase chain reaction
  - High sensitivities
    - May be diagnosed by visual inspection
  - 3% to 5% acetic acid placed on the vulva or penis
  - Will reveal whitish lesions
- Concomittent testing for other STIs
- Tissue biopsy
  - Used when the diagnosis is uncertain
  - Used in the patients who are immune-compromised, if lesions worsen during treatment, or the patient does not respond to standard therapy

Differential Diagnosis

- Benign vulvar lesions
- Benign cervical disease
- Hemorrhoids
- Malignant vulvar lesions
- Penile cancer
- Warts—nongenital
- Folliculitis
- Neoplasm
- Granuloma inguinale

Management

Nonpharmacologic Treatment
- Smoking cessation
- Encourage use of condoms
- Adequate dietary intake of folic acid
- Cryosurgery
- Electrosurgery
- Surgical removal
- Laser surgery
- Cavitron Ultrasonic Surgical Aspirator

Pharmacologic Treatment
- All medications are applied topically on cutaneous surfaces.
- Imiquimod: apply 3 times per week; leave on skin 6 to 10 hours; remove by washing; treatment not to exceed 16 weeks

- Interferon alfa-n3: 0.05 ml (250,000 IU) per wart 2 times/week for up to 8 weeks; maximum recommended dose per treatment is 0.5 ml
- Interferon alfa-2b: 1 million IU injected into each lesion 3 times/week on alternate days for 3 weeks; maximum recommended dose per treatment session is 5 million IU
- Podofilox 0.5% gel or solution applied to anogential warts 2 times daily for 3 consecutive days, then discontinue
  - Repeat cycle until no visible wart tissue or a maximum of 4 cycles
- Podophyllin 25% in benzoin tincture applied by a physician—never dispensed to a patient
  - Reapply each week for up to 6 weeks.
- Cryotherapy with liquid nitrogen, may repeat every 1 to 2 weeks—provider-applied only
- Fluorouracil: 5% applied as a thin layer 1 to 3 times/week; therapy may be required for up to 10 to 12 weeks
- Trichloroacetic acid and bichloracetic acid (TCA & BCA): 80% to 90% solution applied directly by physician per week

Special Considerations

- Pregnancy: Podophyllin, imiquimod, and podofilox are contraindicated.
- Some specialists recommend removal of visible warts during pregnancy.
- Condoms do not eliminate the risk.

When to Consult, Refer, or Hospitalize

- Consult a gynecologist for vaginal and cervical warts—dysplasia must be excluded prior to treatment.
- Refer to colorectal surgeon for perianal condylomata
- Women with large warts (> 2 cm) should be referred to a gynecologist for surgical consideration.
- Consult an infectious disease specialist for assistance in management of HPV disease in patients who are immunocompromised.

Follow-up

Expected Outcomes
- Genital warts may spontaneously regress, remain unchanged, or increase in size.
- Histological evidence of HPV infection on a cervical Pap smear is similar to mild dysplasia.
  - This subclinical disease often spontaneously regresses.

Complications
- Benign vulvar lesions
- Cervical cancer
- Urethral warts
- Penile cancer
- Malignant vulvar lesions
- Anal squamous cell carcinoma
- Treatment procedures may cause scarring.

REFERENCES

Barkley, T., & Myers, C. (2008). *Practice guidelines for acute care nurse practitioners.* St. Louis, MO: Saunders.

Beers, M., Porter, R., Jones, T., Kaplan, J., & Berkwits, M. (Eds.). (2006). *The Merck manual of diagnosis and therapy.* Whitehouse Station, NJ: Merck Research Laboratories.

Centers for Disease Control and Prevention. (2006). Sexually transmitted diseases treatment guidelines. *MMWR: Morbidity and Mortality Weekly Report, 55,* No. RR-11, 1–93.

Donders, G. (2006). Management of genital infections in pregnant women. *Current Opinion in Infectious Disease, 19*(1), 55–61.

Habermann, T., & Ghosh, A. (Eds.). (2008). *Mayo Clinic internal medicine concise textbook.* Rochester, MN: Mayo Clinic Scientific Press.

Fauci, A., Braunwald, E., Kasper, D., Hauser, S., Longo, D., Jameson, J., & Loscalzo, J. (Eds.). (2005). *Harrison's principles of internal medicine.* New York: McGraw Hill.

Marini, J., & Wheeler, A. (2010). *Critical care medicine, the essentials.* Philadelphia: Wolters Kluwer/Lippincott Williams & Wilkins.

McKean, S., Bennett, A., & Halasyamani, L. (Eds.). (2008). *Hospital medicine.* Philadelphia: Wolters Kluwer/Lippincott Williams & Wilkins.

McPhee, S., & Papadakis, M. (Eds.). (2010). *Current medical diagnosis and treatment 2010.* New York: McGraw Hill.

McPhee, S., & Papadakis, M. (Eds.). (2011). *Current medical diagnosis and treatment 2011.* New York: McGraw Hill.

National Guidelines Clearinghouse. (2007). *Gonococcal and chlamydial infections.* Retrieved from http://www.guideline.gov/content.aspx?id=12570&search=gonococcal+and+chlamydial+infections

Rennke, H., & Denker, B. (2007). *Renal pathophysiology, the essentials.* Philadelphia: Lippincott Williams & Wilkins.

15

Palliative Care/End-of-Life Care

Hope Moser, DNP, ANP-BC

PALLIATIVE CARE

- Focused on improving the quality of life of people facing serious illness
- Emphasis on pain and symptom management, communication, and coordinated care
- Palliative care is appropriate from the time of diagnosis and can be provided along with curative treatment.

Quality of Life
- Multidimensional, including physical, social, psychological, and spiritual dimensions
- Patient-driven care
- Palliative care involves a formal assessment of symptoms and collaborative, interdisciplinary decision-making. It is often offered simultaneously with life-prolonging and curative therapies for persons living with serious, complex, and eventually terminal illness.
- Advanced disease progression is characterized by inadequately treated physical distress, disjointed care systems, poor communication, and care giver burden.

Description

The World Health Organization (WHO) defines palliative care as "An approach that improves the quality of life of patients and their families facing problems associated with life-threatening illness, through the prevention and relief of suffering by means of early identification and impeccable assessment and treatment of pain and other problems, physical, psychosocial, and spiritual" (WHO, 2008).

Etiology

- Terminally ill patients have a wide variety of advanced disease.
- Patients require symptom management with noninvasive therapeutic regimes.
- Flexible care settings are necessary.

Incidence and Demographics

- In 2009, 2,436,682 people died in the United States.
- Majority of deaths occurred in those > 65 years of age

Box 15-1. Leading Causes of Death in 2009

Heart disease	Malignant neoplasm
Chronic lower respiratory diseases	Cerebrovascular diseases
Accidents (unintentional injuries)	Motor vehicle accidents
All other accidents	Alzheimer's disease
Diabetes mellitus	Influenza and pneumonia
Nephritis, nephrotic syndrome, and nephrosis	Intentional self-harm (suicide)

Reprinted from "Deaths: Preliminary data for 2009", by K. D. Kochanek, J. Q. Xu, S. L. Murphy, et al., 2011, *National Vital Statistics Reports*, 59(4), 5, retrieved from http://www.cdc.gov/nchs/products/nvsr.htm.

Indications for Palliative Care

- Patients with conditions that are progressive and life-limiting
- Conditions with burdensome symptoms, functional decline, and progressive cognitive deficits
- Assistance in clarification or reorientation of patient or family goals of care
- Assistance in resolution of ethical dilemmas
- Situations in which the patient, family, or both decline further invasive or curative treatments, with stated preference for comfort measures only
- Patients who are expected to die imminently or soon after hospital discharge
- Provision of bereavement support for patient care staff, particularly after loss of a colleague under care

Assessment

- Assessment of physical and mental symptoms
  - Focus on symptoms and impact on quality of life.
  - Standardized assessment is essential.
  - Instruments with good psychometric properties
- Key elements in palliative care:
  - Patient population
  - Patient- and family-centered care
  - Timing of care
  - Comprehensive care
  - Interdisciplinary care
  - Relief from suffering
  - Community involvement
  - Skill in care of dying and bereaved
  - Continuity of care
  - Equitable access
  - High-quality care
- Characteristics of geriatric patients with terminal illness:
  - Frailty
  - Functional dependence
  - Cognitive impairment
  - Multiple comorbidities
  - Symptoms distress
- In frail older adults, disease-specific treatments may ameliorate the burdens of frailty, dependence, and symptom distress but are unlikely to eliminate them.
- Principles of symptom management:
  - Anticipating symptoms before they develop
  - Minimizing technologic interventions
  - Planning alternative routes for medications
- Major symptoms that threaten the comfort of dying patients
  - Respiratory distress
  - Pain
  - Cognitive failure

Delirium Assessment

- **Mini-Mental:** *does not* distinguish between delirium and dementia
- **Delirium Rating Scale:** *does* distinguish between delirium and dementia
- Pharmacologic evaluation: polypharmacy, sedatives, opioids
- **CAM (Confusion Assessment Method):** high sensitivity and specificity for differentiating delirium from dementia in hospitalized, geriatric population; for use by nonpsychiatric practitioners
- **The Diagnostic and Statistical Manual of Mental Disorders (DSM)-IV:** the gold standard for criteria.

Table 15-1. Clinical Practice Guidelines for Symptom Management in Palliative Care

Physical Symptoms	Intervention	Psychological Symptoms	Intervention
Pain	Pharmacologic: opioid analgesics Nonpharmacologic measures (radiotherapy, anesthetia) See section on pain	Anxiety	Supportive therapy and cautious use of short-acting benzodiazepines Monitor for delirium
Fatigue and malaise	Fatigue is subjective. Differentiate between fatigue and acute alteration in mental status. Behavior modifications to conserve energy Minimal pharmacotherapy interventions (glucocorticoids, psychostimulants)	Depression	Psychotherapy, cognitive and behavioral modification techniques Psychiatric consult Monitor for suicidal ideation Pharmacologic therapy dictated by life expectancy
Dyspnea	Energy conservation, oxygen therapy Pharmacologic assistance; see Table 15-4 (p. 638)	Delirium	Distinguish among anxiety, depression, and dementia. Delirium has acute onset, fluctuating consciousness, reversible. Altered LOC is distinguishing feature, which anxiety, dementia, and depression do not have. Identify reversible causes
Anorexia	Pharmacologic approaches such as corticosteroids, megace and cannabinoids		
Constipation	Hydration, increase physical activity, increase fiber (not with use of opioids) Laxative plus stool softener		
Nausea and vomiting	Identify cause see Table 15-5 (p. 639)		
Dyspnea	Adequate oxygenation and protection of airway End of life: opioids and anxiolytics		

Adapted from *Clinical practice guidelines for quality palliative care* by National Consensus Project for Quality Palliative Care, 2004, retrieved from http://www.nationalconsensusproject.org/guideline.pdf

Table 15-2. Symptom Assessment Instruments

Full-Length Instruments to Assess Symptoms		Condensed Instruments to Assess Symptoms	
MSAS	Memorial Symptom Assessment Scale	CMSAS	Condensed Memorial Symptom Assessment Scale
RAI	Rotterdam Assessment Instrument	ESAS	Edmonton Symptom Assessment System
WCQ	Worthing Chemotherapy Questionnaire	MDASAI	MD Anderson Symptom Assessment Inventory
CSAI	Computerized Symptoms Assessment Instrument	SDS	Symptom Distress Scale

Adapted from *Optimizing Cancer Care—The Importance of Symptom Management* by American Society of Clinical Oncology, 2001, Alexandria, VA: Author.

Table 15-3. Management of Dyspnea

Mild dyspnea in opioid-naïve patients	Weak opioids: codeine with or without acetaminophen' hydrocodone
Moderate to severe dyspnea in opioid-naïve patients	Strong opioids: morphine, oxycodone, hydromorphone
Anxiety	Lorazepam, clonazepam, midazolam Give hourly until patient is relaxed, then provide maintenance dose.

Table 15-4. Management of Nausea and Vomiting

Etiology	Causes	Treatment
Chemoreceptor trigger zone stimulation	Pharmacologics such as opioids, digoxin, chemotherapy Electrolyte imbalances (uremia, hypercalcemia) Toxins (tumor-producing peptides, infection)	Haldol, compazine, reglan, zofran, olanzapine
Mechanical causes	Gastric irritation, tumors, gastric distention Nonsurgical bowel obstruction Intracranial processes Vestibular vertigo	Antihistamines, zofran, reglan, H2 blockers, PPIs Octreotide Corticosteroids, benzodiazepines Transdermal scopolamine, meclizine

PAIN: THE FIFTH VITAL SIGN

Definition

Pain is the sensory and emotional experience, associated with actual or potential tissue damage and described in terms of such damage
- Nociceptive pain: results from direct or chemical stimulation of nociceptors and normal neural signaling to the brain
- Visceral pain: results from stimulation of nociceptors in the gastrointestinal, respiratory, or other organ systems
- Neuropathic pain: results from nerve signal disorders
- Pain is subjective. It is what and when the patient says it is.
- OLDCARTS: the mnemonic commonly used for the 7 attributes of a symptom.
  - Onset
  - Location
  - Duration
  - Characteristics
  - Aggravating/Alleviating factors
  - Radiation
  - Timing
  - Severity

Table 15-5. Autonomic Nervous System

Carries nerve impulses to the smooth muscles of organs without thought

Control	Response	Neurotransmitter
Sympathetic	Fight or flight	Norepinephrine
Parasympathetic	Relaxed state	Acetylcholine

Table 15-6. Classifications of Pain

	Acute Pain	Chronic Pain	Chronic Cancer Pain
Onset	Rapid	Constant	Onset varies
Location	Highly localized	Poorly localized	Varies
Duration	Less than 6 months	More than 6 months	More than 6 months
Characteristics	Sharp, radiating, initiated by acute injury	Dull, aching, diffuse, constant, nagging, intractable; chronic pathology or persistent after disease or injury	Impossible to predict when it will begin or end, often gets worse rather than better.
Signs and symptoms	Autonomic nervous system (ANS) response	Exhausted, listless, depressed; hypertension, tachycardia	Acute and chronic

Pharmacologic Treatment

Opioids

Agonist
- Drug that can combine with an opioid receptor on a cell to produce a physiologic reaction typical of a naturally occurring substance. Morphine is the prototypical opioid agonist.

Antagonist
- Drug that interferes with the physiological action of another substance, especially by combining with and blocking its nerve receptor. It typically reverses (and sometimes blocks) effects of an opioid agonist. Naloxone is the prototypical opioid antagonist.

Agonist-Antagonist
- Class of opioid medications that bind to both a receptor that produces pain relief, and to another receptor that does not produce a physiological effect. There is no prototypical agonist-antagonist drug. Some examples include pentazocine and butorphranol.
  - Acute visceral or somatic pain
  - Moderate to severe intensity
  - Not for severe escalating pain
  - May potentiate withdrawal with opiate dependence
  - Tend not to cause respiratory depression

Management of Pain

- Routine and standardized assessment
- Appropriate analgesic prescribing
- Nonpharmacologic modalities
- Management of opioid side effects

Nonpharmacologic Treatment
- Distraction
- Cutaneous stimulation
- Guided image
- Progressive relaxation

Table 15–7. Benefits of Treatment of Pain

Potential Psychological Benefits	Physiologic Benefits
Diminish emotional components of pain	Decrease stimulation of SNS
Strengthen coping abilities	Muscle relaxation
Reduce perceived threat	Lower HR and BP
Give sense of control to patient	Improve oxygenation
Change expectations	
Decrease fatigue	
Restore hope	
Promote sleep	
Improve quality of life	

Patient-Controlled Analgesia (PCA)
- System for the delivery of analgesics
- Allows patient to self-administer medications as needed, with a set rate and a preset limit
- Useful when patient is expected to have severe pain

- Patient must be capable of understanding and operating the PCA button.
- Modes: PCA only, basal only, PCA and basal

Adverse Outcomes of Untreated Pain
- Delirium
- Atelectasis
- Pneumonia
- Deconditioning
- Impaired functional capacity

Box 15-2. Analgesic Groups

Non-opioids	NSAIDs, COX II inhibitors, APAP
Opioids (Narcotics)	Morphine, hydromorphone, fentanyl
Adjuvants	Antidepressants, psychostimulants, corticosteroids

Table 15-8. Opioid Analgesic Equivalents Compared to Morphine

Drug	Oral	Parenteral	Oral Conversion Factor to Oral Morphine
Codeine	200	130	0.15
Hydrocodone	30	NA	1
Hydromorphone	7.5	1.5	4
Morphine	20	NA	1
Oxycodone	20	NA	1.5

Examples of Equivalent Doses:
Hydromorphone 1 mg IV = morphine 6.7 mg IV
Morhpine 10 mg IV = morphine 30 mg p.o. = hydromorphone 1.5 mg IV = hydromorphone 7.5 mg p.o.

Adapted from *Principles of Analgesic Use in the Treatment of Acute Pain and Cancer Pain* (6th ed.), by C. Miaskowski, et al., 2008, Glenview, IL: American Pain Society.

Figure 15-1. WHO Analgesic Ladder

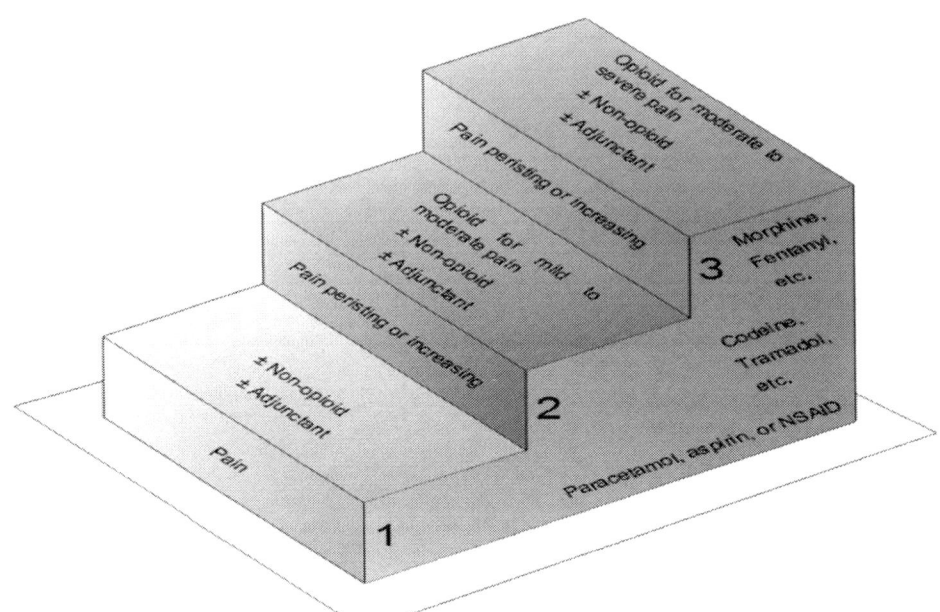

Table 15-9. WHO Analgesic Ladder • Rating on 1-10 scale

1-4 Mild	5-6 Moderate	7-10 Severe
Acetaminophen (APAP)	Opioid combination (oxycodone/APAP, hydrocodone/APAP, codeine/APAP)	Strong pure opioid (morphine, oxycodone, hydromorphone, fentanyl)
NSAIDs/COX-II inhibitors (sparingly because of renal toxicity and GI side effects of NSAIDS and cardiovascular side effects of COX-II inhibitors). Use with extreme caution in low-risk patients (no GI ulcers or bleeding and adequate renal function)	Start after maximal dose of APAP is given and continue until pain relief is achieved. Consider sustained release opioid at that time. Careful consideration while using combination therapy because of danger of APAP toxicity. Nonresponders to APAP should be given one pure opioid (morphine, oxycodone) and titrated until desired pain relief is achieved.	Titrate to desired level of pain relief. High incidence of respiratory depression; monitor carefully.

Figure 15–1 and Table 15–9 reprinted from WHO's *pain relief ladder*, retrieved from http://www.who.int/cancer/palliative/painladder/en/index.html. Reprinted by World Health Organization, (2011), with permission.

Table 15-10. Pharmacologic Treatment for WHO Analgesic Ladder

Mild Pain (oral or parenteral)

Drug	Dose	Max Dose/ 24hours	Precautions
Acetaminophen (APAP)	325–650 mg p.o./ PR q 4–6 hrs	4000 mg Elderly: 2600 mg	Liver disease, renal disease, other APAP
Ibuprofen	400–800mg p.o. q 6–8 hrs	3200 mg	Liver, kidney, GI, and CV disease
Ketorolac	15–30 mg IV (30 mg limit IV) 10 mg p.o. q 4–6 hrs	120 mg IV 40 mg p.o. Older adults 60 mg IV	Dose limit of 5 days Renal function

Moderate Pain (Oral)

Hydrocodone/ APAP	5/325 mg q 4–6 hrs 7.5/325 mg q 4–6 hrs 10/325 mg q 4–6 hrs	4000 mg APAP Older adults: 2600 mg APAP	Liver disease, renal disease Other APAP
Oxycodone/ APAP	5/325 mg q 6 hrs 10/550 mg q 6hrs		Renal, GI (ileus) Other APAP
Tramadol	25–50 mg q 4–6 hrs	400 mg	Seizure or psychological disorders

Severe Pain (Oral)

Fentanyl	100 mcg buccally q 4 hrs	Titrate per need, 24 hours between each escalation	Respiratory eepression. Do not use in opioid nontolerant or acute or postoperative pain.
Hydromorphone	1–2 mg q 4 hrs		GI disease, respiratory distress
Morphine sulfate	5 mg p.o. q 3 hrs		
Oxycodone	5 mg p.o. q 4 hrs		

Continued

Table 15-10. Pharmacologic Treatment for WHO Analgesic Ladder (cont.)

Severe Pain (Parenteral)

Drug	Dose	Max Dose/ 24 hours	Precautions
Fentanyl	20–50 mcg IV q 1–2 hrs	Titrate per need, 24 hours between each escalation	Short duration of action Respiratory distress
Hydromorphone	0.5–1mg IV q 3 hrs		Very potent Good for patients requiring high doses of opiates
Morphine sulfate	2–4 mg IV q 3 hrs		Reduce dose in older adults, those with renal issues, and fragile patients

Adapted from *Principles of analgesic use in the treatment of acute pain and cancer pain* (6th ed.), by C. Miaskowski et al., 2008, Glenview, IL: American Pain Society.

Special Considerations

- Goal of hospice is to provide holistic care at the end of life, focused on relief of patients' suffering.
- Functional status is the most powerful predictor of survival.

Six Themes of Central Importance in Communicating With Patients With Advanced Illness
- Honesty
- Willingness to talk about death and dying
- Deliver bad news in a sensitive way
- Listen
- Encourage questions
- Maintain sensitivity

Principles of Delivering Unfavorable News
- Find a quiet, private place. Sit down close to the patient.
- Listen and clarify patient's and family's understanding of the situation
- Prepare the patient and family ("warning shot"), and obtain their permission to communicate bad news.
- Be silent, pause after giving bad news. Allow the patient and family to absorb and react to the news.
- Encourage and convey hope that is realistic and appropriate for the circumstance.

When to Consult, Refer, or Hospitalize

- The last hours of life can be marked by a constellation of symptoms that can be especially distressing for the patient and caregivers.
- Providing family education regarding expected outcomes at various levels of the death and dying process can improve the family's ability to care for their loved one.

REFERENCES

American Society of Clinical Oncology. (2001). *Optimizing cancer care—The importance of symptom management* (Vol. 1 and 2). Alexandria, VA: ASCO.

Fauci, A. S., Braunwald, E., Kasper, D. L., Hauser, S. L., Longo, D. L., Jameson, J. L., Loscalzo, J. Eds. (2008). *Harrison's principles of internal medicine* (17th ed.). New York: McGraw-Hill.

International Association for the Study of Pain. (2011). *IASP taxonomy.* Retrieved from http://www.iasp-pain.org/AM/Template.cfm?Section=Home&Template=/CM/HTMLDisplay.cfm&ContentID=1728

Kochanek, K. D., Xu, J. Q., Murphy, S. L., et.al. (2011). *Deaths: Preliminary data for 2009. National Vital Statistics Report, 59*(4), 4. Retrieved from http://www.cdc.gov/nchs/products/nvsr.htm

Katzung, B. G., Masters, S. B., & Trevor, A. J. (2009). *Basic & clinical pharmacology* (11th ed.). New York: McGraw Hill.

McCaffery, M., & Passero, C. (1999). *Pain: Clinical manual.* St. Louis, MO: Mosby.

Miaskowski, C., Bair, M., Chou, R., D'Arcy, Y., Hartwick, C., Huffman, L., et al. (2008). *Principles of analgesic use in the treatment of acute pain and cancer pain* (6th ed.). Glenview, IL: American Pain Society.

National Consensus Project for Quality Palliative Care. (2004). *Clinical practice guidelines for quality palliative care.* Retrieved from http://www.nationalconsensusproject.org/guideline.pdf

Radtke, F. M., Franck, M., Schneider, M., Luetz, A., Seeling, M., Heinz, A., et al. (2008). Comparison of three scores to screen for delirium in the recovery room. *British Journal of Anaesthesia, 101*(3), 338–343. Retrieved from http://bja.oxfordjournals.org/content/101/3/338.full.pdf+html

Solomon, D. H., Rassen, J. A., Glynn R. J., Lee, J., Levin, R., & Schneeweiss S. (2010). The comparative safety of analgesics in older adults with arthritis. *Archives of Internal Medicine, 170*(22), 1968–1976.

World Health Organization. (2008). *Definition of palliative care.* Retrieved from www.who.int/cancer/palliative/definition

World Health Organization. (n.d.) *WHO's pain relief ladder.* Retrieved from http://www.who.int/cancer/palliative/painladder/en/index.html

16

Health Promotion
Julie Davey, MSN, RN, ANP-BC, ACNP-BC

DIET AND NUTRITION

Description

- Ideal body weight (IBW) should be used as the goal when diet planning for healthy patients.
- Healthy nutrition is an integral part of health promotion.
- Daily caloric intake should be calculated toward each patient's ideal body weight—overweight patients will lose weight on such a regimen; underweight patients will gain weight.

Determining IBW

- Men: Begin with 106 lbs for first 5 ft., add 6 lbs. for each additional inch of height.
- Women: Begin with 100 lbs for first 5 ft., add 5 lbs. for each additional inch of height.
- IBW for a 5 ft., 6 in. male would be 142 lbs.
- IBW for a 5 ft., 6 in. female would be 130 lbs.
- Regardless of gender, subtract 10% for small body frame; add 10% for large body frame.
- IBW for a large-framed 5 ft., 6 in. male would be 156.2 lbs.
- IBW for a small-framed 5 ft., 6 in. female would be 117 lbs.

Table 16-1. Formula for Determining Ideal Body Weight

Build	Women	Men
Medium	Allow 100 lbs. for first 5 ft. plus 5 lb. for each additional inch. Example: Female patient 5 ft. 4 in. = 120 lbs. (100 + 20)	Allow 106 lbs. for first 5 ft. plus 6 lbs. for each additional inch. Example: Male patient 5 ft. 10 in. = 166 lbs. (106 + 60)
Small	Subtract 10%: 120 − 12 = 108 lbs.	Subtract 10%: 166 − 17 = 149 lbs.
Large	Add 10%: 120 + 12 = 132 lbs.	Add 10%: 166 + 17 = 183 lbs.

Adapted from *Clinician's pocket reference*, by L. Gomella & S. Haist, 2007, New York: McGraw-Hill.

Circumstances When Weight Loss or IBW *Should Not* Be the Goal of Diet Management

- The patient is pregnant.
- Patients suffering from increased physiologic stress, for example, recovering from major surgery
- Patients with uncontrolled chronic illness; control illness before initiating weight loss
- When the goal of diet planning is to maintain present weight, daily caloric needs should be 30 to 35 kcal/kg of body weight.

Healthy Diet Planning

Target weight is determined (IBW vs. maintain present weight).
Daily caloric requirement calculated based upon target weight—patient's weight in kg multiplied by 30 to 35 kcal

Caloric Intake Should Be Divided Among Fuel Sources as Follows:
- 50% to 60% carbohydrate
- 30% or < fats; < 10% from saturated fats
- Remainder of caloric requirement as protein (approximately 0.8 to 1 g protein/kg body weight)

The Food Plate Should Serve as a Foundation
- Bread, rice, cereals: 6 to 11 servings daily
- Vegetables: 3 to 5 servings daily
- Fruits: 2 to 4 servings daily
- Meat, poultry, fish, dry beans, eggs, and nuts: 2 to 3 servings daily
- Milk, yogurt, and cheese: 2 to 3 servings daily
- Fats, oils, and sweets: Use sparingly

Dietary Guidelines for Americans Describes a Healthy Diet as One That:
- Emphasizes a variety of fruits, vegetables, whole grains, and fat-free or low-fat milk and milk products
- Includes lean meats, poultry, fish, beans, eggs, and nuts
- Is low in saturated fats, trans fats, cholesterol, sodium, and added sugars
- Stays within your daily caloric needs

Nutritional Supplements

- Supplemental calcium of 1,000 to 1,500 mg/day is recommended for adolescents and adults.
- 0.4 mg/day of folic acid is recommended for women of childbearing age.
- Other vitamin or supplemental nutrition is not typically necessary in the healthy adult who maintains a healthy diet.

Body Mass Index (BMI)

- BMI measures weight in relation to height: kg of body weight ÷ height in meters, squared
- BMI 18.5 kg/m^2 to 24.9 kg/m^2 is healthy weight.
- BMI of 25 kg/m^2 to 29.9 kg/m^2 is overweight.
- BMI > 30 kg/m^2 is obese.
- BMI must be interpreted as part of the patient presentation—not all patients with a BMI between 18.5 kg/m^2 and 24.9 kg/m^2 are at healthy weight.
- BMI > 25 kg/m^2 carries increased health risks.

PHYSICAL ACTIVITY

- Provides a wide variety of health benefits

Benefits of Physical Activity

- Decreases risk factors for cardiovascular disease, type 2 diabetes mellitus, and colon cancer
- Cardiopulmonary conditioning
- Decreases low-density lipoprotein (LDL) cholesterol
- Increases basal metabolic rate (BMR)
- Improves muscle strength and endurance
- Decreases bone mineral loss
- Promotes psychological well-being
- Increases self-esteem

Risks of Physical Activity

- Risk of musculoskeletal injury increases with more intense and frequent physical activity.
- Incidence of sudden cardiac arrest or myocardial infarction is transiently increased during vigorous physical exertion in those with history of cardiac disease or who are habitually sedentary.

Definition of Physical Activity to Promote and Maintain Health

- Moderately intense aerobic activity (brisk walking or equivalent) for 30 minutes a day, 5 days weekly *or*
- Vigorously intense (jogging or equivalent) aerobic activity for 20 minutes a day, 2 days weekly
- Approaches can be combined; moderately intense activity 2 days weekly combined with vigorously-intense activity 2 days weekly meets recommendations
- All adults should also perform activities that maintain or increase muscular strength and endurance at least 2 days weekly:
  - Resistance training includes 8 to 10 exercises, performed on two or more nonconsecutive days each week using major muscles.
  - Resistance (weight) should be used that results in substantial fatigue after 8 to 12 repetitions.

Before Prescribing a Physical Activity Program

- Patients should have a complete history and physical examination.
- Investigate any symptoms or findings before prescribing exercise:
  - Reports of fatigue, shortness of breath, or chest pain
  - Risk factors for thromboembolic disease
  - Excessive bruising
  - Cardiac murmurs, clicks, or hums
  - Carotid bruits
  - Other physical indicators of undiagnosed vascular disease
- Review current medication list for drugs that may interact with exercise, for example, cardiac or vasoactive medications, or central nervous system agents.
- Maximize control of any chronic illness.
- Emphasize "red flags" for stopping exercise:
  - Shortness of breath
  - Chest pain
  - Nausea or vomiting
  - Dizziness

Evaluation of Physical Activity Program

- Decrease intensity or components if the patient is unable to talk while exercising, is fatigued for > 1 hour after finishing, or develops swelling or pain.
- Increase intensity, time, or both as patient develops tolerance.

SAFETY

- Accidental injury is a leading cause of morbidity and mortality in the adolescent and young adult population.
- Encourage seat belt use.
- Encourage helmet use for bicycles, skateboarding, and motorcycles.
- General home safety is appropriate for all patients.
- Smoke and carbon monoxide detectors
- Common-sense practices regarding door and window locks
- Safe handling and storage of firearms
- Electrical safety in the home
- Avoid environmental hazards and teach fall prevention for older adults.
- Practice personal safety.
  - Use well-lit parking areas at night.
  - Walk and travel with other people after dark.
  - Do not ignore intuition or sensations of unease.

STRESS MANAGEMENT

- Stress becomes pathologic when stressors exceed patients' physiologic and psychological coping mechanisms.
- Whether faced with eustress or distress, when stress input exceeds coping mechanisms, patient will feel stressed.
- Goal of stress management is to restore balance—either decrease stress input or increase coping ability.

Stress May Be Physiologic, Environmental, or Emotional

- Increased metabolic demands of illness
- Anticipation or fear (classic fear, flight or fight response)
- Extremes of environment (heat, cold, precipitation)
- Day-to-day routine environmental stressors (traffic, job-related frustration)
- Personal relationships (significant others, children, parents, siblings)

Stress May Be Good or Bad

- Good stress is "eustress" (e.g., upcoming marriage, trip)—a positive event that places stress on the patient.
- Bad stress is "distress"; the more classic stressors are bad ones.

Assessment of Stress

- The patient may report vague, nonspecific physical symptoms that have no clear organic cause (e.g., "upset" stomach, nausea, headaches, intermittent diarrhea, numbness or tingling in hands or feet).
- The patient may also report difficulty or changes in interpersonal relationships.
- Other patient reports may include:
  - Quick temper
  - Inability to concentrate
  - Withdrawal from social relationships and interactions

Stress Management Techniques and Strategies

- Avoid unnecessary change.
- Manage time using a written calendar with realistic deadlines.
- Avoid triggers—people, places, events
- Increase physical exercise.
- Seek support persons.
- Meditation, guided imagery, biofeedback strategies

DISEASE PREVENTION

Description

- In addition to encouraging the healthy lifestyle practices described previously in this section, providers may promote health among their patient population by recommending and implementing specific disease prevention strategies that promote early detection and treatment. Disease prevention should occur along all levels of the health–illness continuum. *Primary prevention* is the concept of maintaining healthy lifestyle practices to prevent disease from occurring. *Secondary prevention* embodies the principle of routine screening—abnormalities are identified before disease occurs; for example, identifying dyslipidemia before coronary artery disease occurs. *Tertiary preventions* are those practices that prevent deterioration or extension of disease and maximize function—such as control of vascular disease and rehabilitation after stroke.
- Secondary prevention includes the performance of periodic screening questionnaires and laboratory or other tests for high-risk patient populations. It is important to note that there are several different organizations that recommend screening practices and guidelines, and they are not always in agreement. In addition to screening, immunizing patients against a variety of diseases when appropriate further contributes to overall health by preventing the occurrence of a wide variety of infectious diseases.

EPIDEMIOLGOIC PRINCIPLES

Etiology

- Defines the cause or the web of causation of a disease or problem
- Prevalence rates describe a group at a certain point in time and the number within a group that has a particular disease or problem. This description is like a snapshot in time.
- Incidence rates describe the rate of development of a disease in a group over a period of time, the continuing occurrence of new cases of disease. This information is based on large-scale data collection from the Centers for Disease Control and Prevention.

Natural History of Disease

- The course of disease development, expression, and progression. Whether based on the microbiology principles of certain organisms or large-scale research studies of causality, several stages appear to be universally descriptive:
  - Stage of susceptibility
  - Stage of presymptomatic disease
  - Stage of clinical disease
  - Stage of disability
- Goal is to intervene as early as possible to prevent disease or disability

Communicable and Infectious Diseases

- Caused by organisms that attack and invade vulnerable individuals
- Identify of causative agents
- Rely on microbiology principles in understanding life cycle of organism
- Focus on intervention at vulnerable phases in course of disease or life cycle of organism to limit or eradicate disease

Epidemiolgic Concepts

Host–Parasite Relations
- Pathogenicity
- Virulence

Reservoirs of Infection
- Cases
- Carriers

Mechanisms of Transmission of Infection
- Direct
- Indirect through vehicle, vector, or air

Concepts of Epidemic vs. Endemic Infections
- Person-to-person transmission
- Generation time: time between receipt of infection and maximal communicability of that infection
- Herd immunity: resistance of a group to invasion and spread of an infectious agent

Control Measures
- Measures directed against the reservoir: isolation, quarantine
- Measures that interrupt the transmission of organisms: water purification, pasteurization of milk, inspection procedures
- Measures that reduce host susceptibility: immunization

RECOMMENDED ADULT SCREENING PRACTICES

Cholesterol Screening

The National Cholesterol Education Program (NCEP)
- NCEP Adult Treatment Panel (ATP)-III recommendations state that all adults over age 20 should have cholesterol screening every 5 years.
- Screening should include a fasting fractionated lipid profile; those at low risk may be screened with nonfasting total cholesterol/HDL assessment, with a fractionated panel to follow if abnormal.
- Screening may be more frequent if other risk factors for vascular disease are present.

The United States Preventive Services Task Force (USPSTF)
- The USPSTF recommends routine screening to begin at age 35 for men and 45 for women.
- Screening for those aged 20 to 34 is recommended if other risk factors for cardiovascular disease are present.
- Screening should include total cholesterol and high-density lipoprotein (HDL)–cholesterol (HDL-C) fraction.

Hypertension Screening
- Screening recommended for all children and adults at each clinical visit.

Type 2 Diabetes Mellitus

- Screening recommended for all adults with dyslipidemia and hypertension.

Sexually Transmitted Infection Screening

Chlamydia
- All sexually active women aged 25 and younger
- All women at increased risk for infection

Gonorrhea
- All asymptomatic women at high risk of infection
- All high-risk women who are pregnant

Syphilis
- All women who are pregnant
- All persons at increased risk of infection

Human Immunodeficiency Virus (HIV)
- All adolescents and adults at high risk
- All women who are pregnant

Cervical Cancer Screening (Papanicolaou Testing)

- Should be implemented for all sexually active women with a cervix or beginning at no later than age 21
- Should be repeated every 3 years until age 65
- Those with abnormal conditions need more frequent monitoring.
- Screening may be discontinued for women > 65 years of age with consistently normal results and who are not otherwise at high risk for cervical cancer.

Breast Cancer Screening

- Screening mammography alone or with clinical breast examination (CBE) every 1 to 2 years beginning at age 40
- There is insufficient evidence to recommend for or against teaching or performing breast self-examinations (BSE). BSE is an option for women over age 20.
- A variety of professional organizations offer breast cancer screening recommendations that may conflict with these.

Colon Cancer Screening

- Adults aged 50 and older should be periodically screened for colon cancer (every 1 to 2 years).
- Evidence suggests that fecal occult blood testing (FOBT) is adequate.
- There is no evidence to support sigmoidoscopy as superior to FOBT for screening purposes.
- Colonoscopy and double-contrast barium enema are not superior for screening purposes.
- Those with positive FOBT should be further evaluated by colonoscopy.

Prostate Cancer Screening

- There is insufficient evidence to recommend for or against routine screening.
- Digital rectal examination (DRE), tumor markers (prostate-specific antigen; PSA), or transrectal ultrasound are not routinely recommended.
- PSA and DRE should be offered annually to men age 50 and older that have at least a 10-year life expectancy.

Testicular Cancer Screening

- The USPS Task Force recommends against screening for testicular cancer in asymptomatic adolescent and adult males.

Osteoporosis Screening

- Bone density measurements should be performed in all women > 65 years of age.
- Begin at age 60 for those at increased risk:
    - Weight < 70 kg
    - No use of estrogen
    - Long-term corticosteroid use
- Other traditional risk factors such as tobacco use and sedentary lifestyle are less certain and not used in the consideration of screening.

Depression Screening

- Screening recommended for all adults in clinical practices that have systems in place to ensure accurate diagnosis, effective treatment, and follow-up.

RECOMMENDED ADULT IMMUNIZATIONS

Tetanus, Diphtheria, and Pertussis

- Booster every 10 years (once in adulthood for diphtheria)
- Booster dose may be needed at 5 years for wound management
- Administer intramuscularly (IM)

Measles, Mumps, and Rubella (MMR)

- Administer to any person > 18 years of age born after 1957 with no documented proof of immunity
- One or two doses for patients age 19 to 49 years
- One dose > age 50 if other risk factors present
- Administer subcutaneously (SC)

Varicella

- Two doses at week 0, then week 4 to 8 for patients age 19 to 49
- Same schedule for those > 50 if risk factors present
- Persons with a reliable history of chickenpox are immune.

Hepatitis A

- Two doses at month 0, then 6 to 18 months in those at high risk:
    - Illicit drug users
    - Men who have sex with men
    - Persons with clotting disorders
    - Travelers to high-risk areas

Hepatitis B

- Indicated for all adolescents
- Indicated for high-risk adults:
    - Household contacts and sex partners of patients with hepatitis B
    - Heterosexuals with more than one sex partner in 6 months
    - Healthcare workers
    - Patients recently diagnosed with other sexually transmitted infection
- Given as three-dose series at month 0, 1 to 2, and 4 to 6

Influenza

- All adults 65 years of age and older: one dose annually
- All adults aged 19 to 64 at high risk:
  - Chronic medical disease
  - Working or living with persons at high risk
  - Healthy women who are in second or third trimester of pregnancy
  - All pregnant women with medical disease

Pneumococcal Vaccine

- All adults over age 65, once
- All adults aged 19 to 64 at high risk:
  - All adults with chronic medical disease
  - Asplenic persons
  - Persons on immunosuppressive chemotherapy
  - Routinely given as one-time dose
  - Repeat dose at 5 years in those at greatest risk

RISK ASSESSMENT

Description

Risk assessment is another element of wellness promotion that tailors prevention strategies to patient need. Patient education to promote wellness is most effective if it is appropriate to the patient's risk factors. For example, a leading cause of morbidity and mortality in the young adult population is motor vehicle accidents. A risk assessment of any young adult patient would suggest that motor vehicle accidents are a significant threat to wellness—patient education for this population should therefore include accident prevention. Conversely, an older adult who does not drive is at greater risk of injury from falls in the home. Therefore, a risk assessment of this older patient would suggest that education regarding fall prevention is indicated. The leading causes of death, divided by age group, can be found in Table 16–2.

Table 16–2. Leading Causes of Death by Age Groups

Age	Cause of Death	
15–19 years	Motor vehicle injury Homicide Heart disease	Suicide Cancer
20–24 years	Accidents Suicide Heart disease	Homicides Malignant neoplasms
25–34 years	Accidents Homicide Heart disease	Suicide Malignant neoplasms
35–44 years	Malignant neoplasms Heart disease HIV	Accidents Suicide
45–54 years	Malignant neoplasms Accidents CVA	Heart disease Chronic liver disease and cirrhosis
55–64 years	Malignant neoplasms Chronic lower respiratory diseases Diabetes mellitus	Heart disease Cerebrovascular diseases
65 years and older	Heart disease Cerebrovascular diseases Influenza and pneumonia Alzheimer's disease Nephritis, nephrotic syndrome, nephrosis Septicemia	Malignant neoplasms Chronic lower respiratory diseases Diabetes mellitus Accidents

From *Special Reports From the National Vital Statistics Reports, 1999 data,* by the U.S. Department of Health and Human Services, 2004, retrieved from http://www.cdc.gov/nchs/products/pubs/pubd/nvsr/nvsr.htm

ADDITIONAL RISK ASSESSMENT PRINCIPLES

Individual Patient-Specific Issues

- Risks related to disease processes (e.g. injury secondary to seizure disorder)
- Risks related to transient circumstance (e.g. nutritional risks during prolonged illness)
- Psychosocial risk (e.g. domestic violence)

GENERAL INFLUENCES ON HEALTH CARE AND TREATMENT CONSIDERATIONS

Family

- Consider the adults and children with whom the patient lives.
- Family values, beliefs, and patterns of care will influence health promotion, disease prevention, and general healthcare practices.

Ethnicity

- Patient may identify with a race, tribe, or nation.
- Values, social mores, and common law will influence health practices.

Culture

- Learned or socially inherited beliefs or behaviors
- Has both practical and symbolic components
- Certain practices, foods, medicines, and diseases may carry stigma.

Community

- Community resources may have an impact on health practices.
- Availability of public transportation, safety, and other community factors can affect health practices.

Environment

- Climate, altitude, and temperature can affect health.
- Food and water source contamination may lead to disease.

REFERENCES

Barkley, T. W., & Myers, C. (2008). *Practice guidelines for acute care nurse practitioners.* Philadelphia: W. B. Saunders.

Beers, M., Porter, R., Jones, T., Kaplan, J., & Berkwits, M. (Eds.). (2006). *The Merck manual of diagnosis and therapy.* Whitehouse Station, NJ: Merck Research Laboratories.

Buttaro, T., Trybulski, J., Bailey, P., & Sandberg-Cook, J. (2008). *Primary care* (3rd ed.). St. Louis, MO: Mosby

Fauci, A. S., Braunwalk, E., Kasper, D. L., Hauser, S. L., Longo, D. L., Jameson, J. L., et al. (2008). *Harrison's principles of internal medicine* (17th ed.). Philadelphia: McGraw Hill.

Gomella, L. G., & Haist, S. A. (2006). *Clinician's pocket reference* (11th ed.). New York: McGraw-Hill Medical.

McPhee, S., & Papadakis, M. (2010). *Current medical diagnosis and treatment* (49th ed.). New York: Lange/McGraw Hill.

United States Department of Health and Human Services, National Center for Health Statistics. (2004). *Special reports from the National Vital Statistics Reports.* Retrieved from www.cdc.gov/nchs/products/pubs/pubd/nvsr/nvsr.htm

World Health Organization. (2009). *Milestones in health promotion.* Retrieved from http://www.who.int/healthpromotion/en/

Nutritional Imbalances
Pamela Smith, MSN, RN, ACNP-BC, CCRN

Description

- Nutrients are substances that must be supplied by dietary means because they are not manufactured by the body in adequate amounts
  - Essential nutrient requirements
    - Energy
    - Providing 25 to 35 kcal/kg/day will provide adequate nutrition for most patients.
    - The following equations may be used to calculate individual requirements:
      - Resting energy expenditure (REE)
      - Modified for activity with stable weight in kilograms
        - REE = 900 + 10 (weight) for males
        - REE = 700 + 7 (weight) for females
      - Average energy intake is about 2,800 kcal/day for men.
      - Average energy intake is about 1,800 kcal/day for women *or*
      - Harris-Benedict equation (basal energy expenditure or BEE)
        - Weight in kg, height in centimeters
        - BEE (men) = 66 + (13.7 x wt) + (5 x ht) − (6.8 x age)
        - BEE (women) = 655 + (9.6 x wt) + (1.8 x ht) − (4.7 x age)
        - Adjust for additional stress.
          - Minimally active patients may need 1.25 x the BEE.
          - Severely anabolic patient may need up to 1.75 x the BEE.

- Protein
  - Recommended dietary allowance (RDA) is 0.6 g/kg per day.
    - 10% to 14% of calories from protein per day
- Fat and carbohydrate
  - Average fat intake in the United States is 34%.
  - Saturated and trans-fats should be < 10% of calories.
  - Polyunsaturated fats should be < 10% of calories
  - Monosaturated fats should account for majority of fat calories.
- Water
  - 1.0 to 1.5 ml water per kcal of energy expenditure under usual conditions
- Vitamins and trace minerals
- Most healthcare facilities have a nutrition screening process.
- The Joint Commission requires nutritional screening for identifying malnutrition; however, there are no universally recognized standards.
- Factors assessed
  - Abnormal weight for height or body mass index (BMI)
  - Reported weight change (involuntary loss or gain of > 5 kg in the previous 6 months)
  - Diagnoses with known nutritional implications
  - Current therapeutic diet
  - Chronic poor appetite
  - Presence of chewing and swallowing problems or food intolerances
  - Need for assistance preparing or obtaining food or eating
  - Social isolation
  - Reassessment should occur at least once weekly.
- Protein-energy malnutrition (PEM) is a result of a relative or absolute deficiency.
  - Kwashiorkor
    - Malnutrition from acute illness
  - Marasmus
    - End stage of cachexia
    - All available body fat stores have been exhausted because of starvation.
- Obesity is excess adipose tissue with a BMI > 30.
  - National Institutes of Health defines body weight as follows:
    - Normal BMI: 18.5 to 24.9
    - Overweight BMI: 25 to 29.9
    - Class I obesity BMI: 30 to 34.9
    - Class II obesity BMI: 35 to 39.9
    - Class III obesity BMI: > 40
- Anorexia nervosa is a disturbance of body image and intense fear of becoming fat.
  - Weight loss leading to body weight 15% below expected
- Bulimia nervosa is uncontrolled episodes of binge eating at least twice weekly for 3 months.
  - Recurrent activities to prevent weight gain
    - Self-induced vomiting
    - Laxatives
    - Diuretics
    - Fasting
    - Excessive exercise
- Vitamin deficiencies

Etiology

- Protein-energy malnutrition (PEM)
  - Hypermetabolic acute illness (kwashiorkor)
    - Trauma
    - Burns
    - Sepsis
  - Chronic disease (marasmus)
    - Chronic obstructive pulmonary disease (COPD)
    - Congestive heart failure
    - Cancer
    - HIV or AIDS
- Obesity
  - Sedentary lifestyle
  - Ingestion of excess calories
  - Genetic influences
    - Five genes affecting control of appetite
    - Numerous candidate genes for obesity have been identified
  - Medication-induced
    - Hypoglycemic agents
      - Insulin
      - Sulfonylureas
      - Thiazolidinediones
    - Steroid hormones
    - Psychotropic agents
    - Mood stabilizer
      - Lithium
    - Antidepressants
      - Tricyclics
      - Monoamine oxidase inhibitors
      - Paroxetine
      - Mirtazapine
    - Antiepileptic
      - Valproate
      - Gabapentin
      - Carbamazepine
- Anorexia nervosa (AN)
  - Cause not known
  - Multiple endocrinologic abnormalities exist in these patients.
  - Most experts favor a psychiatric etiology; however, no hypothesis explains all cases
- Bulimia nervosa (BN)
  - More difficult to detect that anorexia
  - Psychiatric disorders
  - Psychological and environmental factors

- Chemical etiologies
  - Abnormalities of serotonin
  - Increased levels of peptides involved in mediating appetite
- Vitamin deficiencies
  - Thiamine (B_1)
    - Chronic alcoholism
    - May be precipitated by use of intravenous dextrose solutions in patients with marginal levels
  - Riboflavin (B_2)
    - Dietary inadequacy
    - Medication-induced
      - Oral contraceptives
      - Tetracycline
      - Tricyclic antidepressants
      - Alcohol
      - Antimalarial drugs
      - Probenicid
    - Alcoholism
    - Protein-energy malnutrition
  - Niacin
    - Alcoholism
    - Medication-induced
      - Isoniazid
      - Phenobarbital
      - Chloramphenicol
      - Pyrazinamide ethionamide
      - 6-mercaptopurine
    - Inborn errors of metabolism
  - Vitamin B_6
    - Medication-induced
      - Isoniazid
      - Cycloserine
      - Oral contraceptives
      - Alcohol
      - Inborn errors of metabolism
  - Vitamin B_{12} and folate
    - Vitamin B_{12} deficiency rare
      - Seen in strict vegetarians
      - Abdominal surgery
        - Gastrectomy
        - Blind loop syndrome
        - Surgical resection of the ileum
      - Fish tapeworm
      - Severe Crohn's disease
      - Medication-induced
        - Antacids
        - Metformin

- Folate deficiency because of inadequate dietary intake
- Medication-induced
  - Phenytoin
  - Trimethroprim-sulfamethoxazole
  - Sulfasalazine
- Vitamin C
  - Dietary inadequacy in the urban poor
  - Advanced age
  - Malignancy
  - Chronic kidney disease
- Vitamin A
  - Fat malabsorption syndromes
  - Mineral oil laxative abuse
  - Elderly
- Vitamin D
  - Postmenopausal women
  - Institutionalized older adults
  - Insufficient sun exposure
  - Malnutrition
  - Medication-induced
    - Phenytoin
    - Carbamazepine
    - Valproate
    - Phenobarbital
  - Malabsorption
    - Pancreatic insufficiency
    - Cholestatic liver disease
    - Sprue
    - Inflammatory bowel disease
    - Jejunoilieal bypass
    - Billroth type II gastrectomy
  - Genetic
    - Defective synthesis
    - Defective receptors for vitamin D
- Vitamin E
  - Severe malabsorption
  - Genetic disorder—abetalipoproteinemia
- Vitamin K
  - Deficient dietary intake of green leafy vegetables, soybeans
  - Malabsorption
  - Decreased production by intestinal bacteria
  - Chemotherapy
  - Antibiotics

Incidence and Demographics

- Protein-energy malnutrition
  - About 20% of hospitalized patients suffer from the preceding syndromes.
  - A greater number of patients have risk factors that predispose them to malnutrition.
- Obesity
  - U.S. data suggest that 65% of Americans are overweight and 30.4% are obese.
  - Women are more commonly obese than men.
  - Black and Mexican-American women are more obese than White women.
  - Individuals with lower socioeconomic status are more obese than higher socioeconomic classes regardless of race.
- Anorexia nervosa
  - The lifetime prevalence in the United States is 0.3% to 1%; some studies have numbers as high as 4%
  - The incidence among men is about 0.1%.
  - About 5% of young women show symptoms of anorexia but do not meet full criteria.
  - Female to male ratio is 10 to 20:1 in developed countries.
  - In some professions, the frequency is higher among men (wrestling, running, modeling).
- Bulimia nervosa
  - The lifetime prevalence among women is 1% to 3% and a like percentage of women have less severe variants of the disorder.
  - The lifetime prevalence among men is 0.1%.
  - Primarily occurs in young women, most commonly adolescents and young adults
  - Median age is 18 years
  - Some studies indicate an equal incidence among Blacks and Whites; however, others show a higher incidence in Whites.
  - Some studies estimate the prevalence may as high as 19% in college-aged women.
- Vitamin deficiencies
  - Thiamine (B_1)
    - No accurate statistics
  - Riboflavin (B_2)
    - Isolated deficiency is rare.
  - Niacin
    - Seen in chronic alcoholism
  - Vitamin B_6
    - Rare deficiency
  - Vitamin B_{12}
    - Vitamin B_{12} deficiency affects < 200,000 persons in the United States
  - Vitamin C
    - 10% of females and 14% of males have a vitamin C deficiency.
    - Incidence peaks in the older adult population and at 6 to 12 months of life
    - Non-Hispanic Black males have a slightly higher incidence than White males.
    - Mexican Americans have a lower incidence.
  - Vitamin A
    - Rarely seen

- Vitamin D
  - 70% to 80% of individuals over age 75 have a vitamin D deficiency.
  - Some studies suggest that 70% of the general population may have a vitamin D deficiency.
- Vitamin E
  - Deficiency is rare.
- Vitamin K
  - Deficiency is rare in healthy adults.
  - Seen in:
    - Liver disease
    - Cystic fibrosis
    - Inflammatory bowel disease
    - Abdominal surgeries
    - Anticoagulation
    - Medication-induced
      - Cathartics
        - Bisacodyl
        - Phenolphthalein

Risk Factors

- Protein-energy malnutrition
  - Underweight: BMI < 18.5
  - Recent weight loss ≥ 10% of usual body weight
  - Poor dentition
  - Malabsorption disorders
  - Diarrhea
  - Draining wounds
  - Enteric fistula
  - Nothing by mouth (NPO) status for more than 5 days
  - Fever
  - Surgery
  - Sepsis
  - Advanced age
  - Immunosuppresants
  - Malignancy
  - Burns
  - COPD
  - Congestive heart failure
  - AIDS or HIV
  - Social Isolation
- Obesity
  - Low socioeconomic status
  - Sedentary life style
  - High calorie intake
  - Hypothyroidism

- Cushing's syndrome
- Hypothalmic disease
- Drug-induced weight gain
- Depression
- Anorexia nervosa
  - Highly goal- and achievement-oriented
  - Inadequate interpersonal relationships
  - Depression
  - Anxiety
  - Parents who are concerned with slimness and physical fitness
  - Genetic factors
- Bulimia nervosa
  - Same as anorexia nervosa
- Vitamin deficiencies
  - Alcoholism
  - Inadequate dietary intake
  - Genetic predisposition
  - Advanced age
  - Institutionalized individuals
  - Interaction with medications
  - Smoking
  - Chronic illness

Prevention and Screening

- Nutritional screening in the hospitalized patient
- High index of suspicion in patients with risk factors
- Counseling for suspected eating disorders
- Awareness of medication-induced vitamin deficiencies
- Close follow-up in patients with GI surgeries that affect absorption

Assessment

History
- Protein-energy malnutrition
  - Weight loss
  - History of acute illness, recent trauma, burns, sepsis
  - History of chronic illness
  - Barriers to obtaining nutrition, eating or preparing foods
  - Social situation
- Obesity
  - Age at onset of obesity
  - Family history

- Occupational history
- Eating and exercise behavior
- Cigarette and alcohol use
- Previous weight loss experience
- Assess for depression and eating disorders
- Screen for metabolic disorder
- Is patient motivated to lose weight?
- Evaluate patient's goals for weight loss
- What assistance does the patient need?
- Anorexia
  - Low body weight
  - History of being overachiever
  - Overbearing parents
  - Inadequate interpersonal relationships
  - Low self-esteem
  - Unwillingness to eat
  - Depression
  - Loss of control over body
  - Cold intolerance
  - Constipation
  - Amenorrhea
- Bulimia
  - Obtain dietary history
  - Number and frequency of binge eating episodes
  - Vomiting
  - Use of cathartics
  - Diuretic use
  - Feelings of depression or guilt
  - Intervals of self-imposed starvation
  - Fluctuating body weight
  - Menstruation usually preserved, but amenorrhea may be present
  - Constipation
- Vitamin deficiencies or toxicity
  - Diet history
  - Medication history
  - Availability of food
  - Knowledge of nutrition
  - Social isolation
  - Thiamine (B_1)
    - Paresthesia
    - Irritability
  - Riboflavin (B_2)
    - Weakness
    - Sensitivity to light
    - Tearing, burning of eyes

- Niacin
  - Anorexia
  - Weakness
  - Irritability
  - Mouth soreness
  - Toxicity
    - Gastric irritation
- Vitamin B_6
  - Mouth soreness
  - Weakness
  - Irritability
  - Severe deficiency
    - Peripheral neuropathy
  - Toxicity
    - Sensory neuropathy
- Vitamin B_{12}
  - Anorexia
  - Paresthesias
  - Difficulty with balance
  - Dementia
- Vitamin C
  - Early
    - Malaise
    - Weakness
  - Toxicity
    - Gastric irritation
    - Flatulence
- Vitamin A
  - Night blindness
- Vitamin D
  - Bone pain
  - Muscle weakness
- Vitamin E
  - Gait disturbances
- Vitamin K
  - Easy bruising

Physical Examination
- Protein-energy malnutrition
  - Marasmus
    - Progressive wasting with weight loss
    - Muscle wasting most severe in the temporalis and interosseous muscles
    - Severe cachexia

- Kwashiorkor
  - More rapid onset than marasmus
  - Malnutrition with normal subcutaneous fat and muscle mass; if patient is obese, excess fat and muscle mass
  - Dependent edema
  - Ascites
  - Anasarca
- Combinations of marasmus and kwashiorkor-like syndromes may occur simultaneously when an acute illness is superimposed on a progressively chronic illness.
- Obesity
  - Hypertension
  - Tachycardia
  - Degenerative joint disease
  - Excess abdominal fat—measurement of waist circumference (higher risk for cardiovascular disease)
  - May have excess fat, muscle mass, or both
  - Elevated BMI (see p. 664)
- Anorexia nervosa
  - Loss of body fat
  - Dry, scaly skin
  - Increased lanugo (body hair)
  - Parotid enlargement
  - Edema
  - Severe cases
    - Severe emaciation
    - Bradycardia
    - Hypotension
    - Hypothermia
- Bulimia nervosa
  - May have weight loss if combined with anorexia
  - May have premorbid obesity
  - Gastric dilatation
  - Poor dentition
  - Pharyngitis
  - Esophagitis
  - Aspiration
  - Electrolyte abnormalities
  - Hemorrhoids
  - Dehydration
- Vitamin deficiencies or toxicity
  - Thiamine (B_1)
    - Anorexia
    - Muscle cramps
    - Advanced deficiency
      - Wet beriberi
        - Cardiovascular system
          - Peripheral vasodilation

- High output heart failure
- Dyspnea
- Tachycardia
- Cardiomegaly
- Pulmonary edema
- Peripheral edema
- Warm extremities—may look like cellulitis
- Dry beriberi
  - Nervous system
    - Peripheral nervous system
      - Symmetric motor and sensory neuropathy
      - Pain
      - Paresthesias
      - Loss of reflexes
      - Legs affected more than arms
    - Central nervous system
      - Wernicke-Karskoff syndrome
      - Wernicke's encephalopathy
        - Nystagmus
        - Ophthalmoplegia
        - Truncal ataxia
        - Confusion
      - Korsakoff's syndrome
        - Amnesia
        - Confabulation
        - Impaired learning
- Riboflavin (B_2)
  - Dry, cracked corners of the mouth
  - Stomatitis
  - Glossitis
  - Seborrheic dermatitis
  - Weakness
  - Corneal vascularization
  - Anemia
- Niacin
  - Glossitis
  - Stomatitis
  - Weight loss
  - Advanced deficiency
    - Classic triad of pellagra—advanced pellagra may lead to death
      - Dermatitis
        - Symmetric
        - Involves sun-exposed areas
        - Skin lesions are dark, dry, scaly
    - Diarrhea
      - May be severe
      - May lead to malabsorption because of atrophy of intestinal villi

- Dementia
  - Begins with insomnia, irritability, apathy
  - Progresses to confusion, memory loss, hallucinations, and psychosis
- Toxicity
  - Cutaneous flushing
  - Elevated liver enzymes
  - Hyperglycemia
  - Gout
- Vitamin B_6
  - Glossitis
  - Cheilosis
  - Severe deficiency
    - Anemia
    - Seizures
- Vitamin B_{12} and folate
  - Vitamin B_{12}
    - Megaloblastic anemia
    - In advanced cases, hematocrit may be as low as 10% to 15%
    - Leukopenia
    - Thrombocytopenia
    - Glossitis
    - Diarrhea
    - Usually pale
    - Mildly icteric
    - Decreased vibration and position sense (early stages)
  - Folate
    - Similar to vitamin B_{12} deficiency
    - None of the neurological abnormalities seen with vitamin B_{12} deficiency
- Vitamin C
  - Early
    - Malaise
    - Weakness
  - Advanced stages—signs of scurvy
    - Perifollicular hemorrhages
    - Perifollicular hyperkeratotic papules
    - Petechiae
    - Purpura
    - Splinter hemorrhages
    - Bleeding gums
    - Hemarthroses
    - Subperiosteal hemorrhages
    - Anemia
    - Impaired wound healing

- Late stages
  - Edema
  - Oliguria
  - Neuropathy
  - Intracerebral hemorrhage
  - Death
- Toxicity
  - Diarrhea
  - Oxalate kidney stones
  - False negative for fecal occult blood
  - False-negative or false-positive tests for urine glucose

- Vitamin A
  - Dryness of the conjunctiva
  - Bitot's spots—small white patches on the conjunctiva
  - Ulceration and necrosis of the cornea
  - Late signs
    - Endophthalmitis
    - Blindness
    - Dry skin
    - Hypekeratinization of the skin
    - Loss of taste
  - Toxicity
    - Excess intake of β-carotenes
      - Yellow-orange skin
      - Sclera remain white
    - Excessive vitamin A
      - Dry, scaly skin
      - Hair loss
      - Mouth sores
      - Anorexia
      - Vomiting
      - Excessive bone growth
      - Hypocalcemia
      - Increased intracranial pressure
      - Papilledema
      - Headaches
      - Decreased cognition
      - Hepatomegaly—may lead to cirrhosis
    - Acute toxicity
      - Overdose
      - Consumption of polar bear liver
        - Nausea
        - Vomiting
        - Abdominal pain
        - Headache
        - Papilledema
        - Lethargy

- Vitamin D
  - Osteomalacia
  - Pathological fractures with little or no trauma
  - Toxicity
    - Constipation
    - Anorexia
    - Dehydration
    - Fatigue
    - Irritability
    - Muscle weakness
- Vitamin E
  - Areflexia
  - Disturbances of gait
  - Decreased proprioception and vibration
  - Ophthalmoplegia
  - Toxicity
    - Least toxic of fat-soluble vitamins
    - Nausea
    - Flatulence
    - Diarrhea
    - Can increase the requirement for vitamin K and result in bleeding in patients taking oral anticoagulants
- Vitamin K
  - Prolonged prothrombin time
  - Toxicity
    - Thrombosis

Diagnostic Studies
- PEM, AN, BN
  - Obtain BMI
  - Serum albumin (3.5 to 5.5 g/dL)
    - 2.8 to 3.5: compromised status
    - < 2.8: possible kwashiorkor
    - Increasing value indicates positive protein balance
  - Serum prealbumin (20 to 40 mg/dL)
    - 10 to 15 mg/dL: mild protein depletion
    - 5 to 10 mg/dL: moderate protein depletion
    - < 5 mg/dL: severe protein depletion
    - Increasing value indicates positive protein balance
  - Serum total iron binding capacity (240—450 μg/dL)
    - < 200: compromised protein status, possible kwashiorkor
    - More labile than albumin
    - Increasing value indicates positive protein balance
  - Prothrombin time (12.0—15.5 seconds)
    - Prolonged: vitamin K deficiency

- Serum creatinine (0.6 to 1.6 mg/dl)
  - < 0.6: muscle wasting because of prolonged energy deficiency
  - Reflects muscle mass
- 24-hr urinary creatinine (500 to 1,200 mg/d—standardized for height and sex)
  - Low value: muscle wasting because of prolonged energy deficiency
- 24-hr urinary urea nitrogen—UUN (< 5 g/d—depends on protein intake)
  - Determines level of catabolism
    - 5 to 10 g/d: mild catabolism or normal fed state
    - 10 to 15 g/d: moderate catabolism
    - > 15 g/d: severe catabolism
    - Estimate protein balance
      - Protein balance = protein intake − protein loss
      - Protein loss is protein catabolic rate
      - [24-hr UUN (g) + 4] × 6.25
- Blood urea nitrogen: BUN (8 to 23 mg/dl)
  - < 8: possibly inadequate protein intake
  - 12 to 23: probable adequate protein intake
  - > 23: may be excessive protein intake
  - If serum creatinine is normal, use BUN.
  - If serum creatinine is elevated, use BUN/creatinine ratio.
    - Range same as BUN
- Lymphocyte count
  - Decreased levels-depressed immune function and increased susceptibility to infection
- AN
  - Cholesterol levels may be elevated.
  - Depressed levels of luteinizing and follicle-stimulating hormones
  - Impaired response of luteinizing hormone to luteinizing hormone-releasing hormone
- Obesity
  - Obtain BMI
  - Thyroid panel
  - Dexamethasone suppression testing
  - Serum chemistry panel
    - Elevated glucose
  - Lipid panel
  - Assess PEM, AN, and BN
- Vitamin deficiencies
  - Thiamine (B_1)
    - Erythrocyte transketolase activity
    - A transketolase activity coefficient > 15% to 20% may indicate a thiamine deficiency.
  - Riboflavin (B_2)
    - Riboflavin-dependent enzyme–erythrocyte glutathione
    - Activity coefficients > 1.2 to 1.3 suggestive of riboflavin deficiency
    - Urinary riboflavin excretion and serum levels of plasma and red cell flavins may also be measured.
  - Niacin
    - Urine
      - Niacin metabolites

- *N*-methylnicotinamide
    - Serum and red cell levels of coenzymes nicotinamide adenine dinucleotide and nicotinamide adenine dinucleotide phosphate
- Vitamin B_6
    - Serum pyridoxal phosphate
    - Normal levels are > 50 ng/mL
- Vitamin B_{12}
    - CBC
        - Megaloblastic anemia
            - Elevated mean corpuscular volume (MCV)
                - 110 to 140 fL
            - Occasionally may have normal MCV
        - Leukopenia
        - Thrombocytopenia
        - Pancytopenia
    - Peripheral blood smear
        - Anisocytosis
        - Poikilocytosis
        - Macro-ovalocyte
        - Neutrophils are hypersegmented
    - Bone marrow biopsy
        - Marked erythroid hyperplasia
        - Abnormally large cell size
        - Asynchronous maturation of the nucleus and cytoplasm
    - Liver function studies
        - Elevated serum LDH
        - Slight increase in direct bilirubin
    - Serum cobalamin level
        - Low level indicative of deficiency
        - Normal level > 240 pg/mL
        - A level of 170 to 240 pg/mL is borderline.
        - Low level < 170 pg/mL
        - Symptomatic < 100 pg/mL
        - When B_{12} level is borderline
            - Confirm with elevated level of serum methylmalonic acid > 1,000 nmol/L
- Folate
    - CBC
        - Megaloblastic anemia
- Vitamin C
    - Decreased plasma levels of ascorbic acid < 0.1 mg/dL
    - Diagnosis usually made clinically
- Vitamin A
    - Serum levels < 30 to 65 mg/dL are common with advanced deficiency
- Vitamin D.
    - Serum 25 OH vitamin D < 25 nmol/L

- Vitamin E
  · Serum vitamin E levels < 0.5–0.7 mg/dL
  · Vitamin E is transported by lipoproteins; therefore, the level should be interpreted in relation to the serum lipid levels.
- Vitamin K
  · Prolonged prothrombin time
  · Individual clotting factors low
    - Factors II, VII, IX, X
  · A low factor V activity level is not indicative of isolated vitamin K deficiency and may indicate a underlying defect in liver synthesis function.

Differential Diagnosis

- PEM
  - Any vitamin or trace mineral deficiency
- AN or BN
  - Primary psychiatric disorder
  - Schizophrenia
  - Primary depression
- Obesity
  - Diabetes type 2 or insulin resistance
  - Hypothyroidism
  - Cushing's syndrome
  - Pituitary or hypothalamic lesions
  - Klinefelter's syndrome
- Vitamin deficiencies
  - Thiamine (B_1)
    · Alcoholic fatty liver
    · Alcoholic hepatitis
    · Anemia
    · Folic acid deficiency
    · Uremic encephalopathy
    · Irritable bowel syndrome
  - Riboflavin (B_2)
    · Pyridoxine deficiency
  - Niacin
    · Atopic dermatitis
    · Crohn's disease
    · Drug-induced photosensitivity
    · Lupus erythemotosus—acute, discoid, drug-induced, subacute cutaneous
    · Ulcerative colitis
  - Vitamin (B_6)
    · Pellegra
    · Anemia
    · Malnutrition
    · Homocystinuria

- Vitamin B_{12}
  - Leukemia
  - Folate deficiency
  - Lyme disease
  - Pregnancy
  - Iron deficiency anemia
- Folate
  - Pernicious anemia
- Vitamin C
  - Blood cancers
  - Clotting abnormalities
  - Septic arthritis
  - Ulcerative gingivitis
- Vitamin A
  - Hypothyroidism
- Vitamin D
  - Malabsorptive disorders
    - Celiac sprue
    - Short bowel syndrome
    - Cystic fibrosis
  - End-stage liver disease
- Vitamin E
  - Biliary disease
  - Short bowel syndrome
- Vitamin K
  - Leukemia
    - Acute lymphoblastic
    - Acute myelogenous
    - Chronic myelogenous
    - Chronic lymphocytic
  - DIC
  - von Willebrand's disease
  - Scurvy
  - Thrombotic thrombocytopenia purpura

Management

Nonpharmacologic Treatment
- Nutrition evaluation every 7 days
- Nutrition care plan and patient education
- Maintain hydration
- Daily weights
- Meticulous skin care
- Counseling and behavior modification for selected eating disorders
  - Psychiatry
- Social work consult to evaluate for home safety
- Home health care as needed

- Placement of feeding tube for enteral nutrition as needed
  - Placement confirmed with radiography before use
- Placement of central venous catheter for total parenteral nutrition (TPN) as needed
- Selecting candidates for nutritional support
  - Those unable to eat for long periods of time because of endotracheal intubation or GI tract interruption
  - Patients with high caloric requirements
    - Burns
    - Severe sepsis
    - Major surgery
    - Trauma
  - Patients who sustain high protein losses
    - Corticosteroid or tetracycline use
    - Nephrotic syndrome
    - Draining fistulas
- Enteral feedings
  - Via feeding tube
    - Gastric or postpyloric placement (if at risk for aspiration)
    - Gastric
      - End of tube in the stomach
      - Most similar to route of normal digestion
    - Postpyloric
      - Nasoduodenal
        - End of tube is in the duodenum
        - Acid reflux or aspiration less common
    - Nasojejunal
      - End of tube is in the jejunum
      - Formula type dependent on placement of the tube
    - Surgically placed tube
      - Used when long-term feeding is expected (> 2 to 3 weeks)
      - Percutaneous endoscopic gastrostomy tube
      - Percutaneous jejunostomy tube
      - Complications
        - Perforation
        - Hemorrhage
        - Wound infection
        - Bowel obstruction
        - Bowel necrosis
        - Stomal leakage
  - Preferred to parenteral route
  - GI tract must be functional
    - Begin feedings when residuals are < 100 mL/24 hours
  - Less expensive
  - Deters GI ulceration
  - Preserves small bowel mucosal integrity and function better than parenteral feedings
  - Start with freshly placed tube
  - Continuous feedings are preferable to bolus feedings because they constantly buffer

gastric acid, reduce aspiration risk, produce less bloating, and generate smaller residuals
- Contraindicated in diffuse peritonitis, intestinal obstruction, intractable vomiting, paralytic ileus, intractable diarrhea, gastrointenstinal ischemia
- Bowel sounds and passage of flatus are unreliable predictors for the tolerance of enteral feedings
- Formula selection
  - Polymeric: carbohydrates, fats, proteins in complex, undigested forms
    - Isotonic
    - Lactose-free
    - Available in ready-to-use form
    - Potential for diarrhea low
    - Are most commonly used
  - Elemental: carbohydrate in the form of dextrose or oligosaccharides, protein as crystalline amino acids or short peptides, fats as medium-chain trigylcerides or essential fatty acids
  - Use with patients who have not had enteral nourishment for an extended period of time, have pathology that limits the ability to digest the macronutrient of polymeric formulas, or both
  - May exacerbate diarrhea
- Feeding intolerance is continually assessed until the rate has been advanced to goal
- Patients fed into the small bowel should have an isotonic solution.
- The formula should be started at 25 to 50 mL/hr via an infusion pump
- Head of bed at > 30°
- Intolerance is manifested by emesis, diarrhea, abdominal bloating, high gastric residual ≥ 150 to 200 mL
- Bolus feeding via gastric tube
  - 250 to 500 mL via gravity over 20 to 60 minutes
- Most frequent complication is diarrhea
  - Treated by reducing flow rate, or using a different volume or type of formula
- Other complications include aspiration, esophagitis, emesis, inadequate gastric emptying, hypernatremic dehydration

- TPN
  - TPN alone is indicated in severe gut dysfunction from prolonged ileus, obstruction, or severe hemorraghic pancreatitis
    - Peripheral
      - Lower osmolality for infusion via a peripheral vein
      - Infusions limited to 10 to 14 days to avoid osmolality-related phlebitis
      - Not acceptable for malnourished patients requiring prolonged support, because fewer calories are delivered
    - Central
      - Requires central venous access
      - Placement must be verified by radiography
      - Peripherally inserted central catheter (PICC) most appropriate in the hospitalized patient
      - Catheters inserted in the femoral vein are associated with a higher risk of infection

- For long-term therapy in nonhospital setting, subcutaneously tunneled catheters are used most often.
- Complication of catheter-related sepsis should be treated with catheter removal and antibiotic coverage.
- The TPN prescription is determined by the nutritional assessment.
  - The basic solution is composed of dextrose, amino acids, and water
  - Electrolytes, minerals, trace elements, vitamins, and medications may also be added.
    - Most commercial solutions contain the monohydrate form of glucose that provides 3.4 kcal/g
    - Crystalline amino acids are available in a variety of concentrations, so a broad range of solutions can be made with specific glucose and amino acids to meet individual needs.
    - Typical concentrations for central vein infusion contain 25% to 35% dextrose and 2.75% to 6% amino acids.
      - Osmolality is often in excess of 1,800 mosm/L.
    - Solutions for peripheral infusion contain 5% to 10% dextrose and 2.75% to 4.25% amino acids.
      - Osmolality is between 800 and 1,200 mosm/L.
- Complications of parental nutrition
  - Occur in up to 50% of patients
  - Catheter-related
    - During insertion
      - Pneumothorax
      - Hemothorax
      - Arterial laceration
      - Air embolism
      - Brachial plexus injury
    - While catheter in place
      - Thrombosis
      - Sepsis
  - Metabolic
    - Hyperglycemia
      - Rapid infusion of glucose
      - Stress
      - Corticosteroids
    - Hyperchloremic metabolic acidosis
      - High chloride administration
    - Azotemia
      - Excessive protein administration
    - Hyperosmolar nonketotic dehydration
      - Severe, undetected hyperglycemia
    - Hyperphosphatemia
      - Extracellular to intracellular shifting with refeeding
    - Hypokalemia
      - Same as hyperphosphatemia
    - Hypomagnesemia
      - Same as hyperphosphatemia
    - Liver enzyme abnormalities
      - Lipid trapping in hepatocytes, fatty liver

- Acalculous cholecystitis
  - Biliary stasis
- Zinc deficiency
  - Diarrhea
  - Small bowel fistulas
- Copper deficiency
  - Biliary fistulas
- Types of therapeutic diets
  - Diets that alter consistency
    - Clear liquid
      - Adequate water
      - 500 to 1,000 kcal as simple sugar
      - Some electrolytes
      - Resolving postoperative ileus, acute gastroenteritis, partial intestinal obstruction, preparation for diagnostic gastrointestinal procedures
      - May be initial diet for those that have been NPO for a period of time
    - Full liquid
      - Adequate water, calories, protein
      - Vitamins and minerals should be supplemented
      - Dairy products, soups, eggs, soft cereals
      - Low in residue
      - Used in patients who have difficulty chewing or swallowing, partial obstructions, or preparation for some diagnostic procedures
      - Used after clear liquid diet to advance feedings
    - Soft
      - Used for patients who have difficulty chewing or swallowing
      - Tender foods—usually no raw fruits or vegetables, coarse breads, or cereals
      - Use to progress from full liquid diets
      - Can be designed to meet nutritional needs
  - Diets that restrict or modify nutrients
    - Sodium-restricted
    - Fat-restricted
    - Protein-restricted
    - Carbohydrate-restricted
  - Diets that supplement dietary components
    - High fiber
    - High potassium
    - High calcium
- Bariatric surgery for obesity
  - Roux-en-Y gastric bypass most used
    - May be done laparoscopically
    - Weight loss up to 50% of initial body weight
    - Complications occur in up to 40% of patients.
      - Anastomotic leak or peritonitis
      - Abdominal wall hernias
      - Staple line disruption
      - Gallstones
      - Neuropathy
      - Marginal ulcers

- Stomal stenosis
- Wound infections
- Thromboembolic disease
- GI symptoms
- Nutritional deficiencies
  - Iron
  - Vitamin B_{12}
  - Folate
  - Calcium
  - Vitamin D
- Mortality rates within 30 days are 0% to 1% in low-risk populations.
- Medicare mortality rates are higher: 1-year mortality is as high as 7.5%.
- Gastric banding
  - Less dramatic weight loss
  - Fewer short-term complications
  - Frequent follow-up to adjust the band
  - Long-term follow-up suggests both procedures are associated with significant regaining of weight
  - Surgery is recommended for patients with BMI > 40 or > 35 when obesity-related comorbidities exist.
  - Associated with a significant reduction in deaths at 11-year follow-up

Pharmacologic Treatment
- AN and BN
  - Tricyclic antidepressants
  - Selective serotonin uptake inhibitors (SSRI)
  - Lithium
- Obesity
  - Sibutramine
    - 10 mg orally/day
    - Average weight loss of 3 to 5 kg more than placebo studies over 6 to 12 months
  - Orlistat
    - 120 mg orally three times daily with meals
- Vitamin deficiencies
  - Thiamine (B_1)
    - Thiamine 50 to 100 mg/day IV for 2 to 3 days, then daily oral doses of 5 to 10 mg/day
    - Patients should also be supplemented with therapeutic doses of water-soluble vitamins
- Riboflavin (B_2)
  - 5 to 10 mg/day of riboflavin until clinical findings resolved
- Niacin
  - Oral niacin as nicotinamide 10 to 150 mg/day
- Vitamin B_6
  - Vitamin B_6 10 to 20 mg/day, but if patient taking medications that interferes with vitamin B_6 metabolism, doses of up to 100 mg/day may be required

- Vitamin B_{12}
  - IM injections of 100 mcg daily for the first week, weekly for the first month, then monthly for life
  - Oral cobalamin can provide equivalent results: 100 to 250 mcg/day and continued indefinitely
- Folate
  - Folic acid 1 mg/day
- Vitamin C
  - Scurvy treated with 300 to 1,000 mg of ascorbic acid per day
- Vitamin A
  - Night blindness: 30,000 international units (IU) of vitamin A for 1 week
  - Advanced deficiency: 20,000/kg IU for at least 5 days
- Vitamin D
  - Inadequate sun exposure, aging, pregnant, or lactating
    - 800 to 1,000 IU vitamin D_3 per day *or*
    - 50,000 IU vitamin D_3 per day per month
  - Malabsorption
    - 50,000 IU vitamin D_2 every week
  - Drugs that increase the metabolism of activated vitamin D
    - 50,000 IU vitamin D_2 every 1, 2, or 4 weeks
- Vitamin E
  - Vitamin E 100 to 400 IU/day
  - Optimum therapeutic dose has not been identified
- Vitamin K
  - IV: 1 mg/day, administer over 30 minutes
  - Oral: 5 to 10 mg per day
  - Monitor protime levels

Special Considerations

- Malnutrition is commonly associated with increased complications, length of stay, and healthcare costs.
- In hospitalized patients, it may be the first time their nutrition status has been evaluated.
- A previously healthy patient who is admitted to the hospital and is anticipated to fast for 1 to 2 days does not need nutritional support, but if inadequate nutrition lasts for weeks, weight loss will occur.
- Both overfeeding and underfeeding have complications; therefore, the patient's caloric requirements should be calculated.
- The obese patient may be malnourished.
- Treatment of AN and BN should include the assistance of a psychiatrist or psychologist.

When to Consult, Refer, or Hospitalize

- Adolescents and young adults with otherwise unexplained weight loss should be evaluated by a psychiatrist.
- All patients diagnosed with AN or BN should be comanaged with psychiatry.
- Patients with BMI > 40 should be referred to a bariatric specialist for weight loss surgery.
- Dietary consultation for inpatients
- General surgery or interventional radiology consult for catheter or tube placement for nutritional support
- Endocrinology consult for secondary causes of obesity

Follow-up

Expected Outcomes
- PEM
- Obesity
- AN or BN
- Vitamin deficiencies

Complications
- PEM
  - Multi-organ system failure if not reversed with adequate nutrition
- Obesity
  - Hypertension
  - Diabetes type 2
  - Hyperlipidemia
  - Malignancy
  - Sleep apnea
  - Proteinuria
  - Increased hemoglobin concentration
  - In young and middle-aged adults, mortality from all causes and from cardiovascular disease increases in the obese. After age 75, weight is no longer a risk factor.
- AN or BN
  - Electrolyte abnormalities
  - Amenorrhea
  - Depression or anxiety
  - Multi-organ system failure in advanced cases
- Vitamin deficiencies
  - See Physical examination section

REFERENCES

Bakerman, S. (2002). *ABC's of interpretive laboratory data.* Phoenix: Interpretive Laboratory Data.

Beers, M., Porter, R., Jones, T., Kaplan, J., & Berkwits, M. (Eds.). (2006). *The Merck manual of diagnosis and therapy.* Whitehouse Station, NJ: Merck Research Laboratories.

Cooper, D., Kraink, A., Lubner, S., & Reno, H. (Eds.). (2007). *The Washington manual of medical therapeutics* (32nd ed.). Philadelphia: Wolters Kluwer/Lippincott Williams & Wilkins.

Fauci, A., Braunwald, E., Kasper, D., Hauser, S., Longo, D., Jameson, J., & Loscalzo, J. (Eds.). (2009). *Harrison's principles of internal medicine.* New York: McGraw Hill.

Lopes, A., & Lopes, G. (2009). Reducing serum phosphorus concentrations in patients with end-stage renal disease. *JAMA, 301*(23), 2443–2444.

Schwarz, S., & Freemark, M. (2010). *Obesity.* Retrieved from http://emedicine.medscape.com/article/985333-overview.

Wells, B., DiPiro, J., Schwinghammer, T., & DiPiro, C. (Eds.). (2009). *Pharmacotherapy handbook.* New York: McGraw Hill.

Zempleni, J., Rucker, R. B., McCormick, D. B., & Suttie, J. W. (Eds.). (2007). *Handbook of vitamins* (4th ed.). Boca Raton: CRC Press.

Transplants

Melanie Smith, MSN, ACNP-BC

LIVER TRANSPLANTATION

Description

- Liver transplantation is the surgical procedure to remove a diseased or failing liver, and replace it with a healthy liver or portion of a liver from a donor.

Etiology

- Transplantation is a potential treatment option for any acute or chronic condition resulting in liver failure.
- In the United States, the leading chronic causes of end-stage liver disease are hepatitis C cirrhosis, followed by alcoholic cirrhosis. While there are over 100 types of liver disease, hepatitis C accounts for 40% of chronic liver disease cases.
- Drug-induced liver injury (DILI) is the leading cause of acute liver failure. The most common cause of DILI is acetaminophen overdose.
- Biliary atresia is the leading cause of liver failure in infants and children.

Incidence and Demographics

- The liver is the second most frequently transplanted organ, after kidneys. There is a wide variation in causes of end-stage liver disease among the liver transplant population after hepatitis C cirrhosis and alcoholic cirrhosis: cholestatic disease, hepatocellular carcinoma, Wilson's disease, and genetic disorders such as Crigler-Najjar syndrome and hemochromatosis are common indications for transplant referral.
- According to the United Network for Organ Sharing (UNOS), the private nonprofit organization that manages United States organ donation, about 6,000 liver transplants are performed yearly in the United States, with 16,000 patients on the waiting list. Currently, the average wait for a liver transplant is about 2 years.
- The Model for End-Stage Liver Disease (MELD) is a scoring system used by UNOS to assess the severity of liver disease. The MELD score uses data such as the patient's serum bilirubin, creatinine, and international normalized ratio (INR) to help to predict the probability of death within 3 months without a transplant, and helps prioritize the listing for liver transplantation.
- Hepatitis C is prevalent among drug addicts, war veterans, and the prison population; while the highest prevalence of hepatitis C is among Black men age 30–50; demographically, they also have the highest incidence of poverty, military service, and incarceration.
- Alcoholic cirrhosis develops in 10% to 20% of individuals who drink heavily for 10 years or more.

Risk Factors

- Hepatitis C
  - Blood transfusions or organ transplants before 1992
  - Illegal drug use
  - Long-term hemodialysis.
  - Clotting factor before 1987
  - Sharing personal products with infected people
  - Peripartum
  - Sexual activity
  - Tattooing or body piercing
- Alcoholic cirrhosis
  - Daily alcohol ingestion of 40 g for men, or 20 g for women over 15–20 years' time
  - Protein or calorie malnutrition
  - Concomitant infection with hepatitis B or C virus
- Biliary artesia
  - No clear etiology or risk factors, although infectious and toxic agents are felt to play a role in its development.

Prevention and Screening

- Once hepatitis C or alcoholic cirrhosis develops, the goals of management are to prevent progression to end-stage liver disease or hepatocellular cancer. Guidelines include:
  - Abstaining from alcohol
  - Vitamin and mineral supplementation

- Choosing pain relievers that do not include aspirin
- Hepatitis A and B vaccinations
- Reduced sodium intake
- Medications depend on the condition, but can include: beta blockers, diuretics, antivirals, and corticosteroids.
- Liver transplants are considered when all other surgical and treatment options have been exhausted.
- Candidates are felt to have the best outcome after liver transplantation when:
  - Transplant is **not** performed prior to development of advanced liver disease
  - Hepatocellular cancer (HCC) has not yet developed
  - Timing of referral is based on a MELD score of 15 or above with:
    - Evidence of decompensation
    - Muscle wasting
    - Ascites
    - Encephalopathy
    - Variceal bleeding

Assessment

- Potential transplant candidates are referred by their primary care physician to a hepatologist or transplant center for evaluation. The transplant team then determines what studies should be done prior to listing a patient for transplant and coordinates testing.
- Evaluation includes:
  - Psychiatry or social work evaluation, nutritional counseling, financial evaluation, and a comprehensive medical assessment
  - Blood and tissue typing
  - Transplant candidates over the age of 50 with risk factors for coronary disease, or those with a history of cardiac disease, undergo cardiology consultation with appropriate cardiac studies, often including stress thallium, cardiac catheterization, or both.
  - Cancer screening, including Pap smear and mammogram for women, prostate exam and PSA level for men; fecal occult blood testing, and flexible sigmoidoscopy depending upon age and gender
  - All patients undergo evaluation for identifiable malignancy outside of the liver, including chest CT scan, abdominal and pelvic CT scan, and bone scan. The abdominal cavity is explored carefully at the time of transplantation before proceeding with the hepatectomy and transplantation.
  - Patients with hepatocellular carcinoma undergo an even more exhaustive analysis and sometimes receive adjunctive therapy. In order to improve upon their outcome after transplant, they may undergo adjuvant therapy in the form of chemo-embolization or chemotherapy to control the spread of cancer cells or unrecognized micrometastases.
- Once the pretransplant evaluation is complete, the case is referred to the multidisciplinary selection committee for consideration. Consensus must then be reached to:
  - Accept the patient for transplantation and place him or her on the donor waiting list
  - Accept the patient pending resolution of minor issues
  - Not accept the patient, but recommend reevaluation at a later date
  - Categorically not accept the patient
- Failure to reach consensus in complicated patient scenarios may prompt referral to an ethics committee.

- When it has been determined that transplant is an acceptable treatment option, the patient is listed nationally on the UNOS liver transplant list with ranking prioritized to MELD score and clinical signs and symptoms.
- The transplanted liver may come from a living or deceased donor.
  - Orthotopic transplant entails replacement of the recipient liver with a donor liver; surgery involves multiple surgeons and OR staff and can take up to 4–18 hours to complete.
  - Almost all transplants are done this way.
  - Heterotopic transplantation is considered in cases where the recipient may be too sick to tolerate orthotropic transplant; the native liver is left in place and the donor liver is sewn into an ectopic site; surgery invovles much shorter OR time and fewer anastamoses.
  - In living donor liver transplantation, a piece of liver is removed from a living donor and transplanted into a recipient, often a parent to a child. Surgically, this is the most technically demanding. The procedure is possible because of the regenerative properties of the liver. Despite removal of up to 70% of a healthy liver from a living donor, 100% regeneration is possible within 6 weeks of donation.
- Absolute and relative contraindications to transplantation:
  - Malignancy
  - Active infection
  - Active drug, tobacco, or illicit substance use
  - Inability to comply with medical regimen
  - Acquired immune deficiency syndrome
  - HIV (relative contraindication)
  - Morbid obesity (relative contraindication)

Management

Nonpharmacologic Treatment
- Liver transplantation is major abdominal surgery. General postoperative care of the liver transplant patient entails similar management principles. Monitoring for bleeding, adequate renal perfusion, and stable neurologic function are immediate and ongoing postoperative concerns. Pain control and mobilization are optimized. Complications specific to the liver transplant patient in the immediate postop period include:
  - Right pleural effusion (may affect ventilation necessitating drainage)
  - Hepatic edema secondary to aggressive resuscitation and increased intravascular volume (goal central venous pressure 6–10)
  - Renal failure (secondary to acute tubular necrosis; usually self-limiting)
  - Electrolyte shifts
  - Thrombocytopenia (may respond well to DDAVP)

Pharmacologic Treatment
- Viral, fungal and bacterial infections are common in the transplant patient. Long-term or lifelong prophylaxis therapy includes antivirals such as ganciclovir and antifungals such as oral fluconazole. Bacterial infections are treated based on causative organism. Intra-abdominal infections are seen in liver transplant recipients.

- Immunosuppression is the pharmacological manipulation of the immune system to prevent or suppress rejection. Induction therapy is administered before or after transplant for up to 2 weeks and typically consists of monoclonal or polyclonal antilymphocytic antibodies. Initiated immediately after transplantation and continued for the life of the allograft, it typically consists of triple therapy with a calcineurin inhibitor (tacrolimus, cyclosporine), a corticosteroid taper, and antiproliferative agent (mycophenolate), although this can vary by center.
- Levels are followed daily in the immediate postoperative period and with decreasing frequency once stabilized in desired range.
- No standard guidelines have been developed for transplant recipients related to vaccinations. Protocols differ by transplant centers, but it is recommended that vaccinations be up to date prior to transplantation if possible.
- Hypertension is very common after solid organ transplant. Standard guidelines for BP management should be followed.

Special Considerations

- Important for discharge planning to include patient teaching on preventing exposure to infection, handwashing, good dental hygiene, etc.
- When conducting patient teaching on signs and symptoms of rejection, stress that signs may be insidious because of antirejection medications.
- Compliance with discharge medication regimen and follow-up appointments is essential.
- Transplantation incurs a heavy financial burden; typical costs for medical care 1 year posttransplant approaches $800,000.

When to Consult, Refer, or Hospitalize

- Patients who are experiencing signs and symptoms of rejection or are feeling unwell should be encouraged to call their transplant team or return to the hospital for evaluation.

Follow-up

- Close follow-up and screening are needed after transplant to monitor for rejection and closely evaluate the side effects of the various medications. Because the incidence of rejection is the highest over the first few months, frequent clinic visits are scheduled during the first year after transplant.
- Patient should be instructed on signs and symptoms of rejection, such as fatigue, pruritus, graft tenderness, jaundice, ascites, and dark urine.
- Expect a 3–6 month recovery from surgery.
- Patients may return to work in 2–3 months if progressing without complications.

Expected Outcome
- Prognosis is generally good. There is an 85% 1-year, 70% 5-year, and 58% 15-year survival rate after transplantation.

Complications
- Surgical complications include:
  - Hepatic artery thrombosis (HAT)
  - May occur at any time posttransplant; associated with bile leaks, graft necrosis, and intrahepatic abscesses; diagnosed by CT scan. Treatment may include thrombectomy, thrombolytics, or regrafting.
  - Portal vein thrombosis
  - Biliary leaks
  - Nonsurgical complications:
    - Primary graft dysfunction (failure to function within a week of transplant)
    - Rejection: failure of the new liver occurs in 10%–15% of cases and is due to local and systemic immune responses from preformed antibodies. Rejection is characterized as:
      - Hyperacute: occurs within minutes and causes rapid tissue necrosis
      - Accelerated acute: (1–5 days postoperatively; difficult to treat)
      - Acute: occurs within the first few months but can occur at any time; amenable to treatment
      - Chronic: leads to eventual graft loss; no definitive treatment; gold standard for diagnosis is allograft biopsy
      - Treatment includes high-dose steroids, antilymphocytic therapy, and optimizing the immunosuppressant regimen.
- Infection
- Biliary cast syndrome: the biliary tree becomes clogged with cast sludge; manifests as severe, intractable pruritis
- Recurrence of disease; liver transplant is not a cure for hepatitis C; viral recurrence is almost universal. Predictors of recurrence include:
  - Donor age
  - Recipient HCV viral load
  - Rejection episodes
  - Warm ischemia time greater than 1 hour
  - Cold ischemia time greater than 10 hours

Complications Common to All Solid Organ Transplantation
- Renal insufficiency: the result of nephrotoxicity associated with calcineurin inhibitors. Management includes reducing calcineurin dose, avoiding other nephrotoxic agents such as NSAIDS, and aggressively managing risk factors for renal disease.
- Posttransplant diabetes mellitus: 2.5% to 19% incidence posttransplant and is associated with a higher incidence of graft rejection. Tight glucose control is indicated with oral agents, insulin, or both.
- Hyperlipidemia: occurs in 80% of transplant recipients. Highly associated with immunosuppressive agents, usually sirolimus. Treatment includes dietary modification and pharmacologic therapy with dyslipidemics.
- Bone disease: osteoporosis is common and related to corticosteroid use. Maximum bone loss usually occurs the first 3 months after surgery. Treat with modification of corticosteroid dose, supplemental calcium, bisphosphinates, and hormone replacement when indicated.

- Malignancy: an increased incidence of lymphoma, skin cancer, and Kaposi's sarcoma has been reported. Treatment consists of modification of immunosuppresion, chemotherapy, and radiation, but prognosis is usually poor.

LUNG TRANSPLANTATION

Description

- Lung transplantation is the surgical procedure to replace diseased or failing lungs with a healthy lung, typically from a deceased donor. One or both lungs may be transplanted or a heart-lung transplant may be performed, depending on the nature of the underlying disease. Living donor lung transplant is possible but is usually done for transplantation of a portion of a lung of a healthy adult to a child.

Etiology

- The most common reasons for lung transplantation are end-stage lung disease secondary to chronic obstructive pulmonary disease (COPD), idiopathic pulmonary fibrosis (IPF), and cystic fibrosis (CF).
- Lung transplant candidates typically have symptomatic chronic respiratory failure, are oxygen-dependent, and have exhausted medical treatment options.

Incidence and Demographics

- The first successful single lung transplant was performed in 1983. In 2010, nearly 1,800 lung transplants were performed in the United States. It is estimated that 3,000 patients are on the national waiting list for lung transplant. Transplant candidates with COPD should be under 60 years of age and have a life expectancy without transplantation of 24–36 months.
- Young patients with silicosis and patients with stage III or IV sarcoidosis with cor pulmonale are prioritized for transplant.
- The average wait for a lung transplant is approximately 2 years.

Risk Factors

- COPD is the 4th leading cause of death in the United States; smoking is responsible for 82% of cases.
- The cause of idiopathic pulmonary fibrosis (IPF) is unknown, although an autoimmune response is thought to play a part in its development. The usual age of diagnosis is between 40 and 70, but there is usually radiologic evidence of pulmonary fibrosis 2–5 years prior to diagnosis. Symptoms are progressive and the average life expectancy after diagnosis is 5 years.
- Cystic fibrosis (CF) is a genetically determined disease that occurs in 1 in 2,000 live births, equally distributed between girls and boys. Most CF patients do not live past their twenties.

Prevention and Screening

- Unlike IPF and CF, COPD has a clear path of prevention: smoking cessation.
- The primary objective in recipient evaluation is to select individuals with progressively disabling cardiopulmonary or pulmonary disease who still possess the capacity for full rehabilitation after transplantation.
- Among most heart-lung transplant programs, the upper recipient age limit is 50 years. For bilateral lung transplantation the limit is 55 years, and for single lung transplantation, 60 years.

Assessment

- Potential transplant candidates are identified by their local primary care physician and referred to a transplant center or transplant pulmonologist for evaluation. The transplant team then determines what studies should be done prior to listing a patient for transplant.
- Evaluation includes a psychiatry or social work evaluation, meeting with a financial counselor, and a comprehensive medical assessment individualized to the patient's age and premorbid conditions, including:
  - Pulmonary workup with ventilation perfusion scan, chest CT scan, pulmonary function testing, and arterial blood gas measurement
  - ECG, echocardiography, and right heart catheterization
  - Blood and tissue typing
- Screening for undetected malignancy with mammogram and Pap smear for women, and prostate exam for men.
- Cystic fibrosis recipients should have an otolaryngologic evaluation before being placed on an active waiting list. Most of these patients will require endoscopic maxillary antrostomies for sinus access and monthly antibiotic irrigation to decrease the bacterial load of the upper respiratory tract. This measure has decreased the incidence of serious posttransplant bacterial infections.
- Former smokers must undergo screening to exclude smoking-related illnesses, such as peripheral vascular disease and malignancy. A negative sputum cytology, thoracic CT scan, bronchoscopy, otolaryngologic evaluation, and carotid duplex scan are required. In addition, left heart catheterization and coronary angiography is usually performed in transplant candidates with a history of smoking.
- When the pretransplant evaluation is complete, the case is referred to the multidisciplinary transplant team for consideration. Once it has been determined that transplant is an acceptable treatment option, the patient is listed nationally on the lung transplant list on the basis of clinical urgency, time on the waiting list, ABO blood group, and thoracic cage dimensions.

Management

Nonpharmacologic Treatment
- While single-lung transplants are usually performed off cardiopulmonary bypass (CPB), the majority of double-lung transplants are still performed "on-pump."
- The acute postoperative management for heart-lung and isolated lung graft recipients entails careful hemodynamic, fluid, and ventilatory management in the intensive care unit. The goal of management is to maintain adequate perfusion and gas exchange while minimizing intravenous fluid administration, cardiac work, and barotrauma.
- Because cardiac output is primarily rate-dependent after heart-lung transplantation, the heart rate should be maintained between 90 and 110 beats per minute during the first few postoperative days, using temporary pacing or isoproterenol, as needed.
- 10% to 20% of heart-lung graft recipients experience some degree of transient sinus node dysfunction in the immediate perioperative period, most often sinus bradycardia.
- While bradyarrythmias usually resolve within a week, persistent sinus node dysfunction may require a temporary pacemaker.
- Denervation of the lungs results in a diminished cough reflex and impairment of mucociliary clearance mechanisms. This predisposes recipients to pulmonary infections. Aggressive postoperative pulmonary toilet is critical.
- Bronchial anastamotic complications range from ischemia and anastamotic necrosis to brochial strictures and dehiscence. Endobronchial stents, bronchial dilatation, or retransplantation may be necessary.
- Ischemic-reperfusion syndrome characterized by pulmonary edema, alveolar damage, and hypoxemia usually occurs 72 hours postoperatively and is a major cause of mortality. Ventilatory support, nitric oxide, and extra corporeal membrane oxygen (ECMO) are possible treatment options.

Pharmacologic Treatment
- Immunosuppression begins intraoperatively and continues for life. Cyclosporine/azathioprine/prednisone is a commonly prescribed triple-drug regimen, but protocols may vary by transplant center. Initial high doses are eventually tapered for chronic dosing.
- Cytomegalovirus (CMV) prophylaxis with granciclovir for a several-week course, bactrim for *Pneumocystis carinii*, and nystatin swish and swallow for mucosal *Candida* prophylaxis remain important components of the postoperative management strategy.

Special Considerations

- Strict isolation precautions are no longer required; simple handwashing is deemed sufficient.
- However, patients may be encouraged to wear a mask in public places for the first 3 months following transplantation.
- Teeth and mouth infections can be particularly threatening. Twice-yearly teeth cleaning is recommended with antibiotic prophylaxis prior to cleaning.

When to Consult, Refer, or Hospitalize

- Patients should be encouraged to contact their primary physician or transplant team with any signs or symptoms of infection or rejection, any colds, flu-like symptoms, nausea, vomiting, or diarrhea, and with any questions or concerns.

Follow-up

- Routine clinical follow-up for heart-lung and lung transplant patients is required to monitor graft function and modify immunosuppressive regimens.
- Discharge teaching on the importance of medication compliance, home temperature and vital sign monitoring, and keeping follow-up appointments is critical.
- Most transplant centers have developed protocols for follow-up and monitoring of graft function.
- Serial pulmonary function tests, arterial blood gases, and bronchoscopic evaluation is usually conducted at 2, 4 to 6, and 12 weeks, followed by 6 months after transplantation and yearly thereafter.
- Transbronchial biopsies are obtained from each transplanted lung, and lavage specimens are submitted for staining, culture, and cytology.
- Surveillance endomyocardial biopsies are performed at 3 months and then annually in heart-lung graft recipients.

Expected Outcomes
- 1-, 5-, and 10-year survival rates following lung transplant (single, double, and lobar combined) were 83.6%, 53.4%, and 28.4%, respectively, in 2008.
- 1-, 5-, and 10-year survival rates of heart-lung transplant recipients from the same year were: 73.8%, 46.5%, and 29.3%, respectively.
- Patients may return to nonstrenuous work in 3–6 months.

Complications
- Routine surveillance and follow-up are needed to address changes in the transplant recipient's clinical status. Complications related to transplantation are many, and these must be addressed carefully to prevent long-term graft failure.
- Primary graft failure and infection are the most common early causes of postop mortality. Graft rejection is characterized as:
  - Hyperacute; occurs within minutes and causes rapid tissue necrosis
  - Accelerated acute: 1–5 days postoperatively; difficult to treat
  - Acute: occurs within the first few months but can occur at any time; amenable to treatment
  - Chronic: leads to eventual graft loss; no definitive treatment
- Bronchiolitis obliterans syndrome (BOS) is a manifestation of chronic rejection.
  - Presents as a decrease in FEV_1 with symptoms of cough and progressive exertional dyspnea
  - Therapeutic options are limited; most common cause of late postoperative mortality

Complications Common to All Solid Organ Transplantation
- See page 697.

HEART TRANSPLANT

Description

- Heart transplantation is a surgical transplant procedure that replaces the failing heart of one human being with a healthy heart, usually from a recently deceased or brain-dead donor. Transplantation may be orthotopic, where most of the patient's heart is removed and the donor heart is trimmed and attached to the remaining portions, or heterotopic, where the patient's own heart is left in situ and the donor heart is connected so as to essentially form a "double heart." Heterotopic transplant is usually reserved for situations where the donor heart is not very strong, was harvested from a donor whose body is considerably smaller than the recipient's, or for patients with pulmonary hypertension. Heterotopic grafts can be removed in case of rejection and allow the patient's own heart to begin working again.

Etiology

- The most common indication for heart transplantation is end-stage heart failure. Cardiomyopathy, ischemic heart disease, complex congenital heart disease, and valvular heart disease are among the leading causes of heart failure. Pathological structural changes or "remodeling" of the heart in response to disease or injury leads to severe cardiac dysfunction and high associated morbidity and mortality.

Incidence and Demographics

- Heart failure is a common syndrome in the United States, afflicting 2% of the population, or nearly 5 million people, and is associated with high overall mortality (5% to 20% annually).
- Heart failure is the most common diagnosis in patients older than 65; it is more common in men than women until age 75, and then incidence becomes approximately equal. Estimated death rates among Blacks are 50% higher than Whites.
- The American College of Cardiology and the American Heart Association define patients with marked heart failure symptoms at rest (that is, fluid overload, pulmonary congestion, fatigue, orthopnea, or paroxysmal nocturnal dyspnea, despite optimal medical management) as having stage D or refractory end-stage heart failure. These patients may be treated with palliative care, considered for mechanical circulatory support, or be evaluated for heart transplantation. Treatment options are decided on a case-by-case basis.
- In 2009, it was estimated by the Registry of the International Society for Heart and Lung Transplantation that over 5,000 heart transplants were performed worldwide. This includes more than 2,000 not reported (though the United States legally mandates reporting of heart transplants to this registry, many countries have established their own databases).
- Historically, the number of heart transplant candidates has exceeded the number of donor hearts available by a factor of 10.
- Most heart transplant recipients are between 50 and 59 years of age.

Risk Factors

- Any isolated risk factor or a combination of factors may lead to end-stage heart failure.

    ### Predisposing Factors
    - Hypertension
    - Left ventricular dysfunction from coronary heart disease
    - Diabetes
    - Nicotine abuse
    - Alcohol abuse
    - Obesity

    ### Other Precipitating Factors and Disease States
    - Infections such as pericarditis or viral or bacterial systemic infections
    - Rheumatic or congenital heart disease
    - Valvular heart disease
    - Preeclampsia
    - Alcohol cardiomyopathy
    - Genetic factors leading to hypertrophic cardiomyopathy
    - Autoimmune disorders (such as lupus erythematosus, sarcoidosis, amyloidosis)

Prevention

- Some conditions leading to heart failure are inherited or congenital and, therefore, irreversible; however, risk factors causing disease progression or repeat exacerbations can be modified. Treatment recommendations include:
    - Smoking and alcohol cessation
    - Regular exercise
    - Aggressive blood pressure control
    - Addition of ACE inhibitors to medical therapy
    - Low-sodium, low-fat diet with a 2-liter-a-day fluid restriction.

Assessment

- Assessment of a patient's suitability for heart transplantation entails a multidisciplinary approach and a comprehensive medical, financial, and psychosocial evaluation. The transplant team typically includes the surgeon, an internist, the transplant coordinator, social worker, psychiatrist, and hospital financial administrator. This team works with the patient and family to coordinate diagnostic testing and help the patient resolve modifiable health risk factors, financial problems, and social issues, which can worsen candidacy for transplantation. Diagnostic assessment includes:
    - General: cancer screening, including stool for occult blood, mammograms, breast and pelvic exam for women, PSA and prostate exam for men
    - Cardiac: Right and left heart catheterization with ventriculography and pulmonary hypertension evaluation; echocardiography; radionuclide stress testing. Some patients may require myocardial biopsy or electrophysiology studies.

- Pulmonary: pulmonary function testing, chest x-ray, spirometry, and arterial blood gases.
- Renal: lab tests for kidney function
- GI: lab tests for liver function
- Immunogenetics: for blood and tissue typing and determining human leukocyte antigen level
- Infectious disease: screening, including serology and skin testing
- Absolute and relative contraindications to transplantation:
  - Malignancy
  - Active infection
  - Active drug, tobacco, or illicit substance use
  - Inability to comply with medical regimen
  - Acquired immune deficiency syndrome
  - HIV (relative contraindication)
  - Morbid obesity (relative contraindication)
- After completion of all necessary pretransplant testing, the potential candidate's case is brought before the multidisciplinary transplant team. Consensus must then be reached to:
  - Accept the patient for transplantation and place him or her on the donor waiting list
  - Accept the patient pending resolution of minor issues
  - Not accept the patient, but recommend reevaluation at a later date
  - Categorically not accept the patient
- Failure to reach consensus in complicated patient scenarios may prompt referral to an ethics committee.
- Transplant candidates are listed with UNOS, and a systematic process prioritizes ranking of organ recipients according to organ required, blood group, acceptable donor height range, and the amount of time the patient has been listed, among other factors.

Management

Nonpharmacologic Treatment
- General postoperative care of the heart transplant patient is similar to management of all patients following cardiac surgery. Immediate postoperative complications specific to heart transplant recipients include:
  - Right ventricular dysfunction occurs intraoperatively and in the early postoperative period in 10%–20% of recipients due to elevated pulmonary vascular resistance and is a potentially life threatening complication. Management of right heart failure may require multimodal therapy, including advanced pharmacologic and ventilator support and the use of assist devices.
  - A heart rate below 100–110 bpm should be avoided postoperatively to prevent low cardiac output and inadequate renal perfusion. Isoproterenol may be administered to maintain an acceptable heart rate and to reduce pulmonary vascular resistance. Temporary pacing also may be required to optimize the heart rate.
  - Heart transplant recipients are at high risk for perioperative hemorrhage.
  - Acute organ rejection: allograft rejection occurs when the recipient's immune system recognizes the graft as "nonself" due to local and systemic immune responses. Hyperacute rejection can occur within minutes and cause rapid tissue necrosis.

- Monitoring for cardiac arrhythmias, ability to wean from mechanical ventilation, adequate renal perfusion, and stable neurologic function are immediate and ongoing postoperative concerns. Pain control and mobilization are optimized. Organ rejection is a continuing concern and may be characterized as:
  - Accelerated acute: 1–5 days postoperatively; difficult to treat
  - Acute: generally occurs within the first few months, but can occur at any time; amenable to treatment
  - Chronic: leads to eventual graft loss; no definitive treatment. Symptoms include fatigue, exercise intolerance, shortness of breath. Common signs are atrial arrhythmias, new S3, friction rub, and JVD. Gold standard for diagnosis is allograft biopsy.
- Additional unique surgical and medical issues and complications include:
  - Denervation: the transplanted heart is denervated so response to cardiac medications is altered and cardiac resuscitative/supportive protocols must be modified appropriately.
  - Cardiac allograft vasculopathy (CAV): Accelerated coronary artery disease affecting epicardial and intramyocardial arteries and veins. Presents as heart failure, ventricular arrhythmias, sudden death. There is 11% incidence of CAV at 1 year after transplant and is the leading cause of death in heart recipients. Diagnosed by angiography. Treatment may be angioplasty, revascularization, or retransplantation.
  - Infection: The overall leading cause of death in solid organ transplant. Highest risk for infection is the first 6 months postoperatively.

Pharmacologic Treatment
- Viral, fungal, and bacterial infections are common in the transplant patient. Long-term or lifelong prophylaxis therapy includes antivirals such as ganciclovir and antifungals such as oral fluconazole. Bacterial infections are treated based on causative organism. Nosocomial pneumonia is the most common infection in heart transplant patients.
- Because of denervation (the result of severing the vagus nerve), medications such as atropine and digoxin have minimal effect on the transplanted heart. The inotropic agent used most commonly is isoproteronol.
- Immunosuppression is the pharmacological manipulation of the immune system to prevent or suppress rejection. Induction therapy is administered before or after transplant for up to 2 weeks and typically consists of monoclonal or polyclonal antilymphocytic antibodies. Maintenance therapy must be provided for the life of the allograft and typically consists of a calcineurin inhibitor, a corticosteroid, and an antimetabolite, although this can vary by center.
- No standard guidelines have been developed for transplant recipients related to vaccinations. Protocols differ by transplant centers, but it is recommended that vaccinations be up to date prior to transplantation if possible.
- Hypertension is very common after solid organ transplant. Standard guidelines for BP management should be followed. Calcium channel blockers are frequently used, although single-agent therapy is typically not effective.

Special Considerations

- Important for discharge planning to include patient teaching on preventing exposure to infection, handwashing, good dental hygiene, and so on
- When conducting patient teaching on signs and symptoms of rejection, stress that signs may be insidious because of antirejection medications.

- Compliance with discharge medication regimen and follow-up appointments is essential.
- Patients must continue to work to modify heart disease risk factors.
- Transplantation incurs a heavy financial burden; typical costs for medical care 1 year posttransplant approaches $800,000.

When to Consult, Refer, or Hospitalize

- Patients who are experiencing signs and symptoms of rejection or are feeling unwell should be encouraged to call their transplant team or return to the hospital for evaluation.

Follow-up

- Expect a 3–6 month recovery from surgery.
- Patients may return to work in 2–3 months if progressing without complications.
- Close follow-up and screening are needed after transplant to monitor for rejection and closely evaluate the side effects of the various medications. Since the incidence of rejection is the highest over the first few months, frequent clinic visits and biopsies are scheduled during the first year after transplant. Screening biopsies are currently the only reliable means to predict rejection. Myocardial biopsy may be done weekly for a month, every other week for a month, then monthly for 3–6 months, then yearly with angiography or dobutamine stress testing.

Expected Outcomes
- Approximately 85% to 90% of heart transplant patients are living 1 year after their surgery, with an annual death rate of approximately 4% thereafter. The 3-year survival approaches 75%.
- Factors associated with an increased risk of death up to 1 year after transplantation include:
  - Preoperative need for artificial breathing support (ventilator)
  - If the heart transplantation is the second one for the recipient
  - Heart conditions other than coronary artery disease or cardiomyopathy
  - Preoperative need for heart function assistance with a ventricular assist device
  - Being female
  - Being underweight or obese
  - A female donor is associated with increased 1-year mortality.
  - The age of the donor heart does not affect long-term survival, although coronary artery disease is increased in hearts from donors over 63 years of age because of narrowing in the coronary arteries.
  - Thickening of the left ventricle (left ventricular hypertrophy) in the donor heart is associated with poorer outcomes compared to a heart without thickening.
  - Elevated blood levels of troponin I and T in the donor, which are markers of heart muscle damage, increase the risk of early heart failure

Complications Common to All Solid Organ Transplantation
- See p. 699

KIDNEY (RENAL) TRANSPLANT

Description

- Kidney transplant is surgical replacement of the failed kidneys of a patient in end-stage renal disease with a healthy kidney from a donor. Kidney transplant donors are classified as living (genetically related or non–genetically related), or deceased, depending on the donor source.

Etiology

- Chronic kidney disease (CKD) is the progressive loss of kidney function and is quantified in stages from 1 to 5, according to the glomerular filtration rate (GFR).
- A GFR less than 60 mL/min/1.73m^2 for greater than 3 months meets criteria for chronic kidney disease. Patients with pathologic kidney damage meet criteria for CKD as well, irrespective of GFR.
- Progression to stage 5 CKD (end-stage renal disease or ESRD) or creatinine clearance less than 20 mL/min refractory to medical management indicates referral for dialysis or transplantation.

Incidence and Demographics

- Chronic kidney disease affects 20 million adults age 20 and older in the United States, or approximately 11.5% of the population. Nearly 700,000 of those patients have end-stage renal disease.
- Close to 400,000 patients with ESRD were treated with some form of dialysis in 2007, and approximately 35.3 billion dollars in public and private monies was spent on treatment.
- Just over 17,000 patients received kidney transplants in 2007, compared with 3,785 in 1980. The majority (11,446) of transplanted kidneys came from deceased donors, with living-related, living-unrelated, and spouse or life partner donors coming in 2nd, 3rd, and 4th, respectively. As of March 2010, 83,950 qualified patients were awaiting kidney transplant.

Risk Factors

- Diabetes mellitus (28%)
  - Caused by diabetic nephropathy
  - Progresses to ESRD in 40% of patients with type 1 diabetes, 20% of patients with type 2 (however, type 2 diabetes is 10 times more prevalent than type 1)
- Hypertension (24%)
- Glomerulonephritis (21%)
- Unknown (20%)

- The remaining causes include polycystic kidney disease, vasculitis, drug toxicity, pyelonephritis, and nephrolithiasis

Prevention and Screening

- Prevention of chronic kidney disease progression requires careful management of fluid, electrolytes, and nutrition; avoidance of nephrotoxic drugs and further kidney injury (such as from UTIs, dehydration, nicotine abuse), and management of comorbid conditions, particularly diabetes, hypertension, and hyperlipidemia.
- Nephrology consultation is indicated for the patient with CKD *and:*
  - Single GFR < 30 in the past 12 months
  - Single GFR < 60 in the setting of refractory hypertension, anemia, refractory hyperparathyroidism, proteinuria > 1 g/24 hours, unexplained hematuria, or unexplained GFR > 15 between readings.
- Referral to a renal transplant team may be done by patient's primary care provider or nephrologist. Some patients self-refer.

Assessment

- Screening to determine suitability for transplantation involves a routine preoperative evaluation with cardiac and pulmonary risk assessment, as well as transplant-specific testing. The identification of possible living donors is also part of the screening process because the wait for a donor kidney may be a year or more.
- A multidisciplinary approach is utilized and patients undergo a comprehensive medical, financial, and psychosocial evaluation. The transplant team typically includes the surgeon, an internist, the transplant coordinator, a social worker, a psychiatrist, and the hospital financial administrator. This team works with the patient and family to coordinate diagnostic testing, and to help the patient resolve modifiable health risk factors, financial problems, and social issues, which can worsen candidacy for transplantation. After completion of all necessary pretransplant testing, the potential candidate's case is brought before the multidisciplinary transplant team. Consensus must then be reached to:
  - Accept the patient for transplantation and place him or her on the donor waiting list
  - Accept the patient pending resolution of minor issues
  - Not accept the patient, but recommend reevaluation at a later date
  - Categorically not accept the patient
  - Failure to reach consensus in complicated patient scenarios may prompt referral to an ethics committee.
- Patients are placed on the national list for transplant maintained by UNOS on the basis of their ABO type, PRA (panel reactive antibody), and accrued wait time.
  - Panel reactive antibodies show a patient's level of sensitization to donor antibodies. Patients with high PRA levels have more rejection episodes.
  - Accrued wait time refers to time accrued from the start date patients are listed for transplant. Patients may move on or off transplant lists due to changes in their clinical status.
- A preemptive transplant may be possible before initiation of dialysis, especially if a living donor is available.

- Absolute and relative contraindications to transplantation:
  - Malignancy
  - Active infection
  - Active drug, tobacco, or illicit substance use
  - Inability to comply with medical regimen
  - Acquired immune deficiency syndrome
  - Human immunodeficiency virus (relative contraindication)
  - Morbid obesity (relative contraindication)

Management

Nonpharmacologic Treatment
- General management of the patient after kidney transplant is similar to that of any patient who has undergone major surgery. Postoperative placement may be in an intensive care or intermediate care unit, depending on facility protocols. Optimizing fluid and electrolyte balance, pain control, pulmonary toilet, and early ambulation are emphasized. Foley catheter will usually remain in place for a longer period of time to allow time for healing of the suture line between the ureter and the bladder. Surgical sutures may also stay in place longer to accommodate the slower healing process in the setting of corticosteroids administered for immunosuppresion.
- Surgical complications specific to renal transplant patients include:
  - Graft thrombosis; usually occurs postoperative day 2–3
    - Symptoms include gross hematuria or sudden cessation of urine output
    - Diagnosis confirmed by ultrasound
    - Poor prognosis; usually results in graft loss
  - Urine leak; usually occurs 2–3 days postoperatively; may be caused by surgical technique or necrosis of ureteral anastamosis
    - Symptoms include abdominal pain or fullness, rising serum creatinine
    - Diagnosed by needle aspiration of fluid, analysis will reveal creatinine
    - Treat by replacing Foley catheter, placement of nephrostomy tube, or surgical repair
  - Lymphocele surrounding the allograft
    - Diagnosed with ultrasound guided aspiration
    - May cause ureteral obstruction, iliac vein compression, or scrotal edema
    - Treat by percutaneous aspiration, diversion of fluid into an internal cavity, or chemical sclerosis
  - Bleeding
- Nonsurgical complications include:
  - Delayed graft function (occurs in 10%–15% of transplanted kidneys) secondary to ATN, accelerated acute rejection or ischemic-reperfusion injury
    - Treatment includes dialysis and modification of immunosupresion regimen
  - Organ rejection: Allograft rejection occurs when the recipient's immune system recognizes the graft as "nonself" because of local and systemic immune responses, and is characterized as:
    - Hyperacute; occurs within minutes and causes rapid tissue necrosis
    - Accelerated acute: 1–5 days postoperatively; difficult to treat
    - Acute: occurs within the first few months but can occur at any time; amenable to treatment
    - Chronic: leads to eventual graft loss; no definitive treatment

- Subjective signs and symptoms of rejection can include decreased urine output, chills, myalgias, graft tenderness. Patients may be asymptomatic.
- Objective signs of rejection are elevated BUN and creatinine, and increased resistive indices on ultrasonography.
- Infection-urinary tract infections are common in the renal transplant recipient.

Pharmacologic Treatment
- Viral, fungal, and bacterial infections are common in the transplant patient. Long-term or lifelong prophylaxis therapy includes antivirals such as ganciclovir, and antifungals such as oral fluconazole. Bacterial infections are treated according to causative organism after obtaining culture and sensitivity. BK-type polyoma virus is found primarily in renal transplant patients and can sometimes be confused with acute rejection as it presents with hematuria and elevated serum creatinine. Diagnosis is made by quantitative PCR assays of the blood and urine or by biopsy. BK nephropathy may be treated with intravenous cidofovir or decrease in immunosupression.
- Immunosuppresion is the pharmacological manipulation of the immune system to prevent or suppress rejection. Induction therapy is administered before or after transplant for up to 2 weeks and typically consists of monoclonal or polyclonal antilymphocytic antibodies. Maintenance therapy must be provided for the life of the allograft and typically consists of a calcineurin inhibitor, a corticosteroid, and an antimetabolite, though this can vary by center.
- No standard guidelines have been developed for transplant recipients related to vaccinations. Protocols differ by transplant centers, but it is recommended that vaccinations be up to date prior to transplantation if possible.

Special Considerations

- It is important during discharge planning to include patient teaching on preventing exposure to infection, handwashing, good dental hygiene, etc.
- When conducting patient teaching on signs and symptoms of rejection, stress that signs may be insidious because of antirejection medications.
- Compliance with discharge medication regimen and follow-up appointments is essential.
- Transplantation incurs a heavy financial burden; typical costs for medical care 1 year posttransplant approach $800,000.

When to Consult, Refer, or Hospitalize

- Patients with hypertension, fluid retention, or decreased urine output post discharge should be counseled to seek medical help immediately. Fever, abdominal pain, or redness at the surgical site warrants emergency room evaluation.

Follow-up

- Patient follow-up postoperatively by the transplant team is typically protocol-driven for 3–4 weeks, but care is eventually transferred to the patient's primary care provider.
- Transplant patients will, however, remain under lifelong care of a nephrologist because transplantation is a treatment option and not a cure for kidney disease.
- Lifelong immunosuppressant therapy and prophylactic antibiotics are likely to be required unless the donor organ came from an identical twin.

Expected Outcome
- The outcome of kidney transplantation continues to improve as screening criteria and rejection-specific serologies improve donor–recipient matches. In general, kidney transplantation is superior in recipients receiving a kidney from a living donor. Within this category, recipients of sibling HLA-identical grafts do best. 2010 UNOS data indicate that deceased donor kidney recipients had a 92% 1-year and 71% 5-year survival rate, compared with 96% and 81% for living donor kidney recipients.

Complications Common to All Solid Organ Transplantation
- See p. 699

PANCREAS TRANSPLANTATION

Description

- A pancreas transplant is a surgical treatment option designed to replace the loss of pancreatic insulin-producing cells in patients with diabetes mellitus type 1 with a healthy insulin-producing pancreas.

Etiology

- Type 1 diabetes is an autoimmune disease that destroys the insulin-producing beta cells of the islets of Langerhans in the pancreas.
- Synthetic methods of insulin delivery have still not been developed that replace pancreatic insulin secretion without risk of hypoglycemia. In addition, manual regulation of blood glucose levels via insulin administration does not prevent clinically significant hyperglycemia.
- Hyperglycemia leads to the development and progression of complications of diabetes, such as coronary artery disease, diabetic retinopathy, peripheral vascular disease, stroke, gastroparesis, and diabetic nephropathy. Exogenous insulin typically fails to prevent secondary complications.

Incidence and Demographics

- Diabetes mellitus type 1 is the only indication for pancreas transplantation.
- 1.1 million people in the United States are estimated to have type 1 diabetes mellitus, while only 1,200 pancreas transplants are performed yearly, limited by the availability of donor organs.
- Type 1 diabetes is equally prevalent among males and females, but is more common in Whites than non-Whites.
- Simultaneous kidney and pancreas (SKP) transplant is performed in the majority of cases because most pancreas transplant candidates have end-stage renal disease secondary to diabetic nephropathy.
- Pancreas after kidney transplant (PAK) refers to pancreas transplantation after a previous, successful kidney transplant.
- The transplanted pancreas may consist of the whole pancreas or a pancreatic segment and is almost always from a deceased donor, although some transplant centers are performing live donor transplants.
- Pancreatic islet cell transplantation is also being evaluated as an alternative to pancreas transplantation.
- The native pancreas is left in place after transplantation, because continues to perform functions necessary for the digestive process. In case of rejection, it can prevent life-threatening diabetes. The donor pancreas is attached in a different location and anastamosed to the bladder or small intestine for drainage of exocrine secretions.
- The waiting period for transplantation is typically 1–2 years.
- Pancreas transplant candidates:
  - Are preferred to be under the age of 55, but are typically between the ages of 20 and 40 at the time of transplant
  - Have demonstrated extreme difficulty with glycemic control
  - Characteristically have end-stage renal disease
  - Are in good cardiovascular health

Risk Factors

- Though type 1 diabetes is an autoimmune disease, many factors are being studied for their influence in triggering the immune response.
  - Genetic factors likely influence disease development; there is a strong correlation between parents with type 1 diabetes and type 1 diabetes in a child.
  - There is growing evidence for environmental, dietary, or viral factors, or combination of these, which, combined with genetic predisposition, are thought to trigger type 1 diabetes onset during infancy.
  - Diseases of the pancreas such as pancreatitis, cystic fibrosis, and pancreatic cancer can inhibit insulin production and lead to type 1 diabetes.
  - Congenital rubella, mumps, and cytomegalovirus are infections that can damage the pancreas, leading to type 1 diabetes.

Prevention and Screening

- Currently there is no way to prevent type 1 diabetes, there is no cure, and there is no consensus on a recommended screening process for at-risk children.
- Because of studies showing that children who were exclusively breastfed were less likely to develop type 1 diabetes than those who received cow's milk, some doctors recommend breast milk for infants with a parent or sibling with type 1 diabetes.
- Referral for pancreas or pancreas and kidney transplant is usually considered when the candidate's kidney disease progresses or is refractory to medical management, glycemic control is refractory to medical management, or frequent insulin reactions develop. A referral is made to a transplant center by the primary care provider or nephrologist for a pretransplant assessment.

Assessment

- The transplant candidate undergoes a thorough medical and psychosocial assessment prior to being listed for transplant.
- Transplant evaluation is structured to identify any treatable medical causes that would preclude surgery or adversely affect the outcome, and to ensure the candidate is healthy enough to survive surgery.
- A psychiatry or social work evaluation and meeting with a financial counselor can identify financial constraints or compliance issues
- A comprehensive medical assessment is individualized to the patient's age and premorbid conditions and typically includes:
  - Blood chemistries; liver, coagulation, and hematology profile
  - C-peptide level confirms the candidate has type 1 diabetes.
  - Infectious work-up including hepatitis, HIV, CMV serologies, and TB skin testing.
  - Pulmonary work-up with chest radiography, CT scan, pulmonary function testing, and arterial blood gas measurement.
  - ECG, echocardiography, and stress testing if indicated
  - Blood and tissue typing, including HLA
  - Screening for undetected malignancy with mammogram and Pap smear for women, and prostate exam for men.
  - Former smokers must undergo screening to exclude smoking-related illnesses, such as peripheral vascular disease and malignancy. A negative sputum cytology, thoracic CT scan, bronchoscopy, otolaryngologic evaluation, and carotid duplex scan may be required. Angiography should be performed in recipient candidates who have a history of smoking.
- Once the pretransplant evaluation is complete, the case is referred to the multidisciplinary transplant team for consideration. A decision must be reached to:
  - Accept the patient for transplantation and place him or her on the donor waiting list
  - Accept the patient pending resolution of minor issues
  - Not accept the patient, but recommend reevaluation at a later date
  - Categorically not accept the patient
  - Failure to reach consensus in complicated patient scenarios may prompt referral to an ethics committee.
  - When it has been determined that transplant is an acceptable treatment option, the patient is listed nationally on the UNOS transplant list.

- Absolute and relative contraindications to transplantation:
  - Malignancy
  - Active infection
  - Active drug, tobacco, or illicit substance use
  - Inability to comply with medical regimen
  - Acquired immune deficiency syndrome
  - Human immunodeficiency virus (relative contraindication)
  - Morbid obesity (relative contraindication)

Management

Nonpharmacologic Treatment
- Pancreas or simultaneous pancreas and kidney transplant patients are monitored in the intensive care unit postoperatively.
- General management is similar to that of the patient after any major abdominal surgery with emphasis on optimizing volume and electrolyte status, metabolic function, pulmonary toilet, pain management, thrombosis prophylaxis, and early mobilization.
- Management specific to the transplant procedure is usually protocol-based and often includes lab work as well as imaging studies to monitor graft function or detect possible rejection and includes:
  - Serial measurement of blood chemistry and serum markers, including lipase, amylase, blood glucose for early monitoring of graft function
  - Abdominal sonography or CT scan to detect anastamotic leaks or graft necrosis
  - 12- or 24-hour urine collection for amylase to screen for rejection as indicated by a 50% fall from baseline levels
  - Amylase, HgA1c, and C-peptide levels may be used for long-term monitoring of graft function.
  - Induction of immunosupression
  - Infection prophylaxis

Pharmacologic Treatment
- Immunosuppresion is the pharmacological manipulation of the immune system to prevent or suppress rejection. Induction therapy is administered before or after transplant for up to 2 weeks and typically consists of monoclonal or polyclonal antilymphocytic antibodies such as OKT3. Maintenance therapy must be provided for the life of the allograft and typically consists of a calcineurin inhibitor such as Prograf or Neoral, a corticosteroid, and an antimetabolite such as Cellcept, though specific agents can vary by center.
- Viral, fungal, and bacterial infections are common in the transplant patient. Long-term or lifelong prophylaxis therapy includes antivirals such as ganciclovir and antifungals such as oral fluconazole. Bacterial infections are treated according to the causative organism.

Special Considerations

- Postoperative diet of the pancreas transplant patient need not be restricted because glycemic control after successful transplantation should return to normal.
- Patient teaching on signs and symptoms of rejection should stress that signs may be insidious because of antirejection medications.
- Compliance with discharge medication regimen and follow-up appointments is essential and may be one of the biggest variables influencing graft rejection.
- Transplantation incurs a heavy financial burden; typical costs for medical care 1 year post–pancreas transplant can average over $100,000, not including the costs of antirejection medication costing up to $2,500 a month.

When to Consult, Refer, or Hospitalize

- Patients who are experiencing signs and symptoms of rejection or are feeling unwell should be encouraged to call their transplant team or return to the hospital for evaluation.
- Fever, abdominal pain, and elevated blood glucose levels should always be promptly evaluated, as should any signs or symptoms of opportunistic infections, flu-like symptoms, rashes, or exposures to communicable diseases.
- Subjective signs of graft failure usually include graft tenderness. Pancreas and kidney transplant recipients should also be aware of signs and symptoms of renal failure.
- Elevated serum amylase or lipase or hyperglycemia after transplant are signs of possible rejection.

Follow-up

- Close follow-up and screening are needed after transplant to monitor for rejection and closely evaluate the side effects of the various medications.
- Clinic visits and lab work are usually protocol-based and vary from center to center, but typically include multiple weekly appointments the first few weeks to months following discharge, and gradually taper off by the end of the second year.
- Lifelong immunosuppresion must be taken as long as the graft is functioning
- Resumption of functional capacity depends on the patient's postoperative course, but should follow the same trajectory as any recovery from major abdominal surgery. Patients should be resuming normal activity by 3–6 months after surgery.

    ### Expected Outcomes
    - Immunosuppression to prevent organ rejection is also sufficient for prevention of recurrent autoimmune diabetes.
    - The national 1-year patient, kidney, and pancreas survival rates for recipients of a simultaneous pancreas and kidney transplant are 95%, 91%, and 86%, respectively.
    - Recipients of a pancreas-after-kidney transplant or a pancreas transplant alone have an average 1-year pancreas graft survival rate of 78%–83%.

- Statistically and clinically, the outcome of kidney transplantation is significantly superior in patients receiving simultaneous pancreas and kidney transplantation versus patients with type 1 diabetes receiving kidney transplantation alone, with improved long-term patient and kidney graft survival.

Complications

Surgical
- Anastamotic leaks: present with abdominal pain and elevated serum amylase; usually occur within the first few months after transplant; surgical correction is required
- Bleeding
- Bladder-drained pancreas transplants: hematuria, cystitis, urethritis, metabolic acidosis because of large quantities of alkaline pancreatic secretions being drained
- Small bowel-drained pancreas transplant: intra-abdominal abscess, gastrointestinal bleeding
- Thrombosis

Nonsurgical
- Mild pancreatitis because of transplanted organ manipulation; monitor serum amylase closely; usually self-limiting
- Sepsis: presents as peritonitis; leading cause of death among transplant recipients
- Rejection

Complications Common to All Solid Organ Transplants
- See p. 699

TRANSPLANT TERMINOLOGY

Grafts

- Autograft: transplant of an organ taken from the recipient
- Heterotropic: native organ left in place; donor organ grafted into an ectopic position on the recipient's native organ
- Isograft: organ taken from a genetically identical donor
- Orthotopic: native organ has been removed; donor organ placed at the site from which it has been removed
- Xenograft: transplant from a genetically different donor of the same species

IMMUNOSUPPRESSIVE AGENTS

Prophylaxis of Rejection Agents

Immunophilin Binders
- Calcineurin inhibitors: cyclosporine (Neoral), tacrolimus (FK-506, Prograf)
- Noninhibitors of calcineurin: sirolimus

Antimetabolites
- Inhibitors of novo purine synthesis: azathioprine (Imuran), mycophenolate mofetil (MMF), Cellcept
- Inhibitors of novo pyrimidine synthesis: leflunomide

Others
- Deoxyspergualin
- Corticosteroids
- FTY720

Treatment of Rejection Agents

Biological Immunosuppression
- Polyclonal antibodies: equine antithymocyte globulin (ATG) for treatment and induction
- Rabbit antithymocite globulin (Thymoglobulin)
- Monoclonal antibodies: OKT3, IL-2R (Humanizid)

Induction Agents
- Basiliximab (Simulect)
- Daclizumab (Zenapax)

Types of Transplants

Deceased Donor
- Brain-dead donor
- Non–heart-beating donor

Living Donor
- Related (parent or sibling)

Unrelated Donor
- Spouse or friend
- Paired exchange; altruistic

REFERENCES

Anderson, A., Chan, M., Costanzo, M. R., Dipchand, A. M., Desai, S., Fedson, S., et al. (2010). The International Society of Heart and Lung Transplantation guidelines for the care of heart transplant recipients. *The Journal of Heart and Lung Transplantation, 29*(8), 914–956.

Angulo, P., Brown, R. B., Dove, L. M., & Travis, A. C. (2009). *Patient selection for liver transplantation.* Retrieved from http://www.uptodate.com/contents/patient-selection-for-liver-transplantation/contributors

Barkley, T. W., & Myers, C. M. (Eds.). (2008). *Practice guidelines for acute care nurse practitioners* (2nd ed.). St. Louis, MO: Saunders Elsevier.

Brown, R. S., Cotler, S. J., & Travis, A. C. (2010). *Living donor liver transplantation.* Retrieved from http://www.uptodate.com/contents/living-donor-liver-transplantation?source=search_result&selectedTitle=1%7E14

Brown, R. S., Travis, A. C., Sussman, N. L., & Vierling, J. M. (2010). *Overview of immunosuppression in adult liver transplantation.* Retrieved from http://www.uptodate.com/contents/overview-of-immunosuppression-in-adult-liver-transplantation/contributors

Brennan, D. C., Danovitch, G., & Sheridan, A. M. (2011). *The kidney transplant waiting list.* Retrieved from http://www.uptodate.com/contents/the-kidney-transplant-waiting-list/contributors

Brennan, D. C., Klein, K., Nathan, D. M., Robertson, R. P., & Sheridan, A. M. (2011) *Benefits and complications associated with kidney-pancreas transplantation in diabetes mellitus.* Retrieved from http://www.uptodate.com/contents/benefits-and-complications-associated-with-kidney-pancreas-transplantation-in-diabetes-mellitus/contributors

Brennan, D. C., Murphy, B., Ramos, E., & Sheridan, A. M. (2010). *Evaluation of the potential renal transplant recipient.* Retrieved from http://www.uptodate.com/contents/evaluation-of-the-potential-renal-transplant-recipient/contributors

Brennan, D. C., Post, T. W., Sheridan, A. M., & Vella, J. (2011). *Patient survival after renal transplantation.* Retrieved from http://www.uptodate.com/contents/patient-survival-after-renal-transplantation/contributors

Cohn, L. (Ed.). (2008). *Cardiac surgery in the adult.* New York: McGraw-Hill.

Colucci, W. S., Hunt, S. A., Lien, D., Nador, R. G., & Yeon, S. B. (2011). *Heart-lung transplantation.* Retrieved from http://www.uptodate.com/contents/indications-and-contraindications-for-cardiac-transplantation/contributors

Colucci, W. S., Hunt, S. A., Piña, I. L., & Yeon, S. B. (2011). *Indications and contraindications for cardiac transplantation.* Retrieved from http://www.uptodate.com/contents/indications-and-contraindications-for-cardiac-transplantation/contributors

Eisen, H. J., Ganz, L. I., Hunt, S. A., Rothman, S. A., & Yeon, S. B. (2011). *Arrhythmias following cardiac transplantation.* Retrieved from http://www.uptodate.com/contents/arrhythmias-following-cardiac-transplantation/contributors

Hachem, R. R., Hollingsworth, H., & Trulock, E. P. (2011). *Lung transplantation: An overview.* Retrieved from http://www.uptodate.com/contents/lung-transplantation-an-overview/contributors

Hollingsworth, H., Trulock, E. P., & Reilly, J. J. (2010). *Evaluation and treatment of acute lung transplant rejection.* Retrieved from http://www.uptodate.com/contents/evaluation-and-treatment-of-acute-lung-transplant-rejection?source=search_result&selectedTitle=1%7E10

Hunt, S. A., Lien, D., Nador, R. G., & Yeon, S. B. (2011). *Heart-lung transplantation.* Retrieved from http://www.uptodate.com/contents/heart-lung-transplantation?source=search_result&selectedTitle=1%7E40

Marcelo Cypel, M., Hollingsworth, H., Keshavjee, S., Trulock, E. P., & Waddell, T. (2010). *Lung transplantation: Procedure and postoperative management.* Retrieved from http://www.uptodate.com/contents/lung-transplantation-procedure-and-postoperative-management/contributors

Mulder, J. E., Nathan, D. M., & Robertson, R. P. (2009). *Pancreas and islet transplantation in diabetes mellitus.* Retrieved from http://www.uptodate.com/contents/pancreas-and-islet-transplantation-in-diabetes-mellitus/contributors

United Network for Organ Sharing. (2011). *Data resources.* Retrieved from http://www.unos.org/donation/index.php?topic=data_resources

United Network for Organ Sharing. (2011). *Living donation.* Retrieved from http://www.unos.org/donation/index.php?topic=living_donation

United Network for Organ Sharing. (2011). *Organ allocation.* Retrieved from http://www.unos.org/donation/index.php?topic=organ_allocation

19

Fever and Shock
Pamela Smith, MSN, RN, ACNP-BC, CCRN

GENERAL APPROACH

Fever

- Symptoms are mainly the result of the process causing the fever.
- Fever pattern is of marginal value for most specific diagnoses, except for the relapsing fever of malaria, borreliosis, and some cases of lymphoma such as Hodgkin's disease.
- Markedly elevated temperatures may cause metabolic disturbances, increase insulin requirements, and can alter the metabolism and disposition of medications.

Shock

- Is not defined by hypotension alone
- The four classes of shock are hypovolemic, cardiogenic, distributive, and obstructive.

RED FLAGS

Fever

- Altered mental status
- Headache, stiff neck, or both
- Significant tachycardia or tachypnea
- Temperature > 40° C or < 35° C
- Recent use of immunosuppresants
- Recent travel to area with endemic malaria

Shock

- Extremities may be warm with distributive shock
- Altered mental status may be the first sign of hypoperfusion

FEVER

Description

- Elevation of body temperature that exceeds the normal daily variation, with an increase in the hypothalamic set point
- Once the hypothalamic set point is raised, peripheral vasoconstriction begins.
- For most fevers, body temperature increases by 1 to 2 degrees.
- Shivering may or may not be present at the time the set point is increased.
- The average normal oral body temperature is 36.7° C (range 36° to 37.4° C) for about 95% of the population.
- Normal diurnal variation is 0.5° C to 1° C.
- Normal vaginal or rectal temperature is 0.5° C higher than the oral temperature.
- A fever > 41.5° C is called hyperpyrexia.
- Elevated temperature not due to fever is hyperthermia characterized by an uncontrolled increased in body temperature that exceeds the body's ability to lose heat.
  - The hypothalamic thermoregulatory set point is unchanged.

Etiology

- Noninfectious causes
  - Inflammatory conditions
    - Adverse reaction to medications
    - Reaction to blood products
    - Collagen vascular disorders
    - Acute vasculitis
    - Microcrystalline arthritis
      - Gout
      - Pseudogout
    - Postpericardiotomy syndrome
  - Vascular conditions
    - Deep vein thrombosis
    - Pulmonary embolism
    - Aortic dissection
    - Bowel ischemia
    - Myocardial infarction
    - Hemorrhage
      - Intracerebral
      - Retroperitoneum
      - Joint
      - Lung
      - Bilateral adrenal hemorrhage
  - Metabolic conditions
    - Hyperthyroidism
    - Adrenal insufficiency
    - Delirium tremens
    - Seizures
  - Neoplasia
    - Lymphoma
    - Renal cell carcinoma
    - Hepatoma
    - Metastatic liver disease
  - Colon cancer
- Infectious causes
  - Urinary tract
    - Urosepsis
    - Pyelonephritis
    - Prostatitis with or without abscess
  - Vascular devices
    - Intravenous access site
    - Intraarterial access site

- Respiratory
    - Bronchitis
    - Pneumonia
    - Sinusitis
    - Empyema
    - Lung abscess
- Surgery- or wound-related
- Skin or soft tissue
    - Decubitus
    - Cellulitis
- Gastrointenstinal
    - Antibiotic-associated colitis
    - Ischemic colitis
    - Biliary
        - Cholecysitis
        - Cholangitis
    - Hepatitis
        - B, C
        - Cytomegalovirus
        - Intra-abdominal abscess
    - Diverticulitis
- Prosthetic device infection
    - Cardiac valve, pacemaker, or implanted cardiac defibrillator
    - Joint prosthesis
    - Peritoneal dialysis catheter
    - Intraventricular shunt
- Miscellaneous
    - Pyarthrosis
    - Osteomyelitis
    - Meningitis
- Fever of unknown origin (FUO)
    - Temperature ≥ 38.3° C rectally for 3 weeks or longer without an apparent cause after extensive investigation in three outpatient visits or 3 days of hospitalization (without neutropenia or immunosuppression being present)

Incidence and Demographics

- Approximately one-third of hospitalized patients will develop fever.
- Common in the intensive care unit

Risk Factors

- Exposure to noninfectious and infectious etiologies
- Malignancy
- Immune-compromised patient
- Surgery

Prevention and Screening

- Handwashing between patients
- Isolation of patients with drug-resistant bacterial infections
- Monitoring temperature trends in the hospitalized patient using consistent methods
- Obtain blood, urine, sputum culture, chest x-ray in patients with new onset fever, shivering and chills, or both

Assessment

History
- Fever
- Malaise
- Fatigue
- Confusion
- Angina
- Localizing complaints
- History of renal disease
- Medication allergies
- Previous infections
- Chills
- Sweats or night sweats
- Weight loss
- Arthralgias
- Myalgias
- Recent surgery
- Use of medications
- Travel history, recent exposure to infected individuals, or both
- Recent blood transfusion

Physical Examination
- Vital signs
- Skin, mucous membranes
  - Evidence of drug reaction
  - Vasculitis
  - Endocarditis
  - Soft tissue necrosis

- Enlarged lymph nodes
- Lungs
  - Tachypnea
  - Often nonspecific findings
- Cardiac
  - Tachycardia
  - New murmurs (endocarditis)
  - Dysrythmias (endocarditis)
- Abdomen
  - Local or generalized tenderness
- Head and neck
  - Fundoscopic lesions of disseminated candidiasis
  - Purulent sinusitis
  - Hepetic stomatitis
- Genitalia and rectum
  - Epididymitis
  - Prostatitis
  - Prostatic abscess
  - Perirectal abscess

Diagnostic Studies
- CBC
  - Leukocytosis
  - Anemia
  - Leukopenia may be seen in viral infections
- Urinalysis
- Serum chemistry
- ESR
- Culture and sensitivity
- Blood
  - Two cultures from separate venipuncture sites
- Urine
- Stool
- Lymph node biopsy
- Bone marrow aspirate
- Sputum
  - Expectorant
  - Suction
  - Bronchoalveolar lavage (BAL)
- Abnormal fluid collections
  - Pleural effusion
  - Joint effusion
  - Ascites
  - Cerebrospinal fluid (CSF)
- Immunologic studies

- Rheumatoid and antinuclear antibody factors
- HIV testing
- Anti-DNAase B titers
  - Rheumatic fever
  - Streptococcal infections
- Imaging
  - Chest x-ray
  - Ultrasound
  - Barium enema
  - Upper GI series
  - CT scanning
    - Used to delineate positive or negative findings with ultrasound
  - Radionuclide studies
    - Ventilation-perfusion scan
  - Echocardiography
  - Invasive procedures, biopsy
    - Used for definitive diagnosis in FUO

Differential Diagnosis

- Hyperthermia
- Heat stroke
- Malignant hyperthermia
- Drug-induced hyperthermia

Management

Nonpharmacologic Treatment
- Evaluation of underlying cause to guide treatment decisions
- Cooling blankets: controversial—causes discomfort (for fever > 41° C)
- Fan
- Ice packs

Pharmacologic Treatment
- Antibiotics
  - Empiric broad-spectrum coverage for likely organisms
  - Be familiar with the antibiotogram of the institution.
  - Narrow the antibiotic regimen based on sensitivity results.
- Antifungals
  - Fluconazole dose is variable, depending on source of infection
  - Caspofungin 70 mg IV on day 1, then 50 mg IV every 24 hours (usual dose)
  - Amphotericin B lipid complex 5 mg/kg/day IV (preferred over conventional amphotericin B—more effective, fewer side effects)
- Antipyretics

- Acetaminophen
- Aspirin
- NSAIDS
- Controversy exists regarding the therapeutic value of treating fever; some studies show that fever may enhance the host's defenses.

Special Considerations

- Localized symptoms guide evaluation
- Underlying chronic disorders, especially those involving the immune system, must be considered
- Focal pain may be less prominent in older adults.
- Fever may not meet the usual elevation criteria in older adults.

When to Consult, Refer, or Hospitalize

- Infectious disease consult is desired for multidrug therapy and multidrug-resistant organisms
- For FUO: infectious disease, rheumatology
- Hospitalize for mental status changes, refractory fever, temperature > 41° C

Follow-up

Expected Outcome
- Resolution of fever and underlying cause

Complications
- Related to the underlying cause of the fever
- Hypothermia
  - Inflammation and cellular dysfunction
  - Multi-organ system failure
  - Disseminated intravascular coagulation

SHOCK

Description

- Shock is a clinical syndrome that is the result of inadequate tissue perfusion from a variety of etiologies.
  - One or more of the following mechanisms may be at play:
    - An absolute or relative decrease in oxygen delivery
      - Low cardiac output

- Low blood oxygen content
- Ineffective tissue perfusion
  - Maldistribution of blood flow to tissues
- Impaired utilization of oxygen
  - Cellular or mitochondrial dysfunction
- Shock is not defined by hypotension.
- Stages of shock
  - Initial—Stage 1
    - Early changes at the cellular level
    - Minimal if any signs or symptoms
  - Compensatory—Stage II
    - Cardiac output falls, depending on the cause
      - Decrease contractility
      - Decreased circulating volume
      - Obstruction
      - Altered vascular resistance
    - Three types of compensatory mechanisms
      - Nervous compensation
        - Sympathetic nervous system (SNS) activated
        - Norepinephrine released
      - Cardiac
        - Tachycardia
        - Vasodilation of coronary arteries
        - Vasodilation of skeletal muscles
        - Vasoconstriction of vasculature in the skin, GI tract, kidneys
      - Hormonal
        - Release of adrenocorticotropic hormone
        - Increase of glucocorticoids; glycogenolysis; increased serum glucose
        - Release of aldosterone—increases sodium and water reabsorption
      - Chemical
        - Pulmonary blood flow decreased because of decreased cardiac output
        - Ventilation or perfusion abnormalities
        - Low oxygen tension leads to increased rate and depth of breathing to remove CO_2—respiratory alkalosis, vasoconstriction of cerebral blood vessels
  - Progressive—Stage III
    - Compensatory mechanisms begin to fail and CO_2 rises.
  - Refractory—Stage IV
    - Final, irreversible stage
    - Cardiac failure
    - Acidosis
    - Coagulopathy
    - Inadequate cerebral blood flow
- Four classifications of shock, based on cardiovascular characteristics
  - Hypovolemic
  - Cardiogenic
  - Distributive
  - Obstructive

Etiology

- Hypovolemic
  - Occurs when intravascular volume is depleted relative to the vascular capacity
    - Hemorrhagic
    - Nonhemorrhagic

Table 19-1. Hemorrhage Classification

Variable	Class I	Class II	Class III	Class IV
Systolic BP	Normal	Normal	Decreased	Decreased
Pulse	< 100	> 100	> 120	> 140
Respirations	14–20	20–30	30–40	> 35
Mental status	Anxious	Agitated	Confused	Lethargic
Blood loss (mL)	< 750	750–1500	1500–2000	> 2000
Blood loss (%)	< 15	15–30	30–40	> 40
Urine output	> 30 mL/hr	> 30 mL/hr	< 25–30 mL/hr	Oliguria

Adapted from *Fundamental Critical Care Support*, by B. McLean & J. Zimmerman (Eds.), 2007, Mount Prospect, IL: Society of Critical Care Medicine.

- Cardiogenic
  - Forward blood flow is inadequate as a result of pump failure because of loss of functional myocardium, a mechanical or structural defect, or arrhythmias
  - Suggests that 40% or more of the left ventricle is involved
    - Ischemic
    - Mechanical
    - Valvular
    - Arrhythmic
- Distributive
  - Loss of peripheral vascular tone (vasodilation); may have components of hypovolemic and cardiogenic shock
    - Septic—most common
    - Adrenal crisis
    - Neurogenic
    - Anaphylactic
- Obstructive
  - Obstruction to flow because of impaired cardiac filling and excessive afterload
    - Massive pulmonary embolism
    - Tension pneumothorax
    - Cardiac tamponade
    - Constricive pericarditis
    - Herniation of abdominal viscera through a diaphragmatic hernia

Incidence and Demographics

- The overall incidence of shock is unknown.
- Cardiogenic shock occurs in about 8.6% of patients with ST elevation myocardial infarction, with 29% already in shock when they present to the hospital; mortality rate is 50% to 80%.
- In the United States, septic shock occurs at the rate of three cases per 1,000 population and 2.2 cases per 100 hospital discharges.
- Neurogenic shock only occurs in spinal cord injury above T6.
- Estimated fatal anaphylaxis is 500 to 1,000 individuals per year in the United States
- There are no incidence statistics for hypovolemic shock.

Risk Factors

- Trauma or burn injury
- Hemorrhage
- Myocardial infarction
- Valvular abnormalities
- Infection
- Deep vein thrombosis
- Pericardial effusion
- Cardiovascular or thoracic surgery
- Pericarditis
- Severe dehydration
- GI bleeding
- Ascites
- Bowel obstruction
- Environmental or medication allergies

Prevention and Screening

- Rapid replacement of volume loss
- Treatment of underlying cause
- Early recognition with screening of systemic inflammatory response syndrome criteria (SIRS)
  - Body temperature > 38° C or < 36° C
  - Heart rate > 90 beats per minute
  - Respiratory rate > 20 per minute or $PaCO_2$ level < 32 mm Hg
- Close observation of vital signs
- Monitor intake and output.
- Decrease the workload of the heart.
- Immobilization of spinal cord injuries
- Document allergies with accurate history-taking.
- Comprehensive and supportive care

Assessment

History
- Hypovolemic
  - Nausea
  - Vomiting
  - Diarrhea
  - Trauma
  - Liver disease
  - Peptic ulcer disease
- Cardiogenic
  - Recent myocardial infarction or chest pain
  - Valve disease
  - Recent cardiac or thoracic surgery
- Distributive
  - Medication or environmental allergy
  - Recent critical illness (adrenal insufficiency)
- Obstructive
  - Deep vein thrombosis
  - Recent cardiac surgery
  - Chest trauma
  - Diaphragmatic hernia

Physical Examination
- Hypovolemic
  - Hypotension
  - Tachycardia
  - Tachypnea
  - Oliguria
  - Altered mental status
  - Cool extremities
  - Jugular venous pressure is low
  - Narrow pulse pressure
- Cardiogenic
  - Central venous pressure (CVP) may be elevated
  - Echocardiogram may show reduced ventricular filling, pericardial effusion, or thickened pericardium
  - Dyspnea
  - Altered mental status
  - Weak, rapid pulse or may be bradycardic
  - Narrow pulse pressure
  - Weak apical pulse
  - Soft S1, S3 gallop may be present.
  - Acute mitral regurgitation (MR) and ventricular septal defects (VSD) are associated with systolic murmurs.
  - Rales
  - Oliguria

- Distributive
  - Hyperdynamic heart tones
  - Warm extremities
  - Wide pulse pressure
  - Echocardiogram may show a hyperdynamic left ventricle
  - Tachycardia
  - May be bradycardic in neurogenic shock
- Obstructive
  - Tension pneumothorax
    - Ipsilateral decreased breath sounds
    - Tracheal deviation away from the affected thorax
    - Jugular venous distention
  - Cardiac tamponade
    - Hypotension
    - Neck vein distention
    - Muffled heart tones
      - The preceding three signs are known as Beck's triad.
    - Pulsus parodoxus
    - Inspiratory reduction in systolic pressure > 10 mm Hg
  - Herniation of abdominal viscera through a diaphragmatic hernia
    - Audible bowel sounds in chest

Table 19-2. Hemodynamic Profiles of Shock

Type of Shock	Heart Rate	Cardiac Output	Ventricular Filling Pressures	Systemic Vascular Resistance	Pulse Pressure	$SvO_2/ScvO_2$
Cardiogenic	↑	↓	↑	↑	↓	↓
Hypovolemic	↑	↓	↓	↑	↓	↓
Distributive	↓	↑ or N	↓ or N	↓	↑	↑ or N
Obstructive	↑	↓	↑	↑	↓	↓

N = normal
SvO_2 = mixed venous oxyhemoglobin saturation
$ScvO_2$ = central venous oxygen saturation
Distributive—cardiac output may be decreased prior to or early in resuscitation; left ventricular filling pressures may be normal or low in massive pulmonary embolism

Adapted from *Fundamental Critical Care Support*, by B. McLean & J. Zimmerman (Eds.), 2007, Mount Prospect, IL: Society of Cirtical Care Medicine.

Diagnostic Studies
- Serum chemistry
  - Blood glucose
    - Increased early in shock
    - Decreased late in shock
  - BUN and creatinine
    - Increased—renal hypoperfusion
  - Sodium
    - Increased in early shock
    - Increased or decreased in late shock
  - Potassium
    - Decreased in early shock
    - Increased in late shock
  - Sodium bicarbonate
    - Increased in early shock because of alkalotic state
    - Decreased in late shock—metabolic or respiratory acidosis
  - Liver enzymes
    - Increased
  - Total protein and albumin
    - Low because of leakage from capillaries
    - Decreased synthesis
  - Creatine phosphokinase
    - Increased
- Arterial blood gases
  - Respiratory alkalosis in early stages
  - Respiratory acidosis in late stages
- Amylase and lipase
  - Increased—necrosis of pancreatic cells
- Cultures
  - Blood
  - Urine
  - Sputum
  - Body fluid and tissue
- Complete blood count
  - White blood cell count
    - Increased—infection, stress
  - Hemoglobin
    - Decreased with hemorrhage
  - Hematocrit
    - May be increased early—hemoconcentration
    - Decreased with hemorrhage
  - Platelets
    - Decreased
- Coagulation studies
  - Prolonged
- Thyroid profile
- Urinalysis and urinary indices

- Decreased creatinine clearance
- Osmolality
  - Increased in early stages
  - Decreased in late stages
- Sodium
  - Decreased early because of water retention
  - Decreased or increased in late stages
- Potassium
  - Increased in early stage
  - Increased or decreased in later stages
- Chest x-ray
  - Pulmonary edema
  - Tension pneumothorax
  - Pericardial effusion
  - Adult respiratory distress syndrome
- Electrocardiogram
  - Indentify dysrhythmia
- Echocardiogram
  - Pericardial effusion
  - Valvular abnormalities
  - Left ventricular function
- CT to investigate sources of infection—abscesses, fluid accumulation, pneumonia

Differential Diagnosis

- Acute systolic heart failure
- Acute renal failure
- Diabetic ketoacidosis
- Adrenal crisis
- Aortic aneurysm

Management

Nonpharmacologic Treatment
- Maintain airway and circulation
- Supplemental oxygen
- Invasive hemodynamic monitoring
- Large-bore IVs, central venous catheter, or both
- No IM injections
- Nutritional support
- Correction of acid–base balance
- Intra-aortic balloon pump for cardiogenic shock
- Revascularization for cardiogenic shock
- Pericardiocentesis for cardiac tamponade in obstructive shock
- Needle thoracostomy or chest tube placement for tension pneumothorax in obstructive shock
- Cooling blanket

Pharmacologic Treatment
- Hypovolemic
  - Fluid challenges
    - Crystalloid
    - Colloids
  - Blood products
  - Vasopressors contraindicated until circulating volume restored
- Cardiogenic
  - Morphine sulfate
  - Dopamine 5 to 10 mcg/kg/min IV
  - Dobutamine 2 to 20 mcg/kg/min IV
  - Milrinone 50 mcg/kg bolus followed by maintenance infusion of 3.375 to 0.75 mcg/kg/min IV
  - Amrinone 0.75 mg/kg bolus, repeat in 30 minutes, then 5 to 10 mcg/kg/min IV
  - Norepinephrine 2 to 12 mcg/kg/min IV
  - Diuretics
    - Lasix
    - Nitrates
  - Nitroprusside
  - Lidocaine
- Distributive
  - Septic
    - Fluid resuscitation
    - Antibiotics for septic shock targeting offending organism
    - Drotrecogin alpha (activated protein C) for septic shock
    - Steroids controversial
      - Beneficial in adrenal insufficiency
    - Vasopressors after adequate fluid resuscitation
  - Neurogenic shock
    - Vasopressors
    - Atropine for symptomatic bradycardia
    - Fluid administration
  - Anaphylactic
    - Epinephrine 0.01 mL/kg up to a maximum of 0.2 to 0.5 mL, repeat in 10 to 15-minute intervals until desired effect achieved or adverse affects occur
    - May give epinephrine via endotracheal tube
    - IM or SQ administration may be considered for first-line treatment
    - Inhaled epinephrine is effective for mild to moderate laryngeal edema but not as a substitute for IM or SQ epinephrine.
    - Benadryl 25 to 50 mg IV single dose
    - Treat bronchospasm with β2-agonist intermittently or continuously
      - May consider aminophyllin
    - Hydrocortisone 5 mg/kg or 250 mg IV every 6 hours
    - Inotropic agents may be necessary
- Obstructive
  - Thrombolytics or anticoagulation in massive pulmonary embolism
  - Fluid challenge in cardiac tamponade

Special Considerations

- Shock may develop as an underlying condition progresses or it may the initial presentation.
- Compensatory mechanisms attempt to increase tissue perfusion and oxygenation through complex neuroendocrine responses.
- Initial vasoconstriction can lead to an increase in diastolic pressure and narrowing pulse pressure.
- Hypothermia may be a result of profound vasoconstriction.
- The increased systemic vascular resistance in cardiogenic, hemorrhagic, and obstructive shock is the body's attempt to maintain blood pressure.
- Patients with distributive shock often have warm extremities and vasodilation.

When to Consult, Refer, or Hospitalize

- All patients with any type of shock should be hospitalized.
- Consult subspeciality for the underlying disorder.

Follow-up

Expected Outcomes
- Resolution of the shock state is dependent on the underlying cause and patient's preexisting health.
- Outcomes improve when the hypoperfusion state is treated early.

Complications
- Acute respiratory distress syndrome
- Acute renal failure
- Left ventricular dysfunction, systolic heart failure
- Acute liver failure
- Intestinal ischemia
- Stroke
- Disseminated intravascular coagulation
- Encephalopathy

REFERENCES

Barkley, T., & Myers, C. (2008). *Practice guidelines for acute care nurse practitioners*. St. Louis, MO: Saunders.

Beers, M., Porter, R., Jones, T., Kaplan, J., & Berkwits, M. (Eds.). (2006). *The Merck manual of diagnosis and therapy*. Whitehouse Station, NJ: Merck Research Laboratories.

Bope, E., Kellerman, R., & Rakel, R. (2011). *Conn's current therapy 2011*. Philadelphia: Elsevier/Saunders.

Cooper, D., Kraink, A., Lubner, S., & Reno, H. (Eds.). (2007). *The Washington manual of medical therapeutics* (32nd ed.). Philadelphia: Wolters Kluwer/Lippincott Williams & Wilkins.

Fauci, A., Braunwald, E., Kasper, D., Hauser, S., Longo, D., Jameson, J., & Loscalzo, J. (Eds.). (2009). *Harrison's principles of internal medicine*. New York: McGraw Hill.

Habermann, T., & Ghosh, A. (2008). *Mayo clinic internal medicine concise textbook*. Rochester, MN: Mayo Clinic Scientific Press.

Irwin, R., & Rippe, J. (2008). *Intensive care medicine*. Philadelphia: Wolter Kluwer/Lippincott Williams.

Marini, J., & Wheeler, A. (2010). *Critical care medicine, the essentials*. Philadelphia: Wolters Kluwer/Lippincott Williams & Wilkins.

McKean, S., Bennett, A., & Halasyamani, L. (Eds.). (2008). *Hospital medicine*. Philadelphia: Wolters Kluwer/Lippincott Williams & Wilkins.

McLean, B., & Zimmerman, J. (Eds). (2007). *Fundamental critical care support*. Mount Prospect, IL: Society of Critical Care Medicine.

McPhee, S., & Papadakis, M. (2011). (Eds.). *2011 current medical diagnosis and treatment*. New York: McGraw Hill.

20

Fluid, Electrolyte, and Acid–Base Balance
Pamela Smith, MSN, RN, ACNP-BC, CCRN

HYPONATREMIA

Description

- Defined as a serum sodium (Na^+) < 135 mEq/L and is considered to be severe when the level is < 125 mEq/L
- Reflects an excess of total body water (TBW) relative to total body sodium content
- Hyponatremia is evaluated along with fluid status—hypovolemia, euvolemia, hypervolemia, and osmolality.
- Many cases of hyponatremia are a result of water imbalance and abnormal water handling and not sodium imbalance.

Etiology

- Isotonic hyponatremia (pseudohyponatremia)
- Hypertonic hyponatremia
- Hypotonic hyponatremia
  - Hypovolemia hypotonic hyponatremia
  - Euvolemia hypotonic hyponatremia
  - Hypervolemic hypotonic hyponatremia

Figure 20-1. Hyponatremia

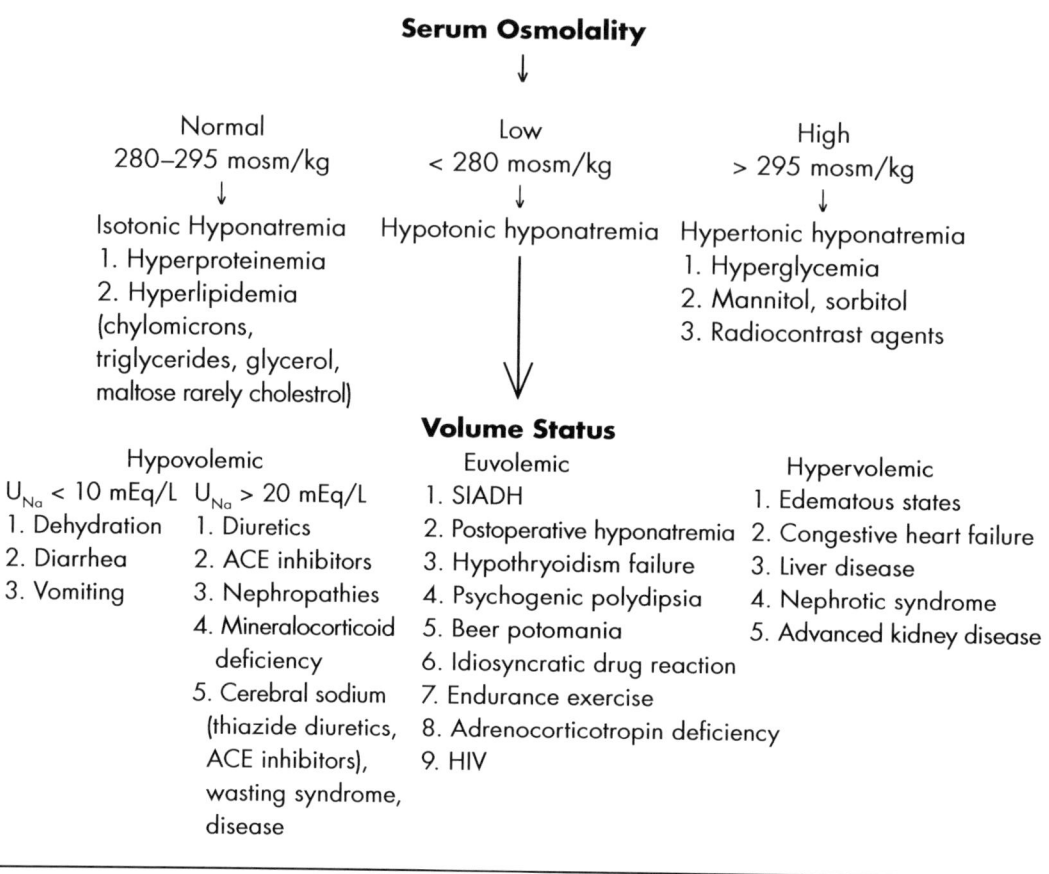

Note. ACE—angiotensin-converting enzyme; SIADH—syndrome of inappropriate antidiuretic hormone Adpated from *Current Medical Diagnosis and Treatment*, by S. McPhee & M. Papadakis, 2011, New York: McGraw Hill.

Incidence and Demographics

- In the hospital approximately 15% to 20% of patients have a serum sodium level < 135 mEq/L.
- 3% to 5% have a level < 130 mEq/L.
- Hyponatremia affects all races and both genders equally.
- Hyponatremia is more common in older adults because of the increased incidence of comorbid conditions.

Risk Factors

- Cardiovascular disease
- Renal disease
- Surgery

- Diuretic use
- Trauma
- Excessive beer intake
- Sepsis
- Dehydration
- Malignancy
- Advanced age
- Intensive exercise
- Low-sodium diet
- Use of SSRIs

Prevention and Screening

- Treat and monitor conditions that cause hyponatremia.
- Educate patients taking medications that predispose them to hyponatremia about the signs and symptoms of the condition.
- Individuals participating in highly intensive exercise—marathons, triathlons, Iron Man competitions, and other demanding physical activities—should drink only as much fluid as they lose in sweat, usually no more than about 1 liter per hour of exercise.
- Use of electrolyte-containing fluids instead of water during exercise
- Monitor intake and output in the hospitalized patient.
- Daily weights for patients with chronic kidney disease and congestive heart failure
- Serial electrolytes while hospitalized

Assessment

History
- Isotonic hyponatremia
  - Elevated lipids
  - Alcoholism
  - Liver disease
    - Hepatitis
    - Autoimmune disease
    - Cirrhosis
- Hypertonic hypnatremia
  - Increased intracranial pressure (ICP)
  - Use of osmotic diuretics to lower ICP
  - Elevated glucose
    - Diabetes
      - Sodium concentration falls 2 mEq/L for every 100 mg/dL rise in glucose when the glucose level is between 200 and 400 mg/dL.
      - If the glucose level is > 400 mg/dL, the sodium concentration falls 4 mEq/L for every 100 mg/dL rise in glucose.
  - Diagnostic studies requiring contrast media

- Hypotonic hyponatremia—most common
  - Hypovolemic
    · Diarrhea
    · Protracted vomiting
    · Replacement of lost volume with hypotonic fluid (water or IVF)
  - Euvolemic
    · Primary polydypsia
      - Acute psychosis
    · Chronic kidney disease
    · Hypothyroidism
    · Adrenal insufficiency
    · Use of thiazide diuretics
    · NSAIDS—increase antidiuretic hormone (ADH) by inhibiting prostaglandin formation
    · Use of SSRIs
    · Abuse of 3,4-methylenedioxymethamphetamine (MDMA, ecstasy)
      - ADH release
      - Primary polydipsia
    · Nausea
    · Pain
    · HIV infection
    · Recent participation in highly intensive sports
    · Hypokalemia
    · SIADH
      - Malignancy
        · CNS
        · Duodenal
        · Lung
        · Lymphoma
        · Pancreatic
      - Pulmonary disorders
        · Aspergillosis
        · Lung abscess
        · Pneumonia
        · Positive-pressure ventilation
        · Tuberculosis
      - Central nervous system (CNS) disorders
        · Abscess
        · Encephalitis
        · Guillain-Barré syndrome
        · Head trauma
        · Meningitis
        · Cerebrovascular accident (CVA)
        · Subdural or subarachnoid hemorrhage
        · Acute psychosis
        · Acute intermittent porphyria

- Endocrine disorders
  - Addison's disease
  - Hypopituitarism
  - Hypothryoidism
- Miscellaneous
  - Protein-energy malnutrition (PEM)
  - Surgery
  - Medications
    - Increased ADH production
      - Antidepressants
      - Antineoplastics
      - MDMA
      - Carbamazepine
      - Clofibrate
      - Neuroleptics
    - Potentiated ADH action
      - Carbamazepine
      - Chlorpropamide
      - Tolbutamide
      - Cyclophosphamide
      - NSAIDS
      - Somatostatin and analogs
      - Amiodarone
- Hypervolemic
  - Cirrhosis
  - Congestive heart failure
  - Nephrotic syndrome
  - Chronic, end-stage renal disease

Physical Examination
- The symptoms of hyponatremia are determined by whether it is acute or chronic.
  - Chronic onset of hyponatremia may be asymptomatic.
  - Mild hyponatremia (130 to 135 mEq/L) is usually asymptomatic.
  - Nausea
  - Malaise
  - Headache
  - Lethargy
  - Disorientation
  - Hypovolemic
  - Flat neck veins
  - Dry skin
  - Dry mucous membranes
  - Positive orthostatic vital signs
  - Postural tachycardia
  - Weight loss
  - Oliguria
  - Ascites
  - Lungs clear
  - No radiographic evidence of volume overload

- Euvolemic
  - No evidence of hypovolemic or hypervolemia
  - Stable weight
- Hypervolemic
  - Distended neck veins
  - Moist mucous membranes
  - Negative orthostatic vital signs
  - Tachcardia
  - Tachypnea
  - Cardiac gallop
  - Weight gain
  - Peripheral edema
  - Dyspnea
  - Crackles on lung exam
  - Radiographic evidence of volume overload

Diagnostic Studies
- Serum electrolytes
- Serum osmolality
- Urine osmolality
- $Urine_{Na}$
- SIADH
  - Hyponatremia
  - Decreased serum osmolality
  - Absence of heart, kidney, or liver disease
  - Normal thyroid and adrenal function
  - Urine sodium over 20 mEq/L
  - May have low BUN (< 10 mg/dL)
  - May have hypouricemia (< 4 mg/dL)

Differential Diagnosis

- Adrenal crisis
- Alcoholism
- Hypothyroidism
- Cardiogenic pulmonary edema
- Hyperlipidemia

Management

- Only hypotonic hyponatremia requires treatment aimed at serum Na^+.
- Isotonic hyponatremia
  - Correction of serum protein and hyperlipidemia
- Hypertonic hyponatremia
  - Correction of serum glucose level
  - Careful use of osmotic diuretics for increased intracranial pressure
- Correction of sodium is determined by the serum level and the rapidity of onset.

Nonpharmacologic Treatment
- Free water restriction regardless of the patient's volume status
  - Free water intake should be < 1 to 1.5 L/d
- Strict intake and output
- Serial serum and urine chemistry and osmolality
- Daily weight
- Determine the duration and magnitude of the hyponatremia, the patient's volume status, and the degree of clinical symptoms.

Pharmacologic Treatment
- Hypovolemic
  - Administer isotonic saline to patients who are hypovolemic to replace contracted intravascular volume—treats the cause of the vasopressin (ADH) release
  - When ADH secretion stops, the kidney excretes the excess water, correcting the hyponatrema.
  - Patients with hypovolemia from diuretic therapy may also need potassium replacement.
- Euvolemic
  - The goal is to remove excess water and is directed at the cause.
    - Calculate the amount of water that must be removed to return the sodium to a safe level: 125 mEq/L.
    - Water excess = weight (kg) x 0.6 x (1 – Na^+/125) for men
      - Use x 0.5 for women.
    - After calculating the water excess, the rate and method of water removal must be determined.
  - Chronic asymptomatic
    - Normovolemic, asymptomatic, and mildly hypovolemic: free water restriction, < 1 liter/day—this approach recommended for asymptomatic SIADH
      - The amount of water ingested must be less that the maximum daily urine volume.
      - Daily water ingestion = maximum daily urine volume (mL) – water excess (mL)/ number of days for correction
      - The number of days depends on the patient's clinical status, but the rate of correction should not exceed 12 mEq/L/d.
        - Example: A patient with water excess of 5 L and a maximum daily urine volume of 1,000 ml must take in less than 750 mL per day to correct serum sodium over 20 days:
          DWI = 1,000 – 5,000/20 = 750 mL
    - The maximum rate of plasma sodium correction is 0.5 mEq/L per hour
      - Correcting the plasma sodium too quickly can cause osmotic demyelination syndrome (formerly called central pontine myelinolysis)—a sudden loss of volume in the brain cells, which leads to shrinkage and destruction of the myeling coatings, causing cell death.
      - Lack of treatment for hyponatremia can also cause neurologic impairment because of increased volume in the brain cells leading to cerebral edema.
    - Do not give patients with SIADH isotonic saline alone—it is the same as giving volume, and the patient does not need volume; it can worsen hyponatremia because the patient retains water because of the ADH and excretes sodium.
      - Use isotonic saline in conjunction with a loop diuretic for net negative loss of sodium with excretion of free water.

- Refractory SIADH
  - Use of pharmacologic agents can allow for more liberal fluid intake.
  - Demeclocycline—increases the diluting capacity of the kidney
    - Treat for 3 to 4 days for maximal effect.
    - Contraindicated in cirrhotic patients
  - Vasopressin 2 antagonists
    - Hospitalized patients
      - Conivaptan—IV loading dose of 20 mg administered over 30 minutes, then as 20 mg continuously over 24 hours
      - Subsequent infusions may be administered every 1 to 3 days at 20 to 40 mg/d by continuous infusion.
- Correct slowly
- Severe symptomatic hyponatremia
  - If serum sodium is < 109 mEq/L
  - (Desired change in serum Na) x TBW
    - TBW = 0.6 × weight in kg for men or 0.5 × weight in kg for women
    - Example: The amount of Na needed to raise the serum Na from 115 mEq to 125 mEq in a 70 kg man is:
      - (125 − 115) × (0.6 × 80) = 480 mEq
      - One liter of 3% saline has 513 mEq of Na—slightly less than one liter will be required to raise the serum Na 10 mEq.
      - Infuse over 24 hours—rate may be increased initially to raise sodium 4 to 6 mEq over 4 to 6 hours in patient with seizures; however, the overall correction should not be more than 10 to 12 mEq over a 24-hour period.

- Hypervolemic
  - Salt and fluid restriction
  - Diuretics
  - Correction of underlying condition
  - Replace lost volume with NS as needed
  - Dialysis for fluid removal
- Psychogenic polydipsia may require psychiatric and pharmacologic intervention
- Pseudohyponatremia because of hyperglyceridemia or hyperproteinemia does not require treatment other than confirmation by serum testing.
- Hyponatremia because of elevated glucose or mannitol use is treated by lower serum glucose levels and discontinuing mannitol use if possible.

Special Considerations

- The brain is able to compensate for hyponatremia when it occurs slowly over days to weeks; the sodium level is not a good indicator of whether or not symptoms will be present. For example, a sodium concentration of 125 mEq/L can cause seizures and coma if it happens quickly (< 48 hours), while a level of 118 mEq/L may be asymptomatic if it has occurred over several weeks.
- Patients at higher risk of acute cerebral edema from hyponatremia are postoperative hospitalized women, older females on thiazide diuretics, and patients with water intoxication from psychogenic polydipsia.
- When infusing 3% saline, electrolytes should be monitored frequently, especially during the first few hours of treatment, then every 6 to 12 hours.

When to Consult, Refer, or Hospitalize

- Hospitalize for symptomatic patients or those who require aggressive therapy and close monitoring of electrolytes and neurological function.
- Consult nephrology or endocrinology in patients with severe, symptomatic, refractory, or complicated cases of hyponatremia.
- Use of hypertonic saline, demeclocycline, vasopressin antagonists, or dialysis requires specialty consultation.
- Gastroenterology or cardiology consultation may be needed in cases where patients have end-stage liver disease or heart disease.
- Critical care consult if ICU required

Follow-up

Expected Outcome
- Resolution of hyponatremia

Complications
- Osmotic demyelination syndrome
- Cerebral edema from lack of treatment

HYPERNATREMIA

Description

- Hypernatremia is defined as serum sodium concentration of > 145 mEq/L.
- It is a common electrolyte disorder is characterized by a decrease in total body water relative to electrolyte content.
- Hypernatremia is a water problem, not a disorder of sodium balance; all patients have hyperosmolality.

Etiology

- Outside of the hospital, it occurs in older adults who are mentally or physically impaired, or both, and who may be infected.
- Inpatients develop hypernatremia from a lack of access to free water, and it is an iatrogenic complication.
  - Hyponatremic patients given excessive hypertonic saline
  - Use of sodium bicarbonate during cardiac resuscitation
  - Patients receiving tube feedings or total parenteral nutrition with inadequate free water
  - Administration of sodium chloride tablets

- Hypernatremia can only develop when the thirst mechanism is impaired and water intake does not respond to hyperosmolality or when water ingestion is restricted.
  - It is rarely the result of an increase in sodium.
  - Mild hypernatremia may be caused by excess mineralocorticoid activity.
    - Primary hyperaldosteronism
    - Congenital adrenal hyperplasia
    - Cushing's syndrome
    - Hyperreninism
- Underlying disorders
  - GI fluid loss
    - Lactulose
    - Persistent diarrhea or emesis
    - Postoperative drainage
  - Central and nephrogenic diabetes insipidous
  - Renal osmotic diuresis
    - Mannitol therapy
    - Urea excretion in burns
    - Relief of urinary obstruction
  - Cutaneous fluid loss
    - Burns
    - Excessive sweating
    - Hypothalmic dysfunction is a rare cause.

Incidence and Demographics

- Occurs in 0.3% to 1% of hospitalized patients

Risk Factors

- Advanced age
- Inability to sense thirst
- Debility following stroke

Prevention and Screening

- Drink when thirsty.
- Administration of free water to hospitalized patients
- Monitor sodium when administering lactulose, mannitol, and sodium bicarbonate.
- Treatment of underlying disorders

Assessment

- The signs and symptoms of hypernatremia result from osmotic shifts of water out of the intracellular compartment into the hypotonic extracellular fluid compartment.
  - Cells shrink, causing dysfunction.

History
- Symptoms in older adults may not be specific and a change in consciousness is associated with a poor prognosis and the severity of the hyponatremia.
- Decreased water intake
- Lactulose or mannitol use
- Acute: > 150 mEq/L
  - Weight loss
  - Lethargy
  - Irritability
  - Weakness
  - Confusion
- Serum sodium > 158 mEq/L (severe hypernatremia)
  - Delirium
- Chronic
  - None to mild CNS symptoms

Physical Examination
- In volume-depleted states
  - Flat neck veins
  - Poor skin turgor
  - Dry mucous membranes
  - No edema
  - Clear lungs
  - Orthostatic hypotension
  - Oliguria
  - Hypotension
  - Tachycardia
- Serum sodium > 158 mEq/L
  - Acute
    - Coma
    - Stupor
  - Chronic
    - None to severe CNS findings
- Awake patients may experience thirst.
- Polyuria or nocturia
  - May indicate renal disorder
    - Diabetes insipidous
    - Osmotic diuresis (glycosuria in hyperglycemia)

Diagnostic Studies
- Serum chemistry
  - Serum Na > 145 mEq/L
- Urine osmolality
  - > 400 mosm/kg: renal water conservation is functioning
    - Nonrenal losses
      - Excessive sweating
      - Water loss via respiratory tract
      - Bowel movements
    - Renal losses
      - Progressive volume depletion from glycosuria
      - Osmotic diuresis
  - < 250 mosm/kg
    - Characteristic of diabetes insipidous
      - Central
        - Inadequate ADH
      - Nephrogenic
        - Renal insensitivity to ADH
        - Lithium
        - Demeclocycline
        - Relief of urinary obstruction
        - Interstitial nephritis
        - Hypercalcemia
        - Hypokalemia

Differential Diagnosis

- Cirrhosis
- Diabetes mellitus type 1
- Hypocalcemia

Management

Nonpharmacologic Treatment
- Correct the cause of fluid loss.

Pharmacologic Treatment
- Calculate free water deficit.
  - $0.4 \times$ body weight (kg) $\times$ [(serum Na^+ /140) − 1]
- Choose correct intravenous fluids
  - Hypernatremia with hypovolemia
    - Isotonic saline
    - After adequate volume resuscitation: 0.45% saline or 5% dextrose or both can be used to replace remaining free water
    - Mild volume deficits can be treated with 0.45 saline and 5% dextrose.

- Hypernatremia with euvolemia
  - Water ingestion or 5% dextrose will result in the excretion of excess sodium.
    - With renal impairment, may use diuretic to increase urinary sodium; however, it will also increase the amount of water that must be replaced
      - With enteral therapy: oral water replacement in conscious patients
- Hypernatremia with hypervolemia
  - 5% dextrose to reduce hyperosmolality
  - Loop diuretics may be needed.
  - Rarely, hemodialysis
- Replace water at rate calculated to reduce serum Na^+ by about 1 mEq/L/hour in acute hypernatremia and by about one-half of the excess > 140 mEq/L over 24 hours in chronic hypernatremia.

Special Considerations

- TBW correlates with muscle mass and decreases with age, cachexia, and dehydration, and is lower in women than men
- Insensible water loss is about 800 to 1,000 mL per day and is increased in those with fever and burns.
  - Respiratory fluid loss is increased by hyperventilation and low humidity.
- Sensible fluid loss is sweat, which contains about 30 mEq/L of sodium.
  - Infections, especially those of the urinary and respiratory tract, are associated with hypernatremia by increasing skin and respiratory water loss from fever, sweating, and hyperventilation.

When to Consult, Refer, or Hospitalize

- Refer to subspecialists for refractory or unexplained hypernatremia.
- Admit patients with symptomatic hypernatremia.
- Critical care consult if ICU required
- Acute illness or significant comorbid conditions along with hypernatremia may require hospitalization for treatment of underlying cause or conditions, as well as the hypernatremia.

Follow-up

Expected Outcomes
- Resolution of hypernatremia
- Serial monitoring of serum sodium
- Avoidance of CNS involvement

Complications
- Altered mental status
- Hyperthermia
- Seizures
- Coma

HYPOKALEMIA

Description

- Defined as a serum potassium level of < 3.5 mEq/L
- Potassium is the most abundant intracellular cation.
- May occur from low dietary intake, intracellular shifting from the vascular compartment, or extrarenal and renal loss
- Cellular uptake of potassium is increased by insulin and β-adrenergic stimulation and blocked by α-stimulation.
- Potassium homeostasis is regulated by the kidney, the important site being the collecting duct where aldosterone receptors are present.
- Excretion is increased by:
  - Aldosterone
  - High levels of sodium at the collecting ducts (for example with diuretic use)
  - Osmotic diuresis
  - Elevated serum potassium levels
  - Negatively charged ions at the collecting duct (for example, bicarbonate)
- Excretion is decreased by:
  - Absence or lack of aldosterone
  - Low levels of sodium at the collecting ducts
  - Low urine flow
  - Low serum potassium level
  - Renal failure

Etiology

- Decreased intake
  - Uncommon since most diets are rich in potassium
  - Intake is usually excessive with a daily intake of 1 mEq/kg/d
  - Eating disorders
  - Tea and toast diet of older adults
  - Potassium poor TPN
- Increased loss
  - Intracellular shift
    - Insulin therapy
    - Intensive catecholamine stimulation
    - Alkalemia
    - Periodic paralysis
      - Rare
      - Because of an abnormality in the alpha 1 subunit of the dihydropyridine-sensitive calcium channel in skeletal muscle
    - Thryotoxic periodic paralysis

- Acquired form of hypokalemic periodic paralysis and occurs most frequently in Asian males
- Mechanism not well understood
  - Refeeding
    - Observed in prolonged starvation, eating disorders, and alcoholism
- GI loss
  - Diarrhea
  - Colonic fistula
  - Surgical drains
  - Villous adenoma
  - Vomiting
- Renal loss
  - Endogenous mineralocorticoid excess
    - Cushing's disease
    - Primary hyperaldosteronism
      - Adenoma
      - Bilateral adrenal hyperplasia
    - Secondary hyperaldosteronism
      - Volume loss, congestive heart failure, cirrhosis
    - Adrenocortical neoplasm
    - Congenital disorders
      - Congenital adrenal hyperplasia
      - Glucocorticoid-remediable hypertension
  - Hyperreninism
  - Medications
    - Diuretics
    - Bicarbonate ingestion
    - Amphotericin B, azole class of antifungal agents, echinocandin class of antifungal agents
    - Gentamicin
    - Cisplatin
    - Stacker 2
    - β-agonist intoxication
  - Exogenous mineralocorticoid excess
    - Steroid therapy for immunosuppresion
    - Glycyrrhizic acid
    - Renal tubular disorders
    - Hypomagnesemia
  - Diabetic ketoacidosis
  - Renal tubular acidosis
    - Type 1 and type 2
  - Congenital disorders
    - Bartter's syndrome
    - Gitelman's syndrome
    - Liddle's syndrome

Incidence and Demographics

- Up to 21% of hospitalized patients have a potassium level < 3.5 mEq/L, and approximately 5% have levels < 3.0 mEq/L.
- In the elderly, about 5% have levels < 3.0 mEq/L.
- In patients taking non–potassium-sparing diuretics, hypokalemia is seen in 20% to 50% of this population.
- Blacks and women are more susceptible to diuretic-induced hypokalemia.
- In patients with eating disorders, the incidence is 4.6% to 19.7%.

Risk Factors

- Poor dietary intake
- Alcoholism
- Cirrhosis
- Presence of an eating disorder
- Bariatric surgery
- Hypomagnesemia
- Presence of congenital disorders
- Congestive heart failure
- Diuretic use
- Diabetes mellitus
- Antibiotic or antifungal therapy
- Use of total parenteral nutrition (TPN)
- Advanced age

Prevention and Screening

- Adequate dietary intake
- Serial monitoring of patients at risk
- Chemistry panel on admission to the hospital
- Potassium supplementation with loop diuretics
- Use of potassium-sparing diuretics
- Use of ACE-I

Assessment

History
- Skeletal muscle cramps
- Muscular weakness
- Shortness of breath
- Constipation
- Abdominal distention
- Exercise intolerance
- Palpitations
- Worsening diabetes control, polyuria

Physical Examination
- Tachycardia, tachypnea may be present
- Hypertension
- Hypotension
- Muscle weakness, flaccid paralysis
- Depressed or absent deep tendon reflexes
- Cardiac rhythm changes

Diagnostic Studies
- Chemistry panel: potassium < 3.5 mEq/L
  - Hyponatremia
    - Suggests thiazide use or marked volume depletion from GI losses
  - Hypernatremia
    - Suggests nephrogenic diabetes from longstanding hypokalemia
    - Presence of primary aldosteronism, especially if hypertension present
  - Increased serum bicarbonate suggests mineralocorticoid excess
  - Serum magnesium level is low (< 1.6 mg/dL) in up to 40% of hypokalemic patients.
  - Hyperglycemia
    - Suggests longstanding hypokalemia may be severe enough to impair glucose tolerance
- Creatine kinase
  - Hypokalemia may produce rhabdomyolysis.
    - Especially in the setting of alcoholism
- Spot urine potassium
  - Urinary potassium concentration: if low, < 20 mEq/L, hypokalemia is from extrarenal losses
  - Urinary potassium concentration: if high, > 40 mEq/L, hypokalemia is from renal loss
- Transtubular K^+ gradient (TTKG) is a rapid means of evaluating net potassium excretion: TTKG = (POsm × UPotassium) / (PPotassium × UOSM)
  - Hypokalemia with a level > 4 suggests renal potassium loss with increased distal K^+ secretion.
  - Plasma renin and aldosterone levels may be helpful in making the differential diagnosis.
  - Presence of nonabsorbed ions (bicarbonate) increases the TTKG.
- 24-hour urine potassium
  - A urine creatinine should also be collected to compare for accuracy.
  - < 20 mEq/L/24 hours indicates appropriate renal excretion and suggests an extrarenal cause for potassium issue
  - > 20 mEq/L/24 hours suggests the hypokalemia is the result of renal wasting
- Electrocardiogram
  - T wave flattening
  - Presence of U waves

Differential Diagnosis

- Hypophosphatemia
- Renovascular hypertension
- Gitelman's syndrome

- Liddle's syndrome
- Bartter syndrome
- See Etiology

Management

Nonpharmacologic Treatment
- High-potassium diet
    - Fruits
    - Raisins
    - Apricots
    - Figs
    - Dried mixed fruit
    - Banana
    - Grains
        - Soya flour
        - Bran wheat
        - Wheatgerm
        - Sultana bran
    - Meats
        - Veal
    - Vegetables
        - Tomato puree
        - Currants
        - Potatoes
- Four goals treatment
    - Identify cause and stop potassium loss
    - Replenish potassium losses
    - Monitor for toxicity from hypokalemia
        - Usually cardiac
    - Prevent further episodes.
- Surgical intervention
    - Required for underlying cause
        - Renal artery stenosis
        - Adrenal adenoma
        - Intestinal obstruction
        - Villous adenoma

Pharmacologic Treatment
- For every decrease in serum K^+ of 1 mEq/L, the estimated potassium deficit is 200 to 400 mEq.
    - This estimation is affected by many factors and may over- or underestimate needs.
- IV potassium
    - For those unable to take oral potassium
    - Symptomatic patients
    - May be added to IV infusion
    - Peripheral vein—maximum concentration is 40 mEq/L

- Central venous access—maximum concentration is 60 mEq/L
- IV piggyback
  - Peripheral vein: 10 mEq/hr
  - Central venous access: 10 to 20 mEq/hr
- Monitor serum potassium levels
- Oral potassium
  - Safest and easiest method
  - May cause GI upsent
  - In the form of potassium chloride
    - 10 to 40 mEq per day in 1 to 2 doses
    - Available in extended release for maintenance dosing
- Correct low serum magnesium
- Potassium-sparing diuretics
  - Spironolactone
  - Amiloride
  - Eplerenone

Special Considerations

- Patients should discontinue strenuous exercise if muscle cramping or pain develops because this could indicate hypokalemia with possible development of rhadomyolysis.
- Body deficits do not correlate well with serum K+ levels because potassium is an intracellular cation.
- Continuous telemetry monitoring to detect cardiac involvement
- Search for underlying cause.
- Hypokalemia contributes to the development of hepatic encephalopathy associated with cirrhosis.

When to Consult, Refer, or Hospitalize

- Refer to endocrinology if Cushing's syndrome, primary hyperaldosteronism, glucocorticoid remediable hypertension, or congenital adrenal hyperplasia is suspected.
- Refer to nephrology for unexplained urinary losses of potassium.
- Psychiatry consult for eating disorders
- Cardiology consult for cardiac involvement
- Critical care consult if ICU required
- Admit patient with severe or symptomatic hypokalemia requiring:
  - Cardiac monitoring
  - Frequent laboratory testing
  - Frequent administration of potassium supplements
- General surgery referral if warranted

Follow-up

Expected Outcomes
- Resolution of the hypokalemic state
- Monitor the patient's laboratory values after resolution to determine if a daily supplement is needed and if the dosage is adequate.
- Prognosis depends on the underlying cause.

Complications
- Atrial and ventricular dysrhythmias
- Hypertension and hypertensive end-organ damage
- Muscle weakness
- Depressed deep-tendon reflexes
- Rhabdomyolysis
- Hypokalemia decreases insulin release and decreases peripheral insulin sensitivity.

HYPERKALEMIA

Description

- Hyperkalemia is defined as an elevated serum potassium level with various high values reported in literature ranging from > 5.0 to 5.3 mEq/L.
- See Hypokalemia.

Etiology

- Increased intake
  - Rare
  - High-potassium, low-sodium diet
  - Ingestion of potassium supplements
  - TPN administration
  - Dietary salt substitutes
  - Penicillin potassium therapy
- Decreased excretion
  - Decreased GFR, especially below 15 to 20 mL/min in acute or chronic renal failure
  - Medications
    - ACE-I
    - Potassium-sparing diurectis
    - NSAIDS
    - Angiotensin receptor blockers (ARBs)
    - Cyclosporin ot tacrolimus
    - Heparin
    - Ketoconazole

- Type IV renal tubular acidosis (RTA)
- Disorders of steroid metabolism
  - Addison's disease
- Kidney transplant
- Interstitial nephritis
- Systemic lupus erythematosus (SLE)
- Sickle cell disease
- Obstructive nephropathy
- Shifting of potassium from the intracellular to the extracellular compartment
  - Metabolic acidosis
    - Does not occur in lactic acidosis, since the organic acid can move across the cell membrane
  - Excessive release of K^+
    - Burns
    - Rhabdomyolysis
    - Hemolysis
    - Severe infection
    - Internal bleeding
    - Vigorous exercise
  - Hypertonicity
  - Insulin deficiency
  - Medications
    - Succinylcholine
    - Arginine
    - Digitalis toxicity
    - β-adrenergic antagonists
- Miscellaneous—pseudohyperkalemia
  - Hemolysis during venipuncture (serum level normal)
  - Marked leukocytosis or thrombocytosis with release of intracellular potassium
  - Repeated fist clenching during venipuncture
  - Specimen drawn from an arm with a K^+ infusion

Incidence and Demographics

- Rare in the general population of healthy individuals
- In the hospitalized patient, the incidence is 1% to 10%.
- Medications are a factor in about 75% of cases involving a hospitalized patient.
- Hyperkalemia in the hospitalized patient is an independent risk factor for death.
- Men are more prone to hyperkalemia than women.
- Individuals at risk for rhabdomyolysis
  - Military recruits
  - Patients with sickle cell trait
  - Drug abuse

Risk Factors

- Extremes of age
- Acute and chronic kidney disease
- Genitourinary disease
- Cancer
- Diabetes
- Polypharmacy
- Use of potassium-sparing medications
- Use of ACE-I
- Male gender
- Congestive heart failure
- Kidney transplant recipients
- Military recruits
- Sickle cell trait
- Abuse of illicit drugs

Prevention and Screening

- Low-potassium diet as needed
- Careful serial monitoring of serum chemistry for at-risk patients
- Avoid medications that raise serum levels in at-risk patients.
- Patient education regarding medications and foods that can potentially raise serum K+ levels
- Periodic review of at-risk patients' medications

Assessment

History
- Symptoms of underlying disorder
- Muscle weakness may progress to paralysis.
- Fatigue
- History of eating disorder
- Use of salt substitutes
- Dietary review
- Medication review
- History of renal disease, diabetes
- Risk factors for rhabdomyolysis
    - Military recruit
    - Alcoholism
    - Sickle cell trait

Physical Examination
- Bradycardia because of heart block
- Tachypnea from muscle weakness
- Signs from underlying condition

Diagnostic Studies
- Serum chemistry
  - Elevated potassium
  - May see elevated BUN and creatinine in renal disease
- 24-hour urine for creatinine clearance
- Estimate GFR
- Measure urine potassium
  - < 20 mEq: impaired renal excretion
- Urine osmolality
  - TTKG: see Hypokalemia
- Complete blood count
- Paired serum renin and aldosterone levels to identify primary or secondary hypoaldosteronism
- Electrocardiogram
  - Peaked T waves
  - Widened QRS complex
  - Flat or absent P waves
  - Fusion of QRS and T wave to form sine wave

Differential Diagnosis

- Pseudohyperkalemia

Management

- Treatment is based on the rapidity of the rise of K+, and the level and evidence of cardiotoxicity
- Five goals:
  - Evaluate for toxicity.
  - Decrease potassium intake.
  - Increase potassium uptake into the cells.
  - Increase potassium excretion.
  - Identify the cause.

Nonpharmacologic Treatment
- Low-potassium diet
  - If hospitalized: 2-gram potassium or low-potassium tube feeding and adjustment in TPN infusion
  - See Hypokalemia section for foods high in potassium.
  - Low-potassium foods
    - Fruits
      - Apples
      - Grapes
      - Watermelon

- Vegetables
  - Alfalfa sprouts
  - Collards
  - Lettuce
  - Popcorn
  - Leeks
- Meat
  - Turkey breast
  - Chicken breast

* Emergent dialysis for patients unresponsive to therapy with life-threatening symptoms or end-stage renal patients not responsive to conservative management

Pharmacologic Treatment
* Normal ECG
  * Loop diuretic
  * Sodium polystyrene resin to increase GI excretion
  * Cardiotoxicity
  * Calcium gluconate 10%, 10 mL over 1 to 2 minutes, may repeat in 3 to 5 minutes in an attempt to normalize ECG
  * Regular insulin 10 units IV over 2 minutes
  * Glucose 50 g if euglycemic
  * Will see effect in 15 to 30 minutes
  * Albuterol via nebulizer over 10 minutes
  * Sodium bicarbonate 50 mEq IV over 1 to 2 minutes
  * Hemodialysis

Special Considerations

* Often occurs in patients with advanced kidney disease but can develop in those with normal renal function
* Generally, the physical examination does not alert the clinician to hyperkalemia unless bradycardia, muscle weakness or tenderness, or both are present.

When to Consult, Refer, or Hospitalize

* Refer to nephrology when renal function is impaired.
* Transplant specialist should be consulted for posttransplant patients—may require adjustment of immunosuppression medications.
* Cardiology consult for cardiac involvement
* Critical care consult if ICU required
* Admit for K^+ levels > 6.0 mEq/L, ECG changes associated with hyperkalemia, or concurrent illness requiring hospitalization

Follow-up

Expected Outcomes
- Resolution of the hyperkalemia
- Once-monthly evaluation of potassium levels
- Prognosis is good for patients with a defined and transient cause.
- Patients with risk factors may have recurrent episodes and require frequent monitoring.
- Patient education regarding:
  - Dietary sources of potassium
  - Medications that affect potassium levels
  - Avoidance of volume depletion

Complications
- Mild ECG changes to cardiac arrest
- Failure to control hyperkalemia
- Hypokalemia from overzealous therapy
- Hypocalcemia from excessive bicarbonate therapy
- Hypo- or hyperglycemia complicating glucose and insulin administration
- Volume depletion, metabolic alkalosis, acute kidney injury, hypomagnesemia, and hypophosphatemia because of aggressive use of loop diuretics
- Colon perforation from sodium polystyrene resin administration

HYPOCALCEMIA

Description

- Hypocalcemia is defined as a serum calcium concentration < 8.6 mg/dL or an ionized calcium level < 4.5 mg/dL.
- Since some calcium is bound to albumin in plasma, the serum calcium concentration can be corrected upward 0.8 mg/dL for each 1 g/dL decrease in serum albumin at a plasma pH of 7.4—known as corrected calcium:
  - Corrected calcium (mg/dL) = Ca^2 (mg/dL) = 0.8 (4 − albumin [g/dL])
- Ionized calcium is physiologically active and not bound to albumin—ionized calcium is not corrected.
- Presentations vary from asymptomatic to life-threatening.
- The calcium ion is required for normal cellular functioning.
  - Neuromuscular signaling
  - Cardiac contractility
  - Hormone secretion
  - Blood coagulation

Etiology

- Hypoparathyroidism (post-thyroidectomy or -parathyroidectomy)
- Pseudohypopathryoidism
  - End-organ resistance to the effects of parathyroid hormone (PTH)
  - Type I
    - Ia
      - Decrease in the Gs alpha-protein
      - Features of Albright hereditary osteodystrophy disorder
        - Short stature
        - Mental retardation
        - Round face
        - Brachymetacarpia
        - Brachymetatarsia
        - Subcutaneous bone formation
    - Ib
      - Normal Gs alpha-protein
      - Hormonal resistance to PTH
    - Ic
      - Resistance to multiple hormonal receptors with normal Gs alpha-protein
    - Type II
      - PTH raises cAMP normally but fails to increase levels of serum calcium or urinary phosphate excretion
        - Check for vitamin D deficiency
- Hypomagnesemia
- Pancreatitis—seen in 40% to 70% of acute pancreatitis cases
- Vitamin D deficiency
  - Chronic renal failure
  - Disturbance in fat absorption
    - Hepatobiliary disease
    - Dysfunction of the pancreas
    - Enteritis
    - Jejunoileal bypass
  - Malnutrition
    - Especially at extremes of age
- Chronic alcoholism
- Medications
  - Phenytoin
  - Cisplatin
  - Estrogen therapy
- Infusion of citrate, phosphate, or calcium-free albumin

Incidence and Prevelance

- Less common than hypercalcemia
- See most commonly with acute and chronic renal failure
- Occurs with equal frequency in both genders

Risk Factors

- Extremes of age
- Chronic renal failure
- History of thyroidectomy
- Alcoholism
- Malnutrition
- Eating disorders
- History of small bowel bypass surgery
- Pancreatitis
- See Etiology

Prevention and Screening

- Patient education regarding dietary sources of calcium and early signs of hypocalcemia
  - Paresthesias
  - Muscle weakness

Assessment

History
- Altered mental status
  - Depression
  - Anxiety
  - Confusion
- Tremors
- Ataxia
- Dystonia
- Weakness

Physical Examination
- Chevostek's sign
  - Facial twitch with tapping of ipsilateral facial nerve
- Trousseau's sign
  - Carpal spasm with brachial artery occlusion with a blood pressure for 3 minutes
- Dry skin
- Brittle hair and nails
- Seizures

Diagnostic Studies
- Serum chemistry
  - Low serum calcium
  - May see low serum magnesium—occurs in about 20% of patients
- Ionized calcium
  - Used frequently in the ICU for guidance with replacement therapy
- Serum albumin
  - Use for corrected calcium value

- Electrocardiogram
  - Prolonged QTc
  - Nonspecific T wave changes

Differential Diagnosis

- Acute or chronic kidney disease
- Anorexia nervosa
- Hyperparathyroidism
- Hyperphosphatemia
- Hypoalbuminemia
- Hypoparathyroidism
- Metabolic alkalosis
- Osteoporosis
- Acute pancreatitis
- Tuberculosis

Management

Nonpharmacologic Treatment
- Parathyroidectomy for patients with severe secondary hyperparathyroidism and renal osteodystrophy
- Diet rich in calcium
- Continuous telemetry monitoring if cardiac involvement present

Pharmacologic Treatment
- Identify the underlying cause.
- Acute
  - Calcium gluconate 10%, 1 to 2 ampules (93 mg/10 mL) in 50 to 100 mL of
  - D5w over 10 minutes *or*
  - Calcium chloride 10% (273 mg/10 mL) in 50 to 100 mL over 10 minutes—infuse via central line
  - Monitor calcium levels every 6 hours if patient symptomatic to guide therapy
    - If serum albumin is low, monitor ionized calcium—common in the ICU
- Chronic
  - Treatment depends on the cause
  - Calcium carbonate or other calcium salt
    - 2 to 3 g elemental calcium/day in divided doses
  - Hypoparathyroidism
    - 0.5 to 2 mcg of calcitriol or 1-alpha-hydroxyvitamin D_3
    - May add a thiazide diuretic for the hypercalcemic effects
  - Dialysis patients
    - Many patients are hypercalcemic; however, postparathyroidectomy it may be difficult to maintain adequate calcium.
    - Oral calcium as described previously
    - Calcitriol enhances the absorption of calcium.

- Vitamin D deficiency
  - Oral calcium as described previously
  - Califerol 750 to 3,000 mcg/day
  - Calcifediol 50 to 200 mcg/day
  - Calcitriol 0.5 to 2 mcg/day

Special Considerations

- Often mistaken as a neurological disorder
- Evaluate for decreased parathyroid hormone or vitamin D depletion
- If the serum calcium is low, but the ionized calcium level is normal, then calcium metabolism is usually normal.

When to Consult, Refer, or Hospitalize

- Refer patients to an endocrinologist or nephrologist if they have hypoparathyroidism, familial hypocalcemia, or chronic kidney disease.
- Critical care consult if ICU required
- Admit patients with tetany, cardiac dysrhythmias, extreme muscle weakness, altered mental status, or a combination of these.

Follow-up

Expected Outcomes
- Resolution of hypocalcemia
- Serial measurements to evaluate therapy

Complications
- Seizures
- Cardiac ventricular dysrhythmias because of the prolonged QTc
- Muscle weakness
- Altered mental status

HYPERCALCEMIA

Description

- Occurs when there are increased serum total and ionized calcium concentrations.
- Value > 10.2 mg/dL total calcium or > 5.3 mg/dL for ionized calcium
- Symptoms usually occur when level is > 12 mg/dL.

Etiology

- Increased intake or absorption
  - Vitamin D or A excess
  - Milk-alkali syndrome
    - Calcium ingestion for osteoporosis
- Endocrine disorders
  - Primary hyperparathyroidism
  - Secondary or tertiary hyperparathyroidism
  - Acromegaly
  - Adrenal insufficiency
  - Thyrotoxicosis
  - Pheochromocytoma
- Malignancy
  - Ovarian, renal, and lung cancers produce PTH-related proteins
  - Multiple myeloma
  - Lymphoma
- Miscellaneous
  - Thiazide diuretics
  - Granulomatous disease
    - Sarcoidosis
    - Tuberculosis
  - Paget's disease (bone)
  - Immobilization
  - Familial hypocalcemic hypercalcemia
  - Kidney transplant
  - Lithium
  - Hypophosphatemia
  - End-stage renal disease, dialysis

Incidence and Prevalence

- Relatively common and is often mild, but may be longstanding
- Incidence of hyperparathyroidism alone is about 1 to 2 cases per 1,000 adults.
- Higher incidence in men than in women but difference decreases with age
- Hypercalcemia from all causes increases with advancing age

Risk Factors

- Elderly
- Male gender
- Presence of malignancy
- Use of thiazide diuretics
- Osteoporosis
- Renal disease

Prevention and Screening

- Educate patients regarding calcium and vitamin D supplements.
- Early detection of underlying cause
- Monitor calcium levels in high-risk patients because mild hypercalcemia is often asymptomatic.
- Educate high-risk patients about signs and symptoms of hypercalcemia.

Assessment

History
- Focus on the duration and presence of a malignancy
- CNS
  - Lethargy
  - Weakness
  - Confusion
  - Depression
  - Coma
- Renal
  - Polyuria
    - Can result in nephrogenic diabetes insipidous
  - Nocturia
  - Dehydration
  - Renal stones
  - Hematuria
- GI
  - Constipation
  - Nausea
  - Anorexia
  - Pancreatitis
  - Gastric ulcer
  - Peptic ulcer disease
- Cardiac effects
  - Ventricular ectopy
  - Idioventricular rhythm
  - Syncope from dysrhythmias

Physical Examination
- CNS
  - Confusion
  - Hypotonia
  - Depressed tendon reflexes
  - Paresis
  - Coma
- Renal
  - Volume depletion
  - Renal failure

- GI
  - Fecal impaction
  - Signs of pancreatitis
  - Signs of malignancy
    - Enlarged liver or masses
- Cardiac
  - Hypertension with chronic hypercalcemia
  - Hypotension with volume depletion
  - Shortened QT interval

Diagnostic Studies
- Serum chemistry
  - Elevated calcium to low phosphate concentration of > 33 to 1 suggests primary hyperparathyroidism.
  - Low serum chloride with high bicarbonate and elevated BUN and creatinine may indicate milk-alkali syndrome.
  - Severe hypercalcemia: > 15 mg/dL, usually occurs in malignancy
- Parathyroid level
- Thyroid panel
  - TSH
  - Free T4 level
- Vitamin D levels
  - 25-OH D_3
  - 1,25-$(OH)_2$ D_3
- Urinary calcium
  - > 200 mg/d of urinary calcium excretion suggest hypercalciuria
  - < 100 mg/d indicates hypocalciuria
  - Hypocalciuric patients may easily develop hypercalcemia in the presence of dehydration.
- Chest radiograph
  - May uncover malignancy or granulomatous disease
- Mammograms to rule out breast cancer
- Bone radiograph
- In primary hyperparathyroidism the following may be used to assist with preoperative localization:
  - CT scan
  - Ultrasound
  - MRI
  - Radionuclide imaging

Differential Diagnosis

- Hyperkalemia
- Hypermagnesemia
- Hypernatremia
- Hyperparathyroidism
- Hyperphosphatemia

Management

Nonpharmacologic Treatment
- Discontinue calcium and vitamin D supplements if applicable.
- Reduce calcium intake to 750 to 1,000 mg/d.

Pharmacologic Treatment
- Acute: Until the underlying cause is identified and treated, renal excretion of calcium is achieved with aggressive hydration and diuresis.
- IV normal saline to restore volume and induce diuresis
    - At least 200 mL/hr
    - Calcitonin, 4 international units (IU)/kg every 12 hours subcutaneously or IM
        - May increase to 8 IU/kg *or*
    - IV biphosphates—treatment of choice with malignancy
        - Pamidronate: 90 mg IV infused over 24 hours—do not repeat for 7 days
        - Etidronate: 7.5 mg/kg in 250 mL NS over 2 to 3 hours for 3 days
    - Plicamycin: 25 mcg/kg in 1 liter of D5W or NS over 24 hours
    - Furosemide: 40 to 80 mg IV every 8 hours to maintain urine output of 150 to 200 mL/hr
        - Use with NS or ½ NS infusion
- Hemodialysis with a low Ca^+ bath
- Chronic
    - Prednisone: 40 to 80 mg/d
        - Sarcoidosis
        - Elevated levels of vitamin D
        - Lymphoma
    - Furosemide: 40 to 80 mg p.o. twice daily
    - Along with a 6 to 8 g sodium diet

Special Considerations

- Hypercalciuria is usually seen before hypercalcemia.
- Asymptomatic, mild hypercalcemia (> 11 mg/dL) is usually the result of hyperparathyroidism, whereas more severe hypercalcemia (> 14 mg/dL) is often the result of malignancy.
- With end-stage renal disease, if dialysis patients don't receive adequate supplementation of calcium and active vitamin D, hypocalcemia may develop; however, hypercalcemia may develop with severe secondary hyperparathyroidism, elevated PTH levels, and release of calcium from the bone.

When to Consult, Refer, or Hospitalize

- Refer to oncology, nephrology, or endocrinology, depending on the underlying cause.
- Patients diagnosed with granulomatous diseases may require referral to an infectious disease specialist, rheumatologist, or pulmonologist.
- Cardiology for dysrhythmias

- Critical care consult if ICU is required
- Admit for symptomatic or severe hypercalemia
- Unexplained hypercalcemia associated with acute kidney injury or malignancy, which may require urgent treatment

Follow-up

Expected Outcomes
- Depends on the underlying cause and the prognosis associated with it
- Resolution of the hypercalcemia
- Hypercalcemia is frequently undiagnosed; all cases need investigation.
- Any sudden rise in calcium levels should prompt further work-up.

Complications
- Hypophosphatemia
- Nephrolithiasis
- Ectopic calcification
- Headache
- Hypertension
- Confusion
- Acute pancreatitis
- Nephrogenic diabetes insipidus
- Cholelithiasis
- Corneal opacity
- Cholelithiasis
- Cardiac arrest
- Renal failure
- QRS prolongation
- QT shortening

HYPOMAGNESEMIA

Description

- Defined as serum magnesium level < 1.6 mEq/L
- Serum magnesium may not be decreased even if there is a depletion of magnesium
- Magnesium is the fourth most abundant cation.
- Functions in energy transfer, storage and use; protein, carbohydrate, and fat metabolism; maintenance of normal cell membrane function; and regulation of PTH secretion

Etiology

- Renal losses
  - Diuretics
    - Loop and thiazides
    - Causes hypomagnesemia in 20% to 40% of patients
  - Chronic alcohol use
    - Seen in about 30% of patients
  - Nephrotoxicity from medications
    - Aminoglycosides
    - Amphotericin B
    - Cisplatin
  - Endocrine
    - Primary aldosteronism from increased renal flow
    - Hypoparathyroidism and hyperthyroidism from renal wasting
  - GI loss
    - Diarrhea
    - Laxatives
    - Malabsorption
    - Inflammatory bowel disease
- Insufficient intake
  - Related to alcohol abuse
  - Protein malnutrition
- Intracellular uptake
  - Alcohol withdrawal
    - Seen in 80% to 85% of patients
  - Acute insulin therapy in diabetic ketoacidosis (DKA)
- Miscellaneous
  - Extracellular volume expansion
  - Pregnancy
  - Excessive lactation
  - Hungry bone syndrome

Incidence and Demographics

- 2% in the general population
- Occurs in 10% to 20% of hospitalized patients
  - 50% to 60% in ICU patients
- 30% to 80% in those who abuse alcohol
- 25% in patients with diabetes
- Incidence equal between genders

Risk Factors

- Hospitalization
- Diabetes mellitus
- Inflammatory bowel disease
- Diuretic use
- Pregnancy
- Malnutrition
- History of bowel resection or small bowel bypass
- Alcoholism
- Thyroid disease

Prevention and Screening

- Education of high-risk patients regarding signs and symptoms of hypomagnesemia
- Daily serial monitoring of lab values in hospitalized patients
- Oral supplementation for patients who do not have a correctable cause
- Maintenance of magnesium-rich diet (see below), eliminating alcohol consumption, and maintaining tight control of diabetes

Assessment

History
- Muscle weakness
- Dysarthria and dysphagia
- Disorentiation
- Psychosis
- Vertigo

Physical Examination
- Trousseau's sign
- Chvostek's sign
- Muscle fasciculations
- Tremors
- Seizures
- Hyperactive deep tendon reflexes
- Ataxia
- Nystagmus

Diagnostic Studies
- Serum chemistry
  - Magnesium < 1.6 mEq/l
  - With severe hypomagnesemia, serum calcium and potassium may be decreased
- Urinary Mg^{++} < 3 mEq/l in 24 hours
  - Indicates deficiency

- Electrocardiogram
  - Prolonged QTc interval
  - Atrial and ventricular dysrhythmias

Differential Diagnosis

- Hypocalemia
- Hypokalemia

Management

Nonpharmacologic Treatment
- Magnesium-rich diet
  - Meat
  - Green vegetables
  - Dairy products
  - Nuts
  - Cereals
  - Seafood

Pharmacologic Treatment
- If patient is symptomatic, is hypcalcemic, or unable to take p.o.
  - 1 to 2 grams of magnesium sulfate
  - May follow with further repletion in 1 liter of IV fluids over 24 hours
- By mouth:
  - Magnesium chloride 100 mg: 2 tablets 3 times daily
  - Magnesium oxide 400 mg: 1 or 2 tablets daily
  - Magnesium lactate, extended release: 2 caps twice daily
- In patients with CKD, replace with caution: 50% to 70% reduction may be required to avoid hypermagnesemia.
- Monitor serum magnesium levels at least daily.

Special Considerations

- Most laboratories measure total serum content of magnesium; however, 30% of magnesium is bound to albumin. Therefore, low albumin states may lead to spuriously low magnesium levels.
- The major role of magnesium occurs intracellularly; the extracellular fluid contains only 2% of total body magnesium and may not always reflect the intracellular magnesium level. Currently, there is no accurate test for intracellular magnesium.

When to Consult, Refer, or Hospitalize

- Refer to endocrinology if underlying cause is endocrine in nature.
- Nephrology consult for patients with chronic kidney disease
- Critical care team consult if ICU required
- Admit symptomatic patients requiring IV therapy.

Follow-up

Expected Outcomes
- Resolution of hypomagnesemia
- Prognosis is excellent once the low level is corrected.
- Symptoms are reversible with treatment.

Complications
- Seizures
- Paroxysmal atrial and ventricular dysrhythmias
- Psychosis
- Nephrocalcinosis
- Hypokalemic distal renal tubular acidosis
- Laryngeal spasm

HYPERMAGNESEMIA

Description

- Defined as serum magnesium level > 2.2 mEq/L
- Usually asymptomatic until levels > 4.0 mEq/L
- Occurs rarely because the kidney is very effective in maintaining magnesium homeostasis

Etiology

- Impaired renal function
- Continued magnesium intake in the presence of renal failure
  - Magnesium sulfate
  - Magnesium hydroxide
  - Magnesium citrate
- IV magnesium administered for preeclampsia
- Decreased GI elimination
  - Narcotics
  - Anticholinergics
  - Bowel obstruction
  - Chronic constipation

- Tumor lysis syndrome
- Adrenal insufficiency
- Rhabdomyolysis
- Milk-alkali syndrome
- Hypothyroidism
- Hypoparathyroidism
- Malignancy with skeletal muscle involvement
- Extracelluar volume contraction

Incidence and Demographics

- Occurs rarely in the United States

Risk Factors

- Exogenous intake of magnesium
- Presence of thyroid disorders
- Narcotic use
- Dehydration
- Adrenal insufficiency
- Preeclampsia

Prevention and Screening

- Daily magnesium level in hospitalized patients at risk
- Educate patients regarding medications that increase magnesium levels:
  - Antacids
  - Laxatives
  - Lithium toxicity

Assessment

History
- Weakness that may progress to paralysis
- Lethargy
- Nausea and vomiting

Physical Examination
- Hypotension
- Diminished or absent deep tendon reflexes—occurs with magnesium levels to 4 to 5 mEq/L
- Weakness to flaccid paralysis with serum Mg++ levels of 8 to 10 mEq/L

Diagnostic Studies
- Serum chemistry
  - Elevated magnesium
  - BUN and creatinine may indicate renal impairment
    - Serum magnesium levels rise when creatinine clearance is < 30 mL/min
  - Hyperkalemia and hypercalcemia may be present
- Creatine phosphokinase or urine myoglobin if rhabdomyolysis is suspected
- Thyroid function tests
- Electrocardiogram
  - Lengthening of PR interval
  - Widening of QRS
  - Complete heart block

Differential Diagnosis

- Adrenal insufficiency or crisis
- Hypercalcemia
- Hyperkalemia
- Hypoparathyroidism
- Hypothyroidism
  - Myxedema coma
- Acute or chronic renal failure
- Rhabdomyolysis
- Lithium toxicity

Management

Nonpharmacologic Treatment
- Stop magnesium intake
- Hemodialysis
  - Consider for symptomatic hypermagnesemia > 4 mEq/L

Pharmacologic Treatment
- IV fluids and diuretics
  - Promote increased excretion by the kidney
  - Normal saline or lactated Ringer's
  - Furosemide
- Calcium
  - 100 to 200 mg 10% solution, continuous infusion, 2 to 4 mg/kg/hr
- Glucose and insulin: may help promote magnesium entry into the cells
  - 10 units IV regular insulin and 50 mL D50W bolus
- ECG changes
  - Calcium gluconate 10% IV 10 to 20 mL IV push over 3 to 5 minutes
  - Furosemide 40 mg with ½ NS at 50 to 100 mL/hr

Special Considerations

- Acute rises in serum magnesium levels are more symptomatic than slow increases.
- Long-term use of magnesium hydroxide and magnesium sulfate should be avoided in patients with advanced CKD.

When to Consult, Refer, or Hospitalize

- Consults are driven by the underlying disorder
  - Renal consult if hemodialysis is required
  - Critical care team consult if ICU required
- Hospitalize for symptomatic hypermagnesemia.

Follow-up

Expected Outcomes
- Resolution of hypermagnesemia
- Prognosis is good once normal levels are restored.

Complications
- Related to level of magnesium
  - 4 mEq/L: hyporeflexia
  - > 5 mEq/L: prolonged AV conduction
  - > 10 mEq/L: complete heart block
  - > 13 mEq/L: cardiac arrest
- Hypotension
- Respiratory failure

HYPOPHOSPHATEMIA

Description

- Defined as a serum phosphorus concentration < 2.5 mg/dL
- Considered severe when phosphorus level is < 1.4 mg/dL
- Major component of the skeleton and provides mineral strength to bone
- Integral component of the nucleic acids that compose DNA and RNA
- Phospate bonds of ATP carry the energy for cellular functions.

Etiology

- Inadequate intake
  - Dietary deficiency
    - Eating disorders
  - Alteration in GI absorption
    - Alcoholism
    - Multifactorial
    - Phosphorus deficient TPN
    - Malabsorption
    - Crohn's disease
    - Celiac sprue
    - Steatorrhea
    - Chronic diarrhea
    - Vitamin D deficiency
- Cellular uptake
  - Acute respiratory alkalosis in association with acute alcohol withdrawal
  - Insulin treatment for diabetic ketoacidosis, refeeding or use of TPN
  - Hungry bone syndrome
  - Post kidney transplant
  - Burns
  - Metabolic acidosis
    - Salicylate poisoning
- Renal losses
  - Diuretics
  - Hyperparathyroidism
  - Hypokalemic nephropathy
  - DKA
    - Osmotic diuresis
  - Renal tubule defects
    - Fanconi's syndrome
  - Genetic renal disorders
    - X-linked hypophosphatemic rickets
    - Autosomal-dominant hypophosphatemic rickets
    - Vitamin D–resistant rickets
  - Acquired phosphate wasting syndromes
    - Vitamin D deficiency
    - Extracelluar volume expansion
    - Oncogenic osteomalacia
- Medication
  - Large quantities of antacids, because of phosphate binding
  - Phosphate binders
    - Aluminum salts
    - Calcium salts
    - Polymer gels

Incidence and Demographics

- In the general hospitalized population, it is seen in 1% to 5% of patients.
  - The percentage is increased in patients with alcoholism, DKA, and sepsis—incidence increases to 40% to 80% in these patients.
- Seen in a significant number of patients post partial hepatectomy for transplantation—up to 55%—and in acute hepatic failure
- Is present in about 30% of kidney transplant patients
- Has also been associated with metabolic syndrome
- X-linked hypophosphatemic rickets is more prevalent in White and males.
- May occur at any age
  - Acquired hypophosphatemia usually occurs in late adolescence to adulthood.
  - With aging, is commonly related to alcoholism, tumors, malabsorption, or vitamin D deficiency

Risk Factors

- Alcoholism
- Diabetes mellitus
- Sepsis
- Hepatic failure
- Kidney transplant
- Genetic predisposition
- Antacid use
- Use of phosphate binders
- Renal failure
- Diuretic use
- Hyperparathyroidism
- COPD
- Asthma
- Metabolic syndrome

Prevention and Screening

- Patients with underlying eating disorders require counseling and dietary therapy.
- Educate patients regarding a balanced diet
- Close monitoring of high-risk patients, including those who have poor socioeconomic status, dental problems, or swallowing difficulties
- Instruct patients to avoid using large quantities of antacids.
- Glucose control in patients with diabetes
- Include phosphate in TPN.

Assessment

History
- Irritability
- Confusion
- Paresthesias
- Diplopia
- Dyasrthria
- Dysphagia
- Weakness of trunk or extremities—especially large muscle groups

Physical Examination
- Muscle weakness
- Diminished respiratory rate and tidal volume
- Hypotension
- Cardiac compromise—impaired contractility and decreased stroke volume
  - Ventricular dysrhythmias
- Rhabdomyolysis—severe levels < 1 mg/dL or less

Diagnostic Studies
- Serum chemistry
  - Phosphorus < 2.5 mg/dL
- Complete blood count
  - Hemolytic anemia
- Creatine kinsase (CK) and urinary myoglobin if rhabdomyolysis is suspected
- Urine phosphate excretion
  - > 20 mg/dL suggests inappropriate renal phosphate loss
  - Tubular phosphate reabsorption can be assessed by TmP/GFR:

    $$\frac{TmP}{GFR} = Serum\ Pi - \frac{(UPi \times UV)}{GFR}$$

    Pi = serum phosphate concentration
    UPi = urine phosphate concentration
    UV = urine volume

    Normal range is 2.5 to 4.5 mg/dL—lower values indicate renal losses (McPhee & Papadakis, 2011, p. 856)
- Serum PTH
- Arterial blood gases
  - Metabolic acidosis
  - Respiratory alkalosis

Differential Diagnosis

- Alcoholic ketoacidosis
- Anxiety
- Diabetic ketoacidosis
- Guillain-Barré syndrome

- Hyperparathyroidism
- Hyperventilation syndrome

Management

Nonpharmacologic Treatment
- Adequate dietary intake

Pharmacologic Treatment
- Oral replacement
  - Mixtures of sodium and potassium phosphate to provide 18 to 32 mmol per day
- IV replacement
  - 9 to 10 mmol/12 hours to raise the level > 1 mg/dL
  - Decrease the infusion if hypotension occurs.
  - Monitor phosphorus, calcium, and potassium every 6 to 12 hours.
  - Result of phosphate supplementation is not predictable.

Special Considerations

- Magnesium deficiency is often present and should be treated.
- Cautious replacement in advanced CKD, hypoparathyroidism, tissue damage and necrosis, and hypercalcemia
- When hyperglycemia is treated, phosphate is shifted intracellularly with glucose.

When to Consult, Refer, or Hospitalize

- Refer to endocrinology or nephrology for refractory hypophosphatemia with increased urinary losses.
- Gastroenterology consult for GI malabsorption
- Critical care team consult if ICU is required
- Admit patients with severe or refractory hypophosphatemia when IV supplementation is required.

Follow-up

Expected Outcomes
- Resolution of hypophosphatemia
- Equilibration with IV replacement therapy may lead to recurrence; therefore, serial monitoring and replacement may be needed over the following 48 hours.
  - Monitor the level every 6 hours to guide further therapy.

Complications
- Mild
  - Usually no complications
- Moderate (1.0 to 2.5 mg/dL)
  - Respiratory muscle depression
    - Can deter weaning from mechanical ventilation
  - Impaired cardiac output
  - Mild metabolic acidosis
  - Hypercalciuria
- Acute hypophosphatemic syndrome (≤ 1 mg/dL)
  - Potentially fatal
  - Seizures
  - Coma
  - Delirium
  - Focal neurological findigs
  - Heart failure
  - Rhabdomyolysis
  - Acute hemolysis
  - Leukocyte dysfunction
  - Abnormal liver function tests
- Chronic
  - Bone pathology
    - Osteomalacia
    - Severe bone pain
    - Fractures

HYPERPHOSPHATEMIA

Description

- Increased serum phosphorus > 5 mg/dL

Etiology

- Increase in extracellular phosphorus
  - Vitamin D therapy
  - Laxatives and enemas containing phosphorus
  - Intravenous phosphate supplement
  - Rhabdomyolyisis
  - Cell lysis from chemotherapy treating malignancy
  - Metabolic acidosis
  - Respiratory acidosis
- Decreased renal excretion—advanced kidney disease is the most common cause

- Chronic kidney disease
- Acute kidney injury
- Hypoparathyroidism
- Pseudohypoparathyroidism
- Acromegaly
- Pseudohyperphosphatemia
  - Multiple myeloma
  - Hyperbilirubinemia
  - Hypertriglyceridemia
  - Hemolysis in vitro
- Medication
  - Liposomal amphotericin B

Incidence and Demographics

- Patients with end-stage renal disease have the highest rates of hyperphosphatemia.
- In the United States, about 250,000 people are affected.
- Chronic hyperphosphatemia is an independent risk factor for the development of cardiovascular disease in the patient with renal failure.

Risk Factors

- Acute and chronic kidney disease
  - Hemodialysis
- Malignancy
- Laxative or enema use
- Antacids
- Crush injury
- Phosphorus supplementation
- Presence of metabolic or respiratory acidosis
- Vitamin D therapy
- Prolonged immobilization
- Ischemic bowel

Prevention and Screening

- Patient education regarding dietary and medication restrictions for at-risk patients
  - Restriction of dietary protein to 0.6 to 0.9 g/d
  - Avoid milk and milk products, meat, fish, poultry, eggs, peanuts, and dark cola.
  - Avoid laxatives, enemas, and antacids because these contain phosphorus.
- Maintain adequate hydration.

Assessment

History
- Related to the underlying disorder
- History of renal disease, malignancy, trauma
- Accurate medication list to include over-the-counter medications
  - Use of nutritional supplements
- Symptoms related to secondary hypocalcemia
  - See Hypocalcemia

Physical Examination
- CNS
  - Altered mental status
  - Delirium
  - Obtundation
  - Seizures
  - Muscle cramping
  - Neuromuscular excitability
  - Paresthesias
- Cardiovascular
  - Hypotension
  - Heart failure
  - Prolongation of the QT interval
- Cataracts
- Ectopic tissue calcification
  - Occurs when serum phosphorus x serum Ca^{++} > 55
  - Areas affected
    - Cornea
    - Skin
    - Joints
    - Vasculature
      - Calcifications seen on radiography
      - Calciphylaxis
      - Medial arterial calcification
    - Heart
      - Valvular calcification
      - Conduction defects

Diagnostic Studies
- Serum chemistry
  - Phosphorus level > 5 mg/dL
  - Evaluate for acute or chronic kidney disease
  - Serum PTH and vitamin D levels
  - Serum calcium to calculate for risk of ectopic tissue calcification—see Physical Examination

- Arterial blood gas to evaluate pH
  - Respiratory acidosis
- CBC
  - For leukocytosis
- Serum CK
  - Elevated with rhabdomyolysis

Differential Diagnosis

- Hypercalcemia
- Hypermagnesemia
- Hypocalcemia
- Tumor lysis syndrome

Management

Nonpharmacologic Treatment
- Maintain adequate hydration.
- Low-phosphorus diet
- Address underlying cause.
- Peritoneal or hemodialysis

Pharmacologic Treatment
- Eliminate medications containing phosphorus.
- Normal renal function
  - Volume repletion and diuresis with a loop diuretic—furosemide
- Renal disease
  - Phosphate binders
    - Aluminum hydroxide
    - Calcium carbonate
    - Calcium acetate
    - Magnesium hydroxide
    - Sevelamer hydrochloride
    - Lanthanum carbonate

Special Considerations

- Hyperphosphatemia associated with hypercalcemia presents a high risk of metastatic calcification.
- Renal failure most often requires phosphorus intake restrictions.
- For unsual cases of hypoparathyroidism, calcium and vitamin D are prescribed (for the treatment of hypocalcemia).

When to Consult, Refer, or Hospitalize

- Nephrology consult to manage the CKD and end-stage renal failure patient
- According to the underlying cause: oncology, endocrinology, general surgery, cardiology, or critical care team if ICU required
- Admission required for severe hyperphosphatemia complicated by hypocalcemic tetany or large extraosseous calcium phosphate crystal deposits
- Hospitalize for treatment of underlying cause if warranted—renal failure, tumor cell lysis.

Follow-up

Expected Outcomes
- Maintenance of phosphorus levels within normal limits
- Serial monitoring of electrolytes

Complications
- Deposition of calcium deposits
  - See Physical examination findings

ACID–BASE DISORDERS

Description

- The body requires a stable concentration of hydrogen ions.
- Acid–base homeostasis maintains the hydrogen ion concentration between 7.35 and 7.45.
- The patient's acid–base balance is measured by arterial pH, PCO_2, and plasma bicarbonate (HCO_3^-).
- Hydrogen ion concentration is expressed as the negative log of its concentration.
  - The symbol for negative log is p.
  - pH is the negative log of the hydrogen ion concentration in mol/L.
- Acidemia
  - Increase in plasma hydrogen ion concentration < 7.35
- Acidosis
  - A process that increases plasma hydrogen ion concentration
- Alkalemia
  - Decrease in plasma hydrogen ion concentration > 7.45
- Alkalosis
  - A process that decreases plasma hydrogen ion concentration
- Acid–base disorders related to respiratory or metabolic disorders
  - Acidosis
  - Alkalosis
  - Mixed acid–base
    - More than one primary disorder occurring simultaneously

- pH points to the dominant disorder
- Analysis for mixed acid–base disorder
  - #1: Determine the primary disorder by evaluating the pH, HCO_3^-, and PCO_2 values.
  - #2: Determine the presence of mixed acid–base disorders by calculating the range of compensatory responses—see Metabolic Acidosis, the next section.
  - #3: Calculate the ion gap—see Metabolic Acidosis.
  - #4: Calculate the corrected HCO_3^- concentration (delta gap) if the anion gap is increased—see Metabolic Acidosis.
  - Examine the patient for clinical signs that indicate the values found.
- Primary changes and compensations for simple acid–base disorders
  - Metabolic acidosis
    - pH < 7.35
    - HCO_3^-—primary decrease
    - PCO_2—compensatory decrease
    - Compensation
      - 1.2 mm Hg decrease in PCO_2 for every 1 mMol/L decrease in HCO_3^-
    - Prediction of compensation
      - $PaCO_2 = (1.5 \times HCO_3^-) + 8 + 2$
  - Metabolic alkalosis
    - pH > 7.45
    - HCO_3^-—primary increase
    - PCO_2—compensatory increase
    - Compensation
      - 0.6 to 0.75 mm Hg increase in PCO_2 for every 1 mMol/L increase in HCO_3^-
      - PCO_2 should not increase > 55 mm Hg with compensation.
    - Prediction of compensation
      - $PaCO_2 = [HCO_3^-] + 15$
  - Respiratory acidosis
    - pH < 7.35
    - HCO_3^-—compensatory increase
    - PCO_2—primary increase
    - Compensation
      - Acute
        - 1 to 2 mMol/L increase in HCO_3^- for every 10 mm Hg increase in PCO_2
        - $\Delta pH = 0.008 \times \Delta PaCO_2$
        - Expected pH = $7.40 - [0.008 \times (PaCO_2 - 40)]$
      - Chronic
        - 3 to 4 mMol/L increase in HCO_3^- for every 10 mm Hg increase in PCO_2
        - $\Delta pH = 0.003 \times \Delta PaCO_2$
        - Expected pH = $7.40 - [0.003 \times (PaCO_2 - 40)]$
    - Predicted compensation
      - Acute
      - Chronic
  - Respiratory alkalosis
    - pH > 7.45
    - HCO_3^-—compensatory decrease
    - PCO_2—primary decrease
    - Compensation

- Acute
  - 1 to 2 mMol/L decrease in HCO_3^- for every 10 mm Hg decrease in PCO_2
  - $\Delta pH = 0.008 \times \Delta PaCO_2$
  - Expected pH = 7.40 + [0.008 × (40 − $PaCO_2$)]
- Chronic
  - 4 to 5 mMol/L decrease in HCO_3^- for every 10 mm Hg decrease in PCO_2
  - $\Delta ph = 0.003 \times \Delta PaCO2$
  - Expected pH = 7.40 + [0.003 × (40 − $PaCO_2$)]

METABOLIC ACIDOSIS

Description

- Metabolic acidosis is characterized by a reduction in serum bicarbonate that results in a pH < 7.35.
- Separated into two categories: anion gap acidosis and normal anion gap acidosis
  - Anion gap is measured as:
    - AG = $Na^+ - (HCO_3^- + Cl^-)$
- Normal AG is 12 ± 4 mEq/L.
- Delta gap
  - The difference between the patient's anion gap and the normal anion gap
  - The amount is considered a bicarbonate equivalent because for every unit rise in the anion gap, the bicarbonate level should decrease by 1 because of buffering.
    - When the delta gap value is added to the measured bicarbonate level, the result should be in the normal bicarbonate range.
    - An elevated result indicates the additional presence of a metabolic alkalosis.
      - To help determine the etiology of metabolic acidosis with normal ion gap, calculate urinary ion gap: $([Na^+] + [K^+]) - ([Cl^-] + [HCO_3])$
  - Differentiates between GI and renal causes

Etiology

- High anion gap ≥ 15 mEq/L
  - Ketoacidosis
    - Diabetes mellitus
    - Alcoholism
    - Starvation
    - Fasting
  - Lactic acidosis
    - Physiological
      - Shock
      - Hypoxia (lung disorder)
      - Seizures

- Exogenous toxins
  - Carbon monoxide
  - Cyanide
  - Iron
  - Toluene
    - Initially high gap, then normal gap after excretion of metabolites
  - Isoniazid
- Renal failure
- Toxins
  - Alcohol
  - Methanol (formic acid)
  - Ethylene glycol (oxalic acid)
  - Paraldehyde (acetate, chloracetate)
  - Salicylates
- Rhabdomyolysis
  - Rare
- Normal anion gap (hyperchloremic acidosis)
  - GI tract bicarbonate loss
    - Colostomy
    - Diarrhea
    - Enteric fistulas
    - Ileostomy
    - Use of ion-exchange resins
  - Urological procedures
    - Ureterosigmoidostomy
    - Ureteroileal conduit
  - Renal bicarbonate loss
    - Tubulointerstitial renal disease
    - RTA types 1, 2, and 4
    - Hyperparathyroidism
  - Infusion
    - Arginine
    - Lysine
    - Ammonium chloride (NH_4CL)
    - Rapid NaCl infusion
  - Ingestion
    - Acetazalamide
    - Calcium chloride
    - Magnesium sulfate
  - Miscellaneous
    - Hypoaldosteronism
    - Hyperkalemia
    - Toluene—late

Incidence and Demographics

- See Etiology to identify high-risk patient populations
- Disorders of acid–base homeostasis can be seen in about 9 of every 10 patients in the ICU.
- May be one of the most common problems encountered in the ICU

Risk Factors

- Diabetes mellitus
- Sepsis
- Hypoxia
- Renal failure
- Massive trauma
- Toxic ingestion
- Diarrhea
- Presence of colostomy, ileostomy
- Endocrine disorders

Prevention and Screening

- Early recognition and treatment of underlying condition

Assessment

History
- Anorexia
- Weakness
- Nausea
- Lethargy
- Symptoms of underlying disorder

Physical Examination
- Kussmaul's respirations
- Hypotension
- Signs of underlying disorder
- Altered mental status—progressing to coma
- Ventricular dysrhythmias in severe, acute acidemia (pH < 7.15)
- Chronic academia
  - Bone demineralization disorders

Diagnostic Studies
- Arterial blood gases
- Serum electrolytes
- Liver function studies
  - Albumin level
    - A 50% reduction in the albumin concentration will result in a 75% reduction in the anion gap.

- Lactic acid level
- Anion gap
- Calculated delta gap
- Calculate predicated compensation
- Urinary anion gap
- Serum and urine ketones in DKA
- Serum salicylate, methanol, or ethylene glycol levels if toxic ingestion is suspected

Differential Diagnosis

- Acute renal failure
- Azotemia
- Chronic renal failure
- Diabetes mellitus type 1 and 2
- Lactic acidosis
- Metabolic alkalosis
- Respiratory alkalosis
- Salicylate toxicity

Management

Nonpharmacologic Treatment
- Supportive nutritional care
- Accurate intake and output
- Treatment is aimed at resolution of the underlying cause and correcting acidemia
- Type IV RTA
  - Low-potassium diet
  - Avoid dehydration.
  - Adjust medication dosage.

Pharmacologic Treatment
- Bicarbonate (alkali) therapy is usually not required until the arterial pH drops < 7.15 to 7.20.
  - An exception is to administer bicarbonate when HCO_3^- levels fall below 10 to 12 mEq/L despite a pH > 7.15.
  - Calculate the amount of bicarbonate to administer.
    - Amount of HCO_3^- deficit = 0.5 x body weight in kg x (24 − Serum HCO_3^-)
    - Half of the calculated deficit should be administered within the first 3 to 4 hours to avoid overcorrection and volume overload.
  - The initial goal of therapy is raise pH to 7.20
  - Usually given when metabolic acidosis is the result of HCO_3^- loss or accumulation of inorganic acids (normal anion gap acidosis)
  - When metabolic acidosis is a result of organic acid accumulation (high anion gap acidosis), the bicarbonate therapy is controversial.
- THAM (Tromethamine)
  - Noncarbonate buffer that corrects pH

- Does not increase CO_2
- Used for patients with metabolic acidosis and adult respiratory distress syndrome (ARDS)
- Administered intravenously
- Dose: base deficit x weight (kg) = amount of 0.3 M THAM solution to give in mL
  - Renal failure
    - Dialysis
    - Alkali administration
      - Insufficient evidence to determine at what pH level $NaHCO_3$ should be given
  - Ketoacidosis
    - Fluid resuscitation
    - Insulin administration
    - Alkali therapy usually not needed
  - Lactic acidosis
    - Correction of underlying disorder
    - Benefit of $NaHCO_3$ is unproven
  - Drug and toxic ingestions
    - Treat underlying cause.
  - Renal tubular acidosis
    - Type 1
      - Treat with HCO_3^- or citrate
      - Usual requirement is 1 to 3 mEq/kg/d
      - Potassium salt may be administered (potassium citrate) to treat the hypokalemia as well.
    - Type 2
      - Find treatable cause
        - Vitamin D deficiency
        - Multiple myeloma
        - Use of carbonic anhydrase inhibitor
    - Type 4
      - Avoiding medications that lead to hyperkalemia

Special Considerations

- With high AG acidosis, the accumulation of organic acids, lactate, and ketones are ions that eventually metabolized to HCO_3^-
  - Once the underlying disorder is treated, the pH corrects, so raise pH only to 7.20.
- The anion gap us a useful tool for the differential diagnosis of metabolic acidosis.
- Hypoalbuminemia can mask an increased concentration of gap by decreasing the value of the anion gap.
- Non–anion-gap acidosis is often the result of infusions of large volumes of chloride fluids.

When to Consult, Refer, or Hospitalize

- Refer to nephrology for patients with renal tubular acidosis and possible alkali therapy
- Admission depends on severity of underlying condition and metabolic acidosis.
- Critical care consult as condition warrants

Follow-up

Expected Outcomes
- Recovery is dependent on the underlying cause.
  - Chronic metabolic acidosis requires serial laboratory monitoring.
- Potassium citrate may be used when acidosis is accompanied by hypokalemia; use with caution in renal impairment—avoid in the presence of hyperkalemia.
- Acute renal failure (urine output < 400 ml/24 hours) can lead to metabolic acidosis.
  - Hyperkalemia may develop rapidly.
- Metabolic acidosis may depress myocardial contractility, leading to worsening heart failure.
- Hypervolemia and salt retention with the administration of $NaHCO_3$ may lead to congestive heart failure.
- The respiratory system may have limited ability to compensate for the metabolic acidosis because of underlying pulmonary disease and ineffective gas exchange.

Complications
- Acute
  - When pH is < 7.20
    - Vasodilatation
    - Myocardial depression
    - Decreased cardiac output
    - Hypotension
- Chronic
  - Bone disease
  - Osteomalacia
  - Osteopenia
  - Loss of body mass
  - Muscle weakness

METABOLIC ALKALOSIS

Description

- Metabolic alkalosis manifests as increased arterial pH, an increase in serum HCO_3^-, and an increase in $PaCO_2$ with hypoventilation as the compensatory mechanism.
- Hypochloremia and hypokalemia are often present.
- Frequently occurs with other acid–base disorders

Etiology

- Occurs from a net gain of HCO_3^- or loss of nonvolatile acid from extracelluar fluid
- It is unusual for alkali to be added to the body.
  - Usually involves loss of acid or inability of kidneys to excrete HCO_3^-
    - Saline-responsive (U_{cl} < 25 mEq/L)

- High body HCO_3^- content
- Renal alkalosis
    - Diuretics
    - Antibiotics that contain a nonreabsorbable anion increase K^+ and H^+
        - Carbenicillin
        - Penicilllin
        - Ticarcillin
    - Posthypercapnia alkalosis
        - In chronic respiratory alkalosis, the kidney decreases bicarbonate excretion.
    - GI alkalosis
        - Vomiting
        - Nasogastric tube (NGT) suction
        - Villous adenoma
        - Chloride diarrhea
        - Antacids
        - Baking soda
        - Sodium citrate, lactate, gluconate, acetate
            - Transfusions
        - Normal body content HCO_3^-
        - Contraction alkalosis
- Saline-unresponsive ($U_{cl} > 40$ mEq/L)
- High body HCO_3^- content
- Renal alkalosis
    - Normotensive
    - Bartter's syndrome
    - Severe potassium depletion
    - Refeeding alkalosis
        - Hypercalcemia and hypoparathyroidism
    - Hypertensive
        - Endogenous mineralocorticoids
    - Primary aldosteronism
    - Hyperreninism
    - Adrenal enzyme deficiency: 11- and 17-hydroxylase
    - Liddle's syndrome
        - Exogenous alkali
        - Exogenous mineralocorticoids
        - Licorice

Incidence and Demographics

- See Metabolic Acidosis

Risk Factors

- Use of diuretics
- NGT suction
- Excessive vomiting

- Antibiotic therapy
- Genetic predisposition
- Hypokalemia
- Massive blood transfusion
- Primary hyperparathryodism
- See Etiology
- Hyperaldosteronism

Prevention and Screening

- Maintenance of adequate volume status
- Identify high-risk patients.
- Early identification and treatment of underlying cause

Assessment

History
- Headache
- Lethargy that may progress to coma
- Weakness or hyporeflexia with hypokalemia
- Paresthesias

Physical Examination
- Postural hypotension
- Tachycardia
- Respiratory depression
- Tetany or seizure associated with hypocalcemia
- Coma

Diagnostic Studies
- Arterial blood gases
  - Elevated pH and HCO_3^-
  - With respiratory compensation, the PCO_2 is increased.
  - Serum chemistry
    - Decreased potassium, chloride, magnesium, and calcium
- Urine chloride—marker of volume status
- < 25 mEq/L
- Saline-responsive
  - Vomiting
  - Low NaCl intake
  - Diuretic use
- > 40 mEq/L
  - Saline-unresponsive
  - Aldosterone excess

Differential Diagnosis

- Respiratory acidosis

Management

Nonpharmacologic Treatment
- Mild metabolic alkalosis does not usually require treatment.
- Severe (pH > 7.6) or symptomatic metabolic alkalosis requires treatment.
- Surgical removal of mineralocorticoid-producing tumors in saline-nonresponsive metabolic acidosis
- Hemodialysis or hemofiltration for patients with a pH > 7.6 with volume overload and renal dysfunction

Pharmacologic Treatment
- Saline-responsive
  - Chloride replacement as NaCl, KCl, or both
  - NaCl infusion is administered at a rate of 50 to 100 mL/hr greater than urinary and other sensible and insensible fluid loss until Cl is > 25 mEq/L and urinary pH normalizes.
  - H2 blockers or PPIs to reduce gastric acid secretion
  - In the presence of heart failure when the volume will not be tolerated
    - Acetazolamide 250 to 375 mg once or twice daily, p.o. or IV
    - Hypokalemia may develop—monitor electrolytes
  - Hydrochloric acid: 0.1 to 0.2 M solution via a central vein catheter at rate not to exceed 0.2 mEq/kg/hr
  - The following equation can be used to determine the amount of HCL needed:
    - HCO_3^- excess = 0.5 x (wt in kg) x (serum HCO_3^- —desired HCO_3^-)
    - Example: for a 70 kg patient with a serum HCO_3^- of 40, the amount of HCL needed to reduce the serum level to 30 is:
      - HCO_3^- excess = 0.5 x 70 x (40 – 30) = 350 mEq
- Saline-nonresponsive
  - Block aldosterone effect with ACE-I or spironolactone
  - Primary aldosteronism
  - Treat with potassium repletion

Special Considerations

- Hypokalemia is both a cause and a consequence of metabolic acidosis.
- Saline-responsive metabolic alkalosis is more common than the nonresponsive disorder.
- The anion gap may be elevated because of the increased "charge equivalency" of albumin and stimulation of organic anion synthesis.

When to Consult, Refer, or Hospitalize

- Referral to nephrology if hemodialysis or hemofiltration needed
- General surgery referral if needed to remove hormone-producing tumor

- Subspecialty consults depend on underlying cause
- Critical care consults as patient condition warrants
- Admit for symptomatic or severe metabolic acidosis that requires inpatient treatment

Follow-up

Expected Outcomes
- Resolution of the metabolic alkalosis
- In the ICU patient, metabolic alkalosis is not easily missed because arterial blood gases and daily chemistry panels are done on these patients.
- Mortality rates may be as high as 45% in patients with an arterial pH > 7.55 and 80% when the pH is > 7.65.

Complications
- Tetany
- Seizures
- Altered mental status
- Refractory dysrhythmias
- Hypokalemia
- Hypoventilation leading to hypoxemia
- Seen in patients with poor respiratory reserve
  - May impede weaning from the ventilator

RESPIRATORY ACIDOSIS

Description

- Also referred to as hypercapnia
- It is a ventilatory process with a primary increase in PCO_2 with or without a compensatory increase in HCO_3^-.
- Respiratory acidosis may be acute or chronic.
- Distinction is made by the degree of metabolic compensation

Etiology

- Respiratory acidosis is caused by a decrease in respiratory rate, respiratory volume (hypoventilation), or both
- Acute
  - CNS depression
  - Opioids, sedatives, anesthetics
  - Cardiac arrest
  - Central sleep apnea

- High-flow oxygen in patients with chronic hypercapnia
- Disorders of the respiratory muscles and chest wall
  - Myasthenia gravis
  - Periodic paralysis
  - Guillain-Barré syndrome
  - Severe hypokalemia or hypophosphatemia
  - Pneumothorax, hemothorax
- Airway obstruction
  - Aspiration
  - Obstructive sleep apnea
  - Laryngospasm
- Gas exchange disturbance
  - ARDS
  - Acute cardiogenic pulmonary edema
  - Pneumonia
- Chronic
  - CNS depression
    - Extreme obesity
    - Pickwickian syndrome
    - Metabolic alkalosis
  - Disorders of the respiratory muscles and chest wall
    - Spinal cord injury
    - Poliomyelitis
    - Amyotrophic lateral sclerosis
    - Multiple sclerosis
    - Myxedema
    - Kyphoscoliosis
    - Extreme obesity
  - Gas exchange disturbances
    - COPD
    - Emphysema
    - Severe asthma
    - Chronic bronchitis
    - Extreme obesity
- Permissive hypercapnia with mechanical ventilation

Incidence and Demographics

- See Metabolic Acidosis
- Patient population corresponds to underlying disorder

Risk Factors

- Smoking
- Obesity
- Presence of CNS disorders

- Trauma
- Cardiac arrest
- Presence of sleep apnea
- History of COPD
- Lung injury or disease
- Anxiety disorders
- Chronic pain
- Presence of stress or tension

Prevention and Screening

- Smoking cessation
- Weight loss
- Caution when administering sedatives, opioids
- Early recognition in high-risk populations

Assessment

- Signs and symptoms depend on the degree of PCO_2 increase
- CO_2 rapidly crosses the blood-brain barrier
- Signs and symptoms are the result of high CNS CO_2 concentration and associated hypoxemia

History
- Acute
- Headache
- Blurred vision
- Restlessness
- Anxiety
- Delirium
- Somnolence
- Shortness of breath
- Chronic
- Memory loss
- Sleep disturbances
  - Excessive daytime sleepiness
- Impaired coordination
- Personality changes

Physical Examination
- Acute
  - Hypertension
  - Altered level of consciousness
  - Papilledema
  - Tremor
  - Gait disturbance

- Blunted deep-tendon reflexes
- Myoclonic jerks
- Asterixis
- Chronic
  - Occasionally mild tremor
  - Cor pulmonale
    - Cyanosis
    - Right ventricular heave
    - Pulmonary diastolic murmur
  - Increased anterior–posterior diameter
  - Expiratory wheezing
  - Use of accessory muscles

Diagnostic Studies
- Arterial blood gases
- Decreased pH
- Increased arterial PCO_2 > 45 mm Hg
- Metabolic alkalosis if compensation has taken place
- Pulmonary function testing
- Decreased forced expiratory volume in 1 second (FEV_1)
- Increased residual volume
- Serum electrolytes
- May see hypochloremia in chronic disease
- Increase in serum bicarbonate
- Calculation of alveolar-arterial (A-a) O_2 gradient helps to distinguish pulmonary from non-pulmonary disease.
- Inspired PO_2: [arterial PO_2 + 5/4 arterial PCO_2]
- Complete blood count
- May have secondary polycythemia
- Drug and toxicology screening

Differential Diagnosis

- Asthma
- Botulism
- Chronic bronchitis
- COPD
- Diaphragm disorders
- Emphysema
- Obesity
- Opioid abuse

Management

Nonpharmacologic Treatment
- Acute
  - Patients are at risk for both hypercapnia and hypoxemia.
  - Supplemental oxygen
  - Mechanical ventilation

- Chronic
  - Maintenance of adequate oxygenation
  - Improve alveolar ventilation.
  - Treat underlying disorder.
  - Supplemental oxygen to keep O_2 saturations in the low 90% range, PaO_2 of 60 to 65 mm Hg

Pharmacologic Treatment
- Acute
  - Control of underlying disease with effective alveolar ventilation
    - Bronchodilators
    - Corticosteroids
  - THAM
    - May be used when the hemodynamic status of the patient is compromised
  - If drug toxicity is suspected, provide appropriate antidote.
    - Naloxone for opioids
    - Flumazenil for benzodiazepines
    - See Poisoning and Drug Toxicities (Chapter 21)
- Chronic
  - Maintenance bronchodilators

Special Considerations

- The body is not well-equipped to compensate for an acute rise in CO_2 concentration.
- Hemoglobin and proteins are the primary modulators of acute respiratory acidosis.
- Caution should be used in correcting chronic hypercapnia.
- Rapid correction can result in metabolic alkalemia.

When to Consult, Refer, or Hospitalize

- Pulmonary consult for management of hypoxemia and hypercapnia
- Ventilator management
- Bronchodilator therapy
- Subspecialty consultations are dictated by the underlying disease process.
- Admit patients who are symptomatic.
- ICU admission
  - Confusion
  - Lethargy
  - Respiratory muscle fatigue
  - Low pH

Follow-up

Expected Outcomes
- Correction of respiratory acidosis
- Treatment of underlying disease
- Prognosis depends on severity of underlying disease process
- Outpatient oxygen therapy when warranted
- PaO_2 < 55 mm Hg or PaO_2 of 59 mm Hg when polycythemia or cor pulmonale is present

Complications
- Chronic hypoxemia
- Pulmonary vasoconstriction
- Confusion
- Papilledema

RESPIRATORY ALKALOSIS

Description

- A ventilator process that, with a decrease in H^+, results in a pH > 7.45 mm Hg
- Arterial PCO_2 is < 36 mm Hg
- Metabolic acidosis is the compensatory mechanism.
- May be acute or chronic
- The chronic form is asymptomatic.
- Distinction is made by the level of metabolic compensation

Etiology

- Respiratory alkalosis results from an increase in respiratory rate or volume (hyperventilation).
- Increased ventilation occurs in response to hypoxia, metabolic acidosis, and increased metabolic demands.
- Increased respiratory rate and volume may also occur in response to pain, anxiety, and some CNS disorders (CVA, head trauma).
- Medications
- Progesterone
- Methylxanthines
- Salicylates
- Catecholamines
- Nicotine

Incidence and Demographics

- The most common acid–base abnormality in critically ill patients is chronic respiratory alkalosis.

Risk Factors

- Pain
- Anxiety
- Fever
- CVA
- High altitude
- Severe anemia
- Pregnancy
- Hyperthyroidism
- Presence of pneumothorax or pneumonia
- Pulmonary edema
- Interstitial lung disease
- Asthma
- Emphysema
- Chronic bronchitis
- Sepsis
- Hepatic failure
- Congestive heart failure
- Mechanical ventilation

Prevention and Screening

- Because of pain and anxiety, patient education in breathing techniques to relieve the hyperventilation may be beneficial.
- Early recognition and treatment of underlying disease

Assessment

History
- Acute
- Confusion
- Lightheadedness
- Paresthesias
- Chest tightness
- Muscle cramps
- Syncope
- Chronic
- Usually asymptomatic

Physical Examination
- Tachypnea
- Hyperpnea
- Carpopedal spasm in severe cases
- Hyperactive deep-tendon reflexes

Diagnostic Studies
- Arterial blood gases
- Serum electrolytes
- Minor hypophosphatemia and hypokalemia from intracellular shifts
- Decreased ionized calcium from an increase in protein binding
- Electrocardiogram
- Tachyarrhythmias
- Ischemic-like ST-T wave changes

Differential Diagnosis

- Asthma
- Atrial fibrillation
- Atrial flutter
- Head trauma
- Hyperthyroidism
- Metabolic acidosis
- Metabolic alkalosis
- Pneumonia
- Pulmonary embolism
- Sepsis
- Salicylate toxicity
- Theophylline toxicity

Management

- Emergent treatment not indicated until pH >7.5

  ### Nonpharmacologic Treatment
  - Acute
    - Correct underlying disorder or stimulus
    - Rebreathing into paper bag
    - Decrease respiratory rate and tidal volume in mechanically ventilated patients.
  - Chronic
    - No treatment generally required

Pharmacologic Treatment
- Acute
  - Ensure adequate pain and anxiety control—especially in the mechanically ventilated patient.
    - Sedatives
    - Antidepressants
  - Beta-adrenergic blockers to combat the hyperadrenergic state

Special Considerations

- If the PCO_2 is corrected rapidly in patients with chronic respiratory alkalosis, metabolic acidosis may develop from the renal compensatory decrease in serum bicarbonate.
- Pseudorespiratory alkalosis
  - Low arterial PCO_2 and high pH in ventilated patients with severe metabolic acidosis from hypoperfusion
  - Occurs when mechanical ventilation eliminates more than normal amounts of exhaled CO_2
  - Respiratory alkalosis is seen in arterial blood, but poor systemic perfusion and cellular ischemia lead to acidosis of venous blood.
  - Diagnosis made by marked arteriovenous differences in PCO_2 and pH, and elevated lactic acid levels
  - Treatment is improvement of hemodynamimcs

When to Consult, Refer, or Hospitalize
- The need for consultants is based on the underlying cause and severity of the condition.
- Consultants may include pulmonology, nephrology, neurology, cardiology, or a combination of these.
- Admit symptomatic patients requiring treatment

Follow-up

Expected Outcomes
- Resolution of acute respiratory acidosis
- Prognosis is related to the underlying cause and severity of illness.

Complications
- Tetany
- Chest pain
- Seizures in severe cases (rare)
- Cardiac dysrhythmias

REFERENCES

Barkley, T., & Myers, C. (2008). *Practice guidelines for acute care nurse practitioners*. St. Louis, MO: Saunders.

Beers, M., Porter, R., Jones, T., Kaplan, J., & Berkwits, M. (Eds.). (2006). *The Merck manual of diagnosis and therapy*. Whitehouse Station, NJ: Merck Research Laboratories.

Bope, E., Kellerman, R., & Rakel, R. (2011). *Conn's current therapy 2011*. Philadelphia: Elsevier/Saunders.

Cooper, D., Kraink, A., Lubner, S., & Reno, H. (Eds.). (2007). *The Washington manual of medical therapeutics* (32nd ed.). Philadelphia: Wolters Kluwer/Lippincott Williams & Wilkins.

Fauci, A., Braunwald, E., Kasper, D., Hauser, S., Longo, D., Jameson, J., & Loscalzo, J. (Eds.). (2009). *Harrison's principles of internal medicine*. New York: McGraw Hill.

Habermann, T., & Ghosh, A. (2008). *Mayo clinic internal medicine concise textbook*. Rochester, MN: Mayo Clinic Scientific Press.

Irwin, R., & Rippe, J. (2008). *Intensive care medicine*. Philadelphia: Wolter Kluwer/Lippincott Williams.

Marini, J., & Wheeler, A. (2010). *Critical care medicine, the essentials*. Philadelphia: Wolters Kluwer/Lippincott Williams & Wilkins.

McKean, S., Bennett, A., & Halasyamani, L. (Eds.). (2008). *Hospital medicine*. Philadelphia: Wolters Kluwer/Lippincott Williams & Wilkins.

McPhee, S. & Papadakis, M. (2011). (Eds.). *2011 current medical diagnosis and treatment*. New York: McGraw Hill.

21

Poisoning and Drug Toxicities

Pamela Smith, MSN, RN, ACNP-BC, CCRN

Description

- A poison is a substance that is harmful to the body when ingested, inhaled, injected, or absorbed through the skin.
- Any substance can be a poison if enough is taken.
- Poisonings are intentional or unintentional.

Etiology

- Unintentional poisoning
  - The use of drugs or chemicals for recreational purposes in excessive amounts—overdose
  - Includes the unknowing excessive use of drugs or chemicals by a child
- Intentional poisoning
  - The result of taking a substance with the intention doing harm
  - Suicide and assault by poisoning
- When the intent is unclear, the poisoning is labeled undetermined.
- In 2004, 95% of unintentional and undetermined poisonings were the result of drugs
  - Opioids most common
  - Cocaine
  - Heroin

Incidence and Demographics

- Unintentional
  - In 2005, 23,618 of the 32,691 poisoning deaths in the United States were unintentional; 10% were undetermined.
  - Unintentional poisoning death rates have steadily risen since 1992.
  - In 2006, unintentional poisoning was second only to motor vehicle accidents as a cause of unintentional injury.
  - Among people 35 to 54, unintentional poisoning caused more deaths than motor vehicle accidents.
  - In 2008, unintentional poisonings accounted for 732,316 emergency department visits.
    - 25% of these visits resulted in hospitalization or transfer to a higher level of care.
  - In 2007, poison control centers reported approximately 2.5 million unintentional poison exposure cases.
  - In 2007, more than 27,600 deaths occurred from unintentional drug poisonings.
- Intentional
  - In 2005, 5,833 of the 32,691 poisoning deaths in the United States were intentional.
    - 5,744 were suicides.
    - 89 were homicides.
  - In 2006, there were about 220,924 emergency department visits because of intentional poisoning.
    - 216,358 involved self-harm.
    - 162,096 resulted in hospitalization or transfer to a higher level of care.
  - Also in 2006, 198,578 cases reported were the result of suspected suicide attempts from poisoning.

Risk Factors

- Men are more likely to die as a result of unintentional poisoning.
- Native Americans have a high death rate from poisoning.
- Peak age: 45 to 49 years of age
- Whites and Blacks had similar rates of unintentional posionings.

Prevention and Screening

- Follow directions on the medication bottle.
- Read all warning labels.
- Turn a light on when taking medications at night.
- Keep medications in their original bottle or container.
- Avoid sharing or selling prescription drugs.
- Properly dispose of unused, unneeded, or expired prescription medications.
- Encourage the use of suicide prevention hot lines.
- Early treatment for depression

Management

- In all cases of overdose or toxicity, initiate advanced cardiac life support measures, two IV lines, electrocardiogram, supplemental oxygen, complete metabolic panel, and complete blood count.
- On all patients with suspected drug overdose, measurement of serum acetaminophen and salicylate levels should be done to rule out co-ingestion.
- Pregnancy testing should be performed on all women of childbearing age.

Special Considerations

- Up to 50% of all poisoning histories are inaccurate.
- The ingestion of multiple drugs is common.
- Try to identify the drug or drugs ingested, the dosage, how many pills are missing, and the timing of ingestion.
- Pay attention to vital signs, neurologic status, pupillary reactions, cardiovascular response, abdominal findings, and unusual odors and excreta.
- For patients who become toxic during chronic therapy, a medication or dosage adjustment, illness, or both may be the reason.

When to Consult, Refer, or Hospitalize

- Consult with a regional poison control center or medical toxicologist if the diagnosis is uncertain or advice is needed regarding specific treatment strategies.
- Admit if the patient has signs and symptoms of drug overdose that are not expected to clear in a 6- to 8-hour observation window.
- Continued administration of an antidote is required
- Psychiatric evaluation, social services evaluation, or both are needed for suicide attempt or drug abuse.
- Subspeciality for specific signs or symptoms; for example, nephrology for renal failure or hemodialysis, cardiology for congestive heart failure or dysrhythmias, critical care intensivists as condition warrants

SPECIFIC POISONINGS/TOXICITIES

ACETAMINOPHEN TOXICITY

Description

- Acetaminophen is the most commonly used analgesic and antipyretic medication in the United States and the world.
- It is combined with other medications in over 100 products.
- Acetaminophen is also known as paracetamol and N-acetyl-p-aminophenol (APAP).
- Hepatotoxicity associated with acetaminophen is well-documented.
- In 2009, the Food and Drug Administration (FDA) issued new restrictions for nonprescription and prescription medication regarding acetaminophen-induced hepatotoxicity.
- There is an increased risk of hepatic injury in the chronic alcoholic, those with liver disease, and those taking hepatotoxic medications.

Assessment

History
- Obtain accurate history of time of ingestion, and quantity and type of acetaminophen product ingested.
- Ask about other medications taken simultaneously—may inhibit acetaminophen absorption
- Phase 1 (0 to 24 hours)
  - Asymptomatic
  - Anorexia
  - Nausea, vomiting, or both
  - Malaise
  - Subclinical rise in serum transaminase levels starts about 12 hours after ingestion
- Phase 2 (18 to 72 hours)
  - RUQ pain
  - Anorexia
  - Nausea, vomiting, or both
  - Continued elevation of serum transaminase levels
- Phase 3 (72 to 96 hours)
  - Continued abdominal pain
    - Due to centrilobular hepatic necrosis
  - Jaundice
    - Coagulopathy
    - Hepatic encephalopathy
    - Nausea and vomiting

- Renal failure
- Death
- Phase 4 (4 days to 3 weeks)
  - Resolution of symptoms

Physical Examination
- Phase 1
  - Pallor
  - Malaise
  - Vomiting
  - Diaphoresis
- Phase 2
  - RUQ tenderness
  - Tachycardia
  - Hypotension
- Phase 3
  - Tender hepatic edge
  - Jaundice
  - Coagulopathy
    - GI bleeding
  - Hepatic encephalopathy
  - Asterixis
- Phase 4
  - Resolution of signs

Diagnostic Studies
- Serum acetaminophen level
  - Draw 4 or more hours after single ingestion
    - Not as reliable with multiple or chronic acetaminophen ingestion
  - Liver injury seen with levels > 7.5 g in adults
- Serum chemistry
  - Monitor and evaluate renal function
- Liver function studies
  - Will be elevated
  - Elevated bilirubin
  - Serial monitoring
- Coagulation studies
  - Prolonged PT
- Type and crossmatch
  - In preparation for GI bleeding
- Urinalysis
  - Renal tubular necrosis
    - Proteinuria
    - Hematuria
- Arterial blood gas
  - pH < 7.3 is predictive of mortality

- Lactic acid
- Monitor liver function studies, coagulopathies, arterial blood gases, and serum chemistry at least every 24 hours until treatment complete.
- CT scan of the head
  - Cerebral edema with late presentation and encephalopathy
- Ultrasound
  - Mild hepatic enlargement in late presentation

Differential Diagnosis

- Cytomegalovirus infection
- Gastroenteritis
- Hepatitis A, B, C
- Hepatorenal syndrome
- Pancreatitis
- Peptic ulcer disease
- Wilson's disease

Management

Nonpharmacologic Treatment
- Supportive therapy
  - Cardiac monitor
  - Supplemental oxygen
  - Placement of nasogastric tube (NGT)

Pharmacologic Treatment
- IV fluids
- Gastric decontamination
  - Oral activated charcoal
    - 25 to 100 g diluted in water
    - Absorbs acetaminophen and is administered if the patient presents within 1 hour of ingestion
    - May be of benefit after 1 hour if ingestion included medications that delay gastric emptying or slow GI motility
    - One study suggests may be administered 4 hours or more after ingestion
- N-acetylcysteine 140 mg/kg loading dose
  - Administered orally within 8 to 10 hours of ingestion
  - Maintenance dose of 70 mg/kg every 4 hours for a total of 17 doses for as long as the acetaminophen level stays in the toxic range (> 20 mcg/ml)
  - Early administration is nearly 100% hepatoprotective and should be given while waiting for an acetaminophen level if the patient presents close to the 8-hour window or if the patient is pregnant.
  - Continuous IV administration (for patients > 40 kg)
    - Loading dose 150 mg/kg infused over 15 minutes (dilute in 200 mL of D5W)—follow with maintenance doses:
  - First maintenance dose 50 mg/kg infused over 4 hours (dilute in 500 mL D5W) followed by second maintenance dose

- Second maintenance dose 100 mg/kg infused over 16 hours (dilute in 1000 mL D5W)
- Intermittent IV administration
  - Late presenting or chronic ingestion
  - > 10 hours after ingestion in patients > 40 kg
  - Loading dose: 140 mg/kg IV over 1 hour (dilute in 500 mL D5W) followed with maintenance dose
  - Maintenance dose: 70 mg/kg IV every 4 hours for at least 12 doses (dilute each dose in 250 mL of D5W), infuse over 1 hour minimum
- Antiemetics
  - Often need to administer N-acetylcysteine
  - Metoclopramide
  - Ondansetron

When to Consult, Refer, or Hospitalize

- Hepatologist if hepatic dysfunction present
- Transplant surgeon when clinical indicators are predictive of death
  - Arterial pH < 7.3 *or*
  - Grade III or IV encephalopathy *and*
  - PT > 100 seconds *and*
  - Serum creatinine > 3.4 mg/dL
- ICU care if signs of hepatic toxicity or other coexisting life-threatening conditions

Follow-up

Expected Outcomes
- Resolution of symptoms
- Psychological counseling as needed
- With aggressive supportive care, the mortality rate is less than 2%.
- Patients who survive should have return normal of liver function.
- Educate patients regarding the potential risks of acetaminophen regarding hepatic toxicity and risk for renal toxicity when used with NSAIDS.

Complications
- Hepatic toxicity leading to liver failure
- Death

ALCOHOL (ETHANOL, METHANOL, ETHYLENE GLYCOL) TOXICITY

Description

- The accidental or deliberate consumption of alcohols is a major cause of health problems in the United States.
- Heavy consumption increases overall mortality from trauma, suicide, cirrhosis, and malignancies.
- Ethanol contributes to about 100,000 deaths in the United States each year and economic costs in excess of $200 billion.
- It is involved in at least 10% of fatalities in U.S. poison centers.
- More than 8 million Americans are dependent on alcohol, and up to 15% of the population is considered to be at risk.
- Ethanol is a central nervous system depressant with an initial phase of excitation as learned social inhibitions are disregarded because of the effects on higher cortical function.
- Tolerance to ethanol's effects develops acutely and after chronic consumption.
- Intolerant individuals may show signs of impaired driving skills at ethanol concentrations as low as 20 mg/dL.
- Ethanol is rapidly absorbed across the gastric mucosa and small intestines, reaching a peak concentration 20 to 60 minutes after ingestion.
  - Once absorbed, it is converted to acetaldehyde, which is then converted to acetate; acetate is converted to acetyl CoA and finally carbon dioxide and water.
- Methanol and ethylene glycol are gradually metabolized to highly toxic organic acids.
  - After a delay of several hours, metabolic acidosis may develop with end-organ injury.

Assessment

History
- Ethanol
  - Determine amount and what was ingested.
    - Found in liquid cold remedies, mouthwashes, rubbing alcohol, aftershave lotion, perfumes, and colognes
    - Common alcoholic beverages: whiskey (40% to 50% ethanol concentration), liqueurs (22% to 50% ethanol concentration), wine (8% to 16% ethanol concentration), beer (3% to 7% ethanol concentration)
  - Patients often underestimate amount of ingestion.
  - History of alcoholism
- Methanol or ethylene glycol
  - Similar clinical picture

Physical Examination
- Depends of ethanol level
  - 50 mg/dL
    - Gross motor control and orientation may be affected.
    - Flushed skin

- Diuresis
- Hypoglycemia
- 150 mg/dL
  - Lethargy
  - Ataxia
  - Muscular incoordination
  - Atrial fibrillation
  - Tachycardia
  - Diplopia
- 250 mg/dL
  - Coma
  - Congestive heart failure
  - Pulmonary edema
  - Respiratory depression
- > 450 mg/dL
  - Death
- Tolerant drinkers can achieve much higher levels than those described before developing similar signs or symptoms.
  - Survival has been reported at serum levels of 1500 mg/dL.
  - At high doses, ethanol acts as an anesthetic.
    - Central nervous system (CNS) depression
    - Autonomic dysfunction
      - Hypotension
      - Hypothermia
    - Coma
    - Death from respiratory depression and cardiovascular collapse
- Ethanol and ethylene glycol
  - Severe metabolic acidosis
    - Ethylene glycol
  - Anion-gap metabolic acidosis
  - Calcium oxalate crystals that precipitate in tissues and kidneys
    - Methanol
  - Formic acid–anion gap metabolic acidosis
  - Blindness
  - Death
- Tachypnea
- Hypotension

Diagnostic Studies
- Ethanol blood level (blood alcohol level)
- Serum chemistry
- Anion gap measurement
- Serum lactate level
  - Low methanol and ethylene glycol toxicity
- Urine pregnancy test in women of childbearing age
- Urine drug screen to exclude other drug ingestions

- Arterial blood gases
  - Metabolic acidosis with methanol or ethylene glycol
- Serum osmolality
  - Can provide additional information about the level of ethanol in the blood
  - An osmolar gap of 22 to 25 mOsm/kg is present for every 100 mg/dL of serum ethanol
- Head CT with altered mental status if trauma cannot be excluded
- Electrocardiogram
  - To identify dysrhythmias

Differential Diagnosis

- Cognitive defects
- Dehydration
- Diabetic ketoacidosis
- Gastroenteritis
- Head trauma
- Hyperammonemia
- Hypoglycemia
- Hyponatremia
- Respiratory distress syndrome

Management

Nonpharmacologic Treatment
- Supportive care
  - Airway
    - Intubate for inadequate ventilation or risk of aspiration
  - Breathing
  - Circulation
  - IV access
  - Maintain body temperature
  - If ingestion occurred within the previous hour, place NGT and evacuate stomach contents.
  - Hemodialysis for clinical deterioration or refractory CNS depression, respiratory depression, or hypotension
    - Also for methanol or ethylene glycol levels > 50 mg/dL

Pharmacologic Treatment
- IV fluid replacement
- Correct hypoglycemia
- For patients with chronic alcohol abuse, administer thiamine 100 mg IV or IM to prevent neurological injury.

- Multivitamin—usually added to IV fluids
- Replenish electrolytes as needed
- Methanol or ethylene glycol—for levels > 50 mg/dL
  - Fomepizole
    - Loading dose 15 mg/kg, then 10 mg/kg every 12 hours x 48 hours
  - Until ethylene glycol level < 20 mg/dL
- Ethanol infusion
  - 750 mg/kg orally or IV
    - Infusion of 100 to 150 mg/kg/hour
  - Folic acid 50 mg IV every 4 hours
  - Vitamin B_1 100 mg IM or IV every 6 hours
  - Pyridoxine 50 mg IV every 6 hours
- The preceding three vitamins enhance the metabolism of the toxic organic acids.

When to Consult, Refer, or Hospitalize

- Nutritionist if malnutrition evident
- Subspeciality consultations dependent on comorbidities
- Counseling for alcohol cessation as needed

Follow-up

Expected Outcomes
- Resolution of symptoms
- Observe patient until mental status has returned to normal.
- Monitor serial electrolytes and blood glucose.
- Evaluate home environment and need for supportive care.
- Daily thiamine administration for chronic alcohol abuse
- Prognosis excellent if patient can avoid complications of short-term use of alcohol and avoid chronic use

Complications
- Risky behavior
- Altered mental status
- Respiratory depression
- Myocardial depression
- Atrial dysrhythmias
- Trauma

ANTIARRHYTHMIC DRUG OVERDOSE

Description
- Class I antiarrhythmics
  - Sodium channel blockers
  - Class Ia
    - Procainamide
    - Qunidine
  - Class Ib
    - Lidocaine
    - Mexiletine
  - Class Ic
    - Flecainide
    - Propafenone
- Class II
  - Beta-adrenergic blockers
    - Propranolol is the most toxic beta-blocker and most frequently used in suicide attempts.
    - Metoprolol
    - Atenolol
    - Carvedilol
    - Labetalol
- Class III
  - Potassium channel blockers
  - Bretyllium
  - Amiodarone
  - Sotolol
  - Ibutilide
  - Dofetilide
- Class IV
  - Calcium channel blockers
  - Dihydropyridine
    - Amlodipine
    - Nifedipine
- Nondihydropyridine
  - Verapamil
  - Diltiazem

Assessment

History
- Class I
  - Procainamide

- Nausea, vomiting, or both
- Headache
- Dizziness
- Hallucinations
- Weakness
- Bitter taste
- In patients with myasthenia gravis
  - Respiratory weaknesss
  - Myasthenia crisis
- In patients with Brugada syndrome
  - Recurrent ventricular tachycardia or fibrillation

- Quinidine
  - Drug fever
  - Systemic lupus erythematosos
  - Asthma
  - Diarrhea
  - Cinchonism syndrome
  - Headache
  - Fever
  - Mydriasis
  - Hearing changes
  - Delirium
  - Nausea and vomiting
  - Hot flushed skin
- Lidocaine
  - Lightheadedness
  - Dizziness
  - Drowsiness
  - Confusion
  - Dysarthria
  - Hearing loss
  - Euphoria
    - Late symptoms
      - Visual disturbances
      - Agitation
      - Muscle fasciculations
      - Coma
      - Seizures
- Mexiletine
  - Paresthesias of tongue
  - Nausea
- Flecainide
  - Nausea and vomiting
- Propafenone
  - Constipation
  - Nausea and vomiting
  - Bitter taste

- Asthma may be exacerbated.
- Visual blurring
- Dizziness
- Paresthesias
- Class II
  - Determine type of beta blocker taken
  - Obtain thorough history
  - Wheezing
  - Blurred vision
  - Lightheadedness
  - Confusion
  - Fever
  - Anxiety
  - Weakness
  - Depressed mental status
- Class III
  - Amiodarone
    - Acute pulmonitis
    - Chronic fibrosis of the lung
  - Bretyllium
    - Depressed gag reflex
    - Nausea and vomiting
  - Sotalol
    - Fatigue
    - Dizziness
    - Chest pain
    - Headache
    - Nausea or vomiting
  - Ibutilide
    - Headache
  - Dofetilide
    - Headache
    - Dyspnea
    - Diarrhea
    - Back pain
    - Abdominal pain
- Class IV
  - Dihydropyridine
    - Amlodipine
      - Chest pain
      - Dizziness
      - Fatigue
      - Flushing
      - Nausea and vomiting
    - Nifedipine
      - Headache
      - Dizziness
      - Nausea

- Nervousness
- Dyspnea
- Nondihydropyridine
  - Verapamil
    - Paralytic ileus
    - Headache
    - Nausea and vomiting
    - Fatigue
  - Diltiazem
    - Syncope
    - Headache

Physical Examination
- Class I
  - Procainamide
    - Hypotension
    - Ventricular fibrillation
    - Seizures
    - Bradycardia
    - Thrombocytopenia
  - Quinidine
    - Torsades de pointes
    - Complete AV block
    - Syncope
    - Respiratory arrest
    - Hypotension
    - QT prolongation
  - Lidocaine
    - Seizures
    - Respiratory arrest
    - Heart block
    - Bradycardia
    - Coma
  - Mexiletine
    - Ventricular dysrhythmias
    - Cardiovascular collapse
  - Flecainide
    - Congestive heart failure
    - Heart block
    - QT prolongation
    - Torsades de pointes
    - Cardiac arrest
    - Hepatic failure
    - Ventricular dysrhythmias
  - Propafenone
    - Ventricular dysrhythmias
    - Asystole
    - Torsades de pointes

- QT prolongation
- Congestive heart failure
- AV block
- Class II
  - Bradycardia
  - Hypotension
  - Seizures
  - Coma
  - Bronchospasm
  - Pulmonary edema
  - Respiratory arrest
- Class III
  - Amiodarone
    - Pulmonary toxicity—may be fatal
    - Pneumonitis—hypersensitivity
    - Pneumonitis—alveolar or interstitial
    - Pulmonary fibrosis
    - Pulmonary hemorrhage
    - Hepatotoxicity—may be fatal
    - Ventricular dysrhythmias
    - Severe bradycardia
    - Complete heart block
    - Cardiogenic shock
    - Thyrotoxicosis
    - Hypotension—severe
    - Irreversible blindness
    - Pancreatitis
    - Acute renal failure
  - Bretylium
    - Hypotension
    - Asystole
    - Anuria
    - Neurologic depression
  - Sotalol
    - Torsades de pointes
    - QT prolongation
    - Congestive heart failure
    - Heart block
    - Severe bradycardia
    - Bronchospasm
  - Ibutilide
    - Polymorphic ventricular tachycardia
    - Torsades de pointes
    - QT prolongation
    - AV block
    - Bradycardia
  - Dofetilide
    - Ventricular dysrhythmias
    - Torsades de pointes

- QT prolongation
- Class IV
  - Dihydropyridine
    - Amlodipine
      - Angina
      - Acute myocardial infarction
      - Acute hypotension
      - Reflex tachycardia
      - Acute lung injury
    - Nifedipine
      - Congestive heart failure
      - Pulmonary edema
      - Acute myocardial infarction
      - Severe hypotension
      - Reflex tachycardia
      - Acute lung injury
  - Nondihydropyridine
    - Verapamil
      - Severe bradycardia
      - AV block
      - Severe hypotension
      - Congestive heart failure
    - Dilitazem
      - Severe bradycardia
      - AV block
      - Severe hypotension
      - Acute hepatic injury
      - Congestive heart failure

Diagnostic Studies
- Class I
  - Procainamide
    - Total procainamide serum level: 5 to 20 mg/L
  - Junctional tachycardia and conduction defects at 42 mg/L
  - Severe hypotension and lethargy at levels > 60 mg/L
  - Qunidine
    - Therepeutic levels: 2 to 6 mg/L
    - Toxic levels > 8 mg/L
    - Levels > 14 mg/L produce cardiac toxicity
  - Lidocaine
    - Therapeutic plasma level is 1.5 to 5 mg/L
    - CNS toxicity is seen at 7 mg/L
    - Fatal concentration is > 15 mg/L in an adult
  - No useful laboratory testing in the clinical setting for the following medications; most levels are obtained postmortem
    - Mexiletine
    - Flecainide
    - Propafenone

- Class II
  - Serum chemistry
    - Hypoglycemia
    - Hypokalemia
    - Cardiac enzymes
    - Arterial blood gases
- Class III
  - Amiodarone
    - Obtain sputum culture if patient presents with ARDS or pulmonary fibrosis or pneumonitis
    - Thyroid function tests
    - Liver function tests
    - Serum chemistry
  - Bretylium—serum concentrations do have a role in the clinical setting
  - No specific testing for sotalol, ibutilide, and dofetilide; currently under investigation
- Class IV
  - Serum chemistry
    - Hypoglycemia
  - Lactic acid level
  - Digoxin level to exclude co-ingestion
- Chest radiograph for patients with cardiopulmonary signs and symptoms
- Electrocardiogram
- Urinalysis

Differential Diagnosis

- Myocardial infarction
- Torsade de pointes
- Anticholinergic toxicity
- Antidepressant toxicity
- Antihistamine toxicity
- Hyperkalemia
- Plant poisoning—cardiac glycosides
- Cocaine toxicity
- Carbon monoxide poisoning

Management

Nonpharmacologic Treatment
- GI decontamination
  - Beta blockers
  - Controversial for calcium channel blocker
  - Qunidine
  - Flecainide
  - Propafenone
  - Amiodarone

- Hemodialysis
  - Procainamide
  - Mexiletine
  - Bretylium
  - Beta blockers
- Pacemaker
  - Procainamide
  - Quinidine
  - Propafenone
  - Amiodarone
  - Beta blockers
- Intra-aortic balloon pump
  - Same as for pacemaker
- Extracorporeal pump for massive lidocaine overdose

Pharmacologic Treatment
- Airway, breathing, circulatory support, IV access, and telemetry monitoring
- Class I
  - Procainamide
    - GI decontamination and activated charcoal
    - Avoid use of quinidine for dysrhythmias
  - Quinidine
    - Seizures may be treated with diazepam or other benzodiazepines.
    - Activated charcoal, 50 to 100 g
    - Treat hypotension with IV fluids and vasopressor agents if needed.
  - Norepinephrine
    - Use class Ib agents for dysrhythmias.
    - Avoid class Ia medications.
    - Correct electrolyte deficiencies.
    - Dialysis is not helpful.
  - Lidocaine
    - Avoid using phenytoin for seizures because of its synergistic cardiac effects.
    - Use benzodiazpines for seizures.
  - Mexiletine
    - GI decontamination contraindicated
  - Flecainide
    - Gastric emptying if ingestion within 1 hour
    - Seizures can develop within 2 hours of the overdose.
    - Hemodialysis not effective
  - Propafenone
    - Activated charcoal
    - Hemodialysis not useful
    - No antidote
    - Diazepam for seizures
    - Vasopressors as needed for cardiovascular support.
- Class II
  - IV fluids—cystalloids to maintain blood pressure
  - Epinephrine for hypertension

- Glucagon: 5 to 10 mg
- Activated charcoal may be beneficial.
- Benzodiazepines for seizures
- High-dose insulin infusion with glucose administration has been reported to improve outcomes.
  - Insulin is a positive inotrope.
  - Suggested dosing 0.5 to 1 U/kg/hr with frequent boluses of dextrose
- Class III
  - Amiodarone
    - Activated charcoal
    - Beta-adrenergic agonist for bradycardia
    - Cholestyramine to decrease the enterohepatic recirculation of amiodarone
    - Corticosteroids for pulmonary toxicity
  - Bretylium
    - Supportive and symptomatic
  - Procainamide
    - Activated charcoal within 3–4 hours
  - Sotalol
    - Atropine for bradycardia
- Class IV
  - Avoid ipecac
  - Activated charcoal
  - Atropine for significant bradycardia
  - Calcium gluconate IV 4 g or calcium chloride IV 1 g
  - Dopamine to improve heart rate and contractility: 5 to 10 mcg/kg/min

When to Consult, Refer, or Hospitalize

- Admit for evaluation of cardiac dysrhythmias until signs and symptoms have abated and medication(s) have cleared the system—at least 48 hours.
- Cardiology consultation

Follow-up

Expected Outcomes
- Recovery from effects of the drug toxicity
- Patients should be observed with continuous telemetry until ECG changes have resolved.
- Continued monitoring for noncardiac adverse effects of the drug toxicity

Complications
- Dysrhythmias
- Congestive heart failure
- Cardiovascular collapse
- Seizures
- AV block
- Death

ANTICHOLINERGIC AGENTS

Description

- The anticholinergic syndrome has been described with the mnemonic "Blind as a bat, Hot as Hades, Dry as a bone, Red as a beet, and Mad as a hatter."
- Selected examples
  - Atropine
  - Scopolamine
  - Belladonna and other plant derivatives
  - Diphenoxylate with atropine
  - Tricyclic antidepressants
  - Antihistamines
  - Antipsychotics

Assessment

History
- Dry mouth
- Thirst
- Difficulty in swallowing
- Blurred vision
- Agitation

Physical Examination
- Dilated pupils
- Flushed skin
- Tachycardia
- Fever
- Delirium
- Hallucinations
- Myoclonus
- Ileus
- Convulsions
- Tachycardia
- Coma

Diagnostic Studies
- There are no specific diagnostic studies for anticholinergic drug toxicity.
- Serum drug levels are not useful in the clinical setting.
- Draw serum acetaminophen and salicylate levels to determine if a combination medication has been ingested.
- Serum chemistry
- Serum creatine kinase to rule out rhabdomyolysis
- Urine pregnancy test for women of childbearing age
- CT of the head for altered mental status for changes not explained by the ingested agent
- Electrocardiogram to rule out dysrhythmias

Differential Diagnosis

- Hypoglycemia
- Meningitis
- Neuroleptic malignant syndrome
- Schizophrenia
- Toxicity
- Amphetamine
- Antidepressant
- Carbamazepine
- Lithium
- Methamphetamine
- Mushrooms
  - Gyromitra
  - Hallucinogens
- Thyroid hormone

Management

Nonpharmacologic Treatment
- GI decontamination
  - Gastric lavage
- Hemodialysis and hemoperfusion are not effective treatment strategies.
- Foley catheter for urinary retention
- Cooling blanket for severe hyperthermia

Pharmacologic Treatment
- Activated charcoal 1 g/kg without a cathartic, may repeat if needed
- Tachycardia and hypotension are treated with crystalloid infusion.
- Physostigmine salicylate is the only reversible acetycholinesterase inhibitor that can directly treat the CNS effects associated with anticholinergic toxicity.
  - Indicated by the following signs and symptoms
    - Supraventricular tachycardia with hemodynamic compromise
    - Intractable seizures
    - Severe agitation, hallucinations, or psychosis (when the patient is considered a threat to self or others)

- Dose range: 0.5 to 2 mg low IV push at a rate of 0.5 mg/min
- Contraindications
  - May cause seizures in tricyclic overdose
  - Do not administer if prolonged PR or QRS intervals are present on the ECG
  - Bronchospasm
  - Mechanical obstruction of GI or urinary tract
- Sodium bicarbonate
  - For treating antihistamine-induced QRS prolongation (> 100 ms) with a quinidine-like pattern
  - 1 to 2 mEq/kg IV push, may repeat as needed
  - Monitor pH—do not increase > 7.55
  - Monitor for resolution of widened QRS
- Benzodiazepines for control of seizures

When to Consult, Refer, or Hospitalize

- Hospitalize to monitor for resolution of cardiovascular and neurological symptoms.
- Cardiology consult for abnormal ECG and/or dysrhythmias
- Neurology and psychiatry consults as warranted

Follow-up

Expected Outcomes
- Resolution of symptoms
- Patients with severe CNS manifestations have the highest morbidity rates.

Complications
- Seizures
- Cardiovascular collapse
- ECG abnormalities, dysrhythmias
- Coma
- Death

ANTICONVULSANT AGENTS

Description
- Use in the management of seizure disorders. Carbamazepine and valproic acid are also used for mood disorders.
- Examples
  - Phenytoin
    - May be given IV or p.o.
    - Most commonly used anticonvulsant medication

- Iatrogenic intoxications may occur with drug interactions.
- Chronic intoxication may occur with only slightly increased doses because of zero-order kinetics and a small therapeutic window.
- Carbamazepine
  - Used for treatment of trigeminal neuralgia, temporal lobe epilepsy, and other seizure disorders
- Valproic acid
  - Commonly used for the treatment of acute manic episodes, mood stabilization, and prophylaxis for migraine and affective disorders
- Newer agents
  - Gabapentin
  - Levetiracetam
  - Vigabatrin
  - Zonisimade
  - Felbamate
  - Lamotrigine
  - Topiramate
  - Tiagabine

Assessment

History
- Phenytoin
  - With levels of 20 to 40 µcg/ml
    - Nausea
    - Vomiting
    - Blurred vision
    - Diplopia
    - Dizziness
  - As concentration increases
    - Confusion
    - Hallucinations
    - Psychosis may develop
- Carbamazepine
  - Toxicity may be seen with serum levels > 20 mg/L, but severe poisoning is associated with concentrations > 30 to 40 mg/L.
  - Because of erratic and slow absorption, intoxication may progress over several hours to days.
  - Drowsiness
- Valproic acid
  - Confusion
  - Disorientation
  - Hallucinations
  - Hyperactivity
- Newer agents
  - Gapabentin
  - Levetriacetam

- Vigabatrin
- Zonisamide
  - The following symptoms are associated with the preceding four medications:
    - Confusion
    - Dizziness
    - Blurred vision
    - Headache
    - Weight gain
    - Felbamate
  - Nausea
  - Vomiting
  - Abdominal pain
  - Headache
  - Insomnia
- Lamotrigine
- Topiramate
- Tiagabine
  - The following symptoms are associated with preceding three medications:
    - Drowsiness
    - Dizziness
    - Headache
    - Nausea
    - Paresthesias
    - Fatigue

Physical Examination

- Phenytoin
  - With levels of 20 to 40 μcg/mL
    - Normal to dilated pupils
    - Tremor
    - Excitement or agitation
    - Ataxia
    - Nystagmus
    - Drowsiness
  - As concentration increases
    - Progressive CNS depression
    - Sluggish pupillary response
    - Diminished deep tendon reflexes
  - Serum concentration > 90 μ/mL
    - Myocardial depression
    - Respiratory depression
    - Cardiac arrest from the solvent, propylene glycol
  - Carbamazepine
    - Stupor
    - Dilated pupils
    - Tachycardia
    - Nystagmus
    - Ataxia
    - Hypertension
    - Urinary retention

- Ileus
- Neuroleptic-type movements
- High levels: coma and seizures
• Valproic acid
  - Hypotension
  - Tachycardia
  - Miosis
  - Metabolic acidosis
  - With higher levels, coma and respiratory depression
    - Encephalopathy
    - Cerebral edema
  - Patients with underlying seizure disorder may have breakthrough seizures.
  - CNS effects may last at least 24 hours.
• Newer agents
  - Gabapentin
    - Dysarthria
    - Ataxia
    - Slurred speech
  - Levetiracetam
    - Aggression
    - Shallow respirations
    - Syncope
  - Vigabatrin
    - Agitation
    - Ataxia
    - Sedation
  - Zonisamide
    - Stevens-Johnson syndrome
    - Hyperthermia
    - Pancreatitis
    - Metabolic acidosis
  - Felbamate
    - Crystalluria
    - Renal dysfunction
    - Idiosyncratic aplastic anemia
    - Hepatic failure
  - Lamotrigine
    - Stevens-Johnson syndrome
    - Ataxia
    - Tremor
    - Unsteady gain
  - Topiramate
    - Metabolic acidosis
    - Urolithiasis
  - Tiagabine
    - Hypertension
    - Tachycardia
    - Seizures

Diagnostic Studies
- Draw levels for acetaminophen, salicylate, and other anticonvulsant agents.
  - Phenytoin
    - Serum levels
    - Complete blood count
    - Serum chemistry
    - Liver function tests
    - Electrocardiogram
  - Carbamazepine
    - Sequential serum carbamazepine levels
    - Serum chemistry
    - Electrocardiogram
    - Liver function tests
  - Valproic acid
    - Serum sequential valproic acid levels
    - Complete blood count
    - Reticulocyte cell count
    - Ammonia level
  - Elevated serum sodium
    - Serum chemistry level
  - Hypoglycemia
    - Liver function studies
  - Mild liver aminotransferase elevations
    - Arterial blood gases
  - Metabolic acidosis
  - Newer agents
    - Gabapentin
      - Serum chemistry levels
      - No therapeutic serum concentration
      - Draw level to confirm ingestion
    - Levetiracetam
      - Complete blood count
      - No therapeutic serum concentration
    - Draw level to confirm ingestion
    - Vigabatrin
    - No therapeutic serum concentration
      - Draw level to confirm ingestion
    - Zonisamide
  - Arterial blood gases
      - No therapeutic serum concentration
    - Draw level to confirm ingestion
    - Felbamate
    - Urinalysis
      - Crystals
    - Serum chemistry panel
      - Acute renal failure
    - Complete blood count

- No therapeutic serum concentration
  - Draw level to confirm ingestion
- Lamotrigine
- Complete blood count
- No therapeutic serum concentration
  - Draw level on confirm ingestion
- Topiramate
  - Serum chemistry
  - Urinalysis
  - Arterial blood gases
  - No therapeutic serum concentration
    - Draw level to confirm ingestion
- Tiagabine
- Serum chemistry
- Electrocardiogram
- No therapeutic serum concentration
  - Draw level to confirm ingestion

Differential Diagnosis

- Alcohol intoxication
- Wernicke's encephalopathy
- CNS infection
- Occult trauma
- CVA
- Toxicity
- Antidysrhythmics
- Anticholinergics
- Antihistamines
- Opiates
- Tricyclic antidepressants

Management

Nonpharmacologic Treatment
- GI decontamination
  - Whole-bowel irrigation for sustained-release medications
  - Carbamazepine
- Valproic acid
- Hemodialysis
  - Valproic acid
    - For levels > 800 mg/L
- Hemoperfusion
  - Carbamazepine
    - For levels > 60 mg/L
- For all newer agent medications
  - Supportive care for sign/symptoms

Pharmacologic Treatment
- Multiple dose activated charcoal (MDAC) 1 g/kg, repeat as needed
- No specific antidotes
- Supportive care for signs and symptoms
- Carnitine may be used with valproic-acid–induced hyperammonemia.

When to Consult, Refer, or Hospitalize

- Admit for supportive care until resolution of symptoms.
- Neurology consult for seizure activity

Follow-up

Expected Outcome
- Recovery from intoxication

Complications
- Seizures
- Coma
- Cardiovascular collapse
- Stevens-Johnson syndrome

ANTIDEPRESSANT TOXICITY

Description

- Classifications of antidepressants include tricyclic antidepressants, selective serotonin reuptake inhibitors (SSRIs), and monoamine oxidase inhibitors (MOAIs).
- Atypical antidepressants include bupropion and the SSRIs.
- Tetracyclic antidepressants include maprotiline and mirtazapine.
- Trazodone and nefazodone are triazolopyridine derivatives.

Assessment

History
- Hallucinations
- Confusion
- Blurred vision
- Urinary retention
- Altered mental status

Physical Examination
- Tachycardia
- Hypotension
- Arrhythmias
- Seizures
- Hypothermia
- Anticholinergic effects
- Serotinin syndrome
- Agitation or restlessness
- Confusion
- Tachycardia
- Dilated pupils
- Ataxia
- Diaphoresis
- Diarrhea
- Headache
- Shivering

Diagnostic Studies
- Complete metabolic panel
- Complete blood count
- Creatine kinase
- Rhabdomyolysis may occur with seizures.
- Urinalysis
- Electrocardiogram
- Arterial blood gases and chest x-ray as warranted
- Serum levels are not helpful for management.

Differential Diagnosis

- Alcoholic ketoacidosis
- Anaphylaxis
- Anxiety
- Delirum tremens
- Heart block
- Hyperkalemia
- Toxicity
    - Anticholinergic
    - Antidysrhythmic
    - Antihistamine
    - Beta blocker
    - Calcium channel blocker
    - Clonidine
    - Cocaine
    - Digitalis
    - Isoniazid

Management

Nonpharmacologic Treatment
- Airway management, IV, supplemental oxygen

Pharmacologic Treatment
- Tricyclic antidepressants
- Activated charcoal 1 g/kg
- MAOIs
- Muscular hyperactivity and seizures—treat with benzodiazepines
- Nitroprusside, nitroglycerine, and esmolol are recommended for hypertension.
- For hypotension—epinephrine, norepinephrine, isoproterenol
- Hypotension responds to fluid resuscitation.
- Abnormal conduction (QRS > 100 ms in the limb leads) is treated with alkalinization and hyperventilation
  - Sodium bicarbonate IV 0.5 to 2 mEq/L, additional boluses every 3 to 5 minutes until QRS intervals narrow
  - Target pH 7.5 to 7.55
- Serotonin syndrome
  - Sedation, paralytics, intubation and ventilation, anticonvulsants, antihypertensives, and rapid cooling as needed

When to Consult, Refer, or Hospitalize

- Admission to the ICU for symptoms of toxicity
- MAOI overdose patients with or without persistent signs and symptoms of food or drug interactions should be admitted to an ICU for at least 24 hours.

Follow-up

Expected Outcomes
- Resolution of symptoms
- Asymptomatic patients who have ingested classic cyclic antidepressants may be observed in the emergency department for at least 6 hours with continuous cardiac monitoring and an IV in place.
- *Asymptomatic* is defined as a patient with a normal ECG throughout the observation period, a mild sinus tachycardia that resolves in 1 to 2 hours, clear mental status, and a nontoxic acetaminophen level.
- Patients must have had adequate GI decontamination and at least one charcoal stool.
- Patients with bupropion, trazodone, nefazodone, venlafaxine, or SSRI overdose may also be observed for 6 to 8 hours or until the ECG returns to baseline.

Complications
- Respiratory failure requiring intubation
- Prolonged seizures
- Metabolic acidosis
- Hyperthermia
- ECG changes

ANTIPSYCHOTIC DRUG TOXICITY

Description

- Antipsychotic drugs are also known as neuroleptics and major tranquilizers.
- They are used to treat schizophrenia, the manic phase of bipolar disorder, and agitated behavior.
- In addition, they are used as preanesthetics and to treat drug-associated delirium and hallucinations, nausea, vomiting, headaches, hiccups, pruritus, Tourette's syndrome, and several extrapyramidal movement disorders (chorea, dystonias, spasms, tics, torticollis).
- One way to classify antipsychotics is to place them in two categories—typical and atypical.
  - Typical
    - Traditional medications produce extrapyramidal side effects at clinical antipsychotic doses.
  - Atypical
    - Newer agents have minimal extrapyramidal side effects at clinical doses and are capable of treating the negative symptoms of schizophrenia.
    - Low incidence of causing tardive dyskinesia with long-term treatment

Assessment

History
- Lethargy
- Deep sleep
- Confusion
- Nausea
- Vomiting
- Neuroleptic malignant syndrome
- Cardiovascular alterations
- Urinary retention
- Decreased bowel sounds

Physical Examination
- Slurred speech
- Hypotension
- Orthostatic hypotension

- Dry skin and mucosa
- Dystonias and extrapyramidal symptoms
- Rigidity
- Stiff neck
- Hyperreflexia
- Cardiovascular involvement
- AV block
- Atrial and ventricular dysrhythmias
- Widened QRS complexes
- Prolonged QT interval
- ST depression
- T-wave abnormalities
- Tachycardia
- Coma
- Respiratory depression
- Miosis
- Seizures

Diagnostic Studies
- Electrocardiogram
- Prolonged QRS, QT intervals
- Arterial blood gases
- Chest x-ray
- Abdominal x-ray
  - May show densities in the GI tract associated with butyrophenone or phenothiazine poisoning
- Complete blood count
- Complete metabolic panel
- Serum and urinalysis drug screen to identify ingested substances
- Quantitative drug levels are not useful in the clinical setting.

Differential Diagnosis

- Delirium tremens
- Heat exhaustion
- Heat stroke
- Rhabdomyolysis
- Status epilepticus
- Torsades de pointes
- Withdrawal syndrome
- Parkinson's disease
- Toxicity
- Anticholinergic
- Antidepressant
- Antihistamine
- Cocaine
- Lithium
- Methamphetamine
- Salicylate

Management

Nonpharmacologic Treatment
- Continuous cardiac, respiratory, and temperature monitoring
- Supplemental oxygen
- Central venous, pulmonary arterial, and arterial pressure monitoring may be indicated.
- GI decontamination

Pharmacologic Treatment
- Activated charcoal 1 g/kg without cathartic, may repeat every 6 hours
- Hypotension is treated with crystalloid infusions
    - Vasopressors as needed
        - Norepinephrine
        - Phenylephrine
- Sodium bicarbonate, 1 to 2 mEq/kg IV for widened QRS complexes
- Lidocaine and electrical cardioversion for ventricular tachyarrhythmias
    - Type IA, Type IC, and Type III antiarrhythmic medications are not recommended
    - Torsades de pointes should be treated with magnesium
- Seizures are treated with benzodiazepines
- Physostigmine may be used for peripheral or central anticholinergic symptoms
    - 2 mg IV over 3 minutes
- Acute dystonic reactions
    - Benztropine mesylate 1 to 2 mg IV over 1 to 2 minutes
    - Diphenhydramine 50 to 100 mg IV over 1 to 2 minutes
    - Therapy with an oral anticholinergic agent should be continued for 48 to 72 hours.

When to Consult, Refer, or Hospitalize

- Admit patients with protracted hypotension, significant CNS depression, agitation, seizures, acid–base abnormalities, nonsinus dysrhythmias, and cardiac conduction disturbances to the ICU.

Follow-up

Expected Outcomes
- Resolution of symptoms
- Permanent deficits are unusual.
- The outcome is usually favorable.

Complications
- Permanent neurologic disability

CARBON MONOXIDE POISONING

Description

- Carbon monoxide is a colorless, odorless, nonirritating gas.
- Poisoning is the result of intentional or accidental exposure.
  - Automobile exhaust
  - Smoke inhalation
  - Fire
  - Accidental exposure via faulty gas heater, generator, wood or gas stoves
- Binds to hemoglobin
- Much greater affinity than oxygen, > 250 times
- Decreases the oxygen-carrying capacity of RBCs
- Causes tissue hypoxia

Assessment

History
- Headache
- Dizziness
- Abdominal pain
- Nausea
- Confusion

Physical Examination
- Tachycardia
- Tachypnea
- Hypoxia
  - Respiratory depression
- Syncope
- Hypotension
- Seizures
- Coma
- Cardiac arrest
- Mild cases may be mistaken for influenza, whereas high-level exposure may present with rapid unconsciousness, seizures, and death.

Diagnostic Studies
- Elevated carboxyhemoglobin level (CoHb): 10% to 50% or greater.
  - Levels > 20% to 30% are associated with moderate symptoms.
  - Levels > 50% to 60% are associated with a serious or fatal outcome.
  - There can be variability between symptoms and level of carbyoxyhemoglobin.
- Electrocardiogram
- Complete metabolic panel
- Arterial blood gases to determine metabolic acidosis
  - Not reliable for PO_2

Differential Diagnosis

- Altitude sickness
- Encephalitis
- Gastroenteritis
- Headache—cluster, tension
- Hypothyroidism
- Lactic acidosis
- Meningitis
- Toxicity
  - Narcotics
  - Alcohol

Management

Nonpharmacologic Treatment
- Remove from site of exposure
- If associated with smoke inhalation, consider the presence of other toxic gases.
- Administer 100% oxygen by tight-fitting, high-flow reservoir face mask or endotracheal tube.
- Hyperbaric oxygen chamber therapy
  - 100% oxygen at higher than atmospheric pressures
  - May reduce the incidence of neurologic or neuropsychiatric effects resulting from toxic exposure
  - Treatment controversial
  - Indications
    - Loss of consciousness
    - CoHb > 25%
    - Metabolic acidosis
    - Age > 50 years
    - Cerebellar deficits on neurological examination

Pharmacologic Treatment
- IV fluids, vasopressors for hypotension as needed

When to Consult, Refer, or Hospitalize

- Admit patients with CoHb levels > 10%.
- Admit to telemetry unit or cardiac care unit
- ICU care for cerebral edema, cardiovascular instability

Follow-up

Expected Outcomes
- Resolution of symptoms
- Cardiac arrest, coma, metabolic acidosis, and high CoHb levels are associated with a poor outcome.
- Neuropsychiatric testing may be able to determine delayed neurological deficits.
- Minimize physical activity for 2 to 4 weeks after exposure.

Complications
- Survivors of severe poisoning may develop permanent neurological deficits.

CARDIAC GLYCOSIDE POISONING

Description
- Digoxin is the major cardiac glycoside used in medicine.
- Used for atrial fibrilliation with rapid ventricular response and in congestive heart failure

Assessment

History
- Acute
  - Nausea
  - Vomiting
  - Abdominal pain
  - Headache
  - Weakness
  - Dizziness
  - Confusion
  - Coma
  - Ventricular dysrhythmias uncommon
- Chronic
  - Nausea
  - Vomiting
  - Confusion
  - Blurred vision
    - Yellow-green halos
  - Delirium
  - Hallucinations
  - Fatigue
  - Anorexia

Physical Examination
- Acute
  - Bradydysrhythmias
  - Supraventricular dysrhythmias with AV block
- Chronic
  - Coma
  - Various dysrhythmias

Diagnostic Studies
- Serum chemistry
  - Elevated potassium with acute toxicity
  - Hypokalemia with chronic toxicity
- Digoxin level
  - Markedly elevated with acute toxicity (> 2.4 nanograms/mL)
  - May be in therapeutic range or slightly elevated with chronic toxicity
  - After treatment, free digoxin levels are decreased within 0 to 1 minute of digoxin immune FAB administration; however, total serum levels are markedly increased and have no correlation with toxicity.
- Electrocardiogram

Differential Diagnosis

- Abdominal pain—older adults
- Acute coronary syndrome
- Aystole
- Atrial fibrillation or flutter
- Benign positional vertigo
- Dilated cardiomyopathy
- Congestive heart failure
- Delirium
- Dementia
- Amnesia
- Depression
- Aortic dissection
- Heart block
- Mesenteric ischemia
- Myocardial infarction
- Pulmonary embolism
- Cardiogenic shock
- Septic shock

Management

Nonpharmacologic Treatment
- Continuous cardiac monitoring
- IV access

Pharmacologic Treatment
- Activated charcoal 1 g/kg every 6 hours
- Digoxin immune FAB
  - Dosing varies according to digoxin level.
  - Available as 38 mg/vial
  - Digoxin intoxication
    - # vials = digoxin level (ng/mL) × wt (kg)/100
  - Give as IV bolus if cardiac arrest is imminent
  - Average dose in adults is six vials IV over 30 minutes
  - Skin testing should be done for known hypersensitivity or history of digoxin immune FAB administration
  - Acute digoxin toxicity
    - # vials = digoxin load (mg) × 0.8/0.5
    - Alternative: administer 10 vials IV for each 25 tablets ingested
    - Give as IV bolus if cardiac arrest imminent
    - For acute ingestion of unknown amount, give 10 to 20 vials IV
      - 380–760 mg
- Skin testing—see preceding

When to Consult, Refer, or Hospitalize

- Admit for new cardiac dysrhythmias, severe bradyarrhythmias, advanced AV block, acute prolonged QRS interval, severe electrolyte abnormalities, dehydration, inability of the patient to care for himself or herself, suicidal ideation
- ICU admission
  - Hemodynamic instability, refractory dysrhythmias, hyperkalemia, and renal failure
  - Administration of digoxin immune FAB

Follow-up

Expected Outcomes
- Resolution of symptoms
- Adjustment of digoxin dose in chronic toxicity (or discontinuation)
- Morbidity and mortality are increased if the patient has a new dysrhythmia, advanced AV block, or other significant ECG abnormality.

Complications
- Cardiac arrest
- From digoxin immune FAB therapy
  - Allergic reactions
  - Worsening congestive heart failure
  - Tachyarrhythmias
  - Hypokalemia

CHOLINERGIC TOXICITY

Description

- Cholinergic agents are used in clinical medicine, as insecticides, and as weapons of mass destruction.
- Many poisonings occur during the agricultural use of pesticides.
- Suicide attempts involve ingestion.
- Medicinal cholinergic medications
  - Edrophonium
  - Neostigmine
  - Physostigmine
  - Donepezil
  - Rivastigmine
  - Tacrine

Assessment

History
- Mild poisoning
  - Fatigue
  - Headache
  - Dizziness
  - Nausea
  - Vomiting
  - Numbness
  - Chest tightness
  - Abdominal cramps
  - Diarrhea
- Moderate poisoning
  - Weakness
  - Fasciculations
- Severe poisoning
  - Unconscious
  - Fasciculations

Physical Examination
- Mild poisoning
  - Able to walk
  - Sweating
  - Salivation
- Moderate poisoning
  - Not able to walk
  - Difficulty speaking
  - Miosis

- Severe poisoning
  - Unreactive pupils
  - Flaccid paralysis
  - Secretions of mouth and nose
  - Moist rales
  - Respiratory distress
  - Cardiac depression
  - Seizures

Diagnostic Studies
- Primary laboratory studies are plasma cholinesterase and butyrl-cholinersterase
- Red blood cell acetylcholinesterase
  - Acute exposures are classified according to the degree of depression of the RBC cholinesterase.
- Mild poisoning
  - RBC cholinesterase 20% to 50% of normal
- Moderate poisoning
  - RBC cholinesterase 10% to 20% of normal
- Severe poisoning
  - RBC cholinesterase < 10% of normal

Differential Diagnosis

- Gastroenteritis
- Influenza
- Mental illness
- Diabetic ketoacidosis
- Pneumonia
- Myasthenia crisis
- Nicotine poisoning
- Opiate overdose
- Hypertensive encephalopathy
- Asthma attack
- Coronary ischemia

Management

- For ingestion toxicity

  Nonpharmacologic Treatment
  - Gastric lavage

  Pharmacologic Treatment
  - Activated charcoal
  - IV fluids
  - Blood pressure support with vasopressors

- Norepinephrine
- Phenylephrine
- Epinephrine
- Cardiac depression may be treated with dobutamine.
- Seizures should be treated with atropine followed by benzodiazepines.
- Benzodiazepines may be beneficial for CNS effects even in the absence of seizures.
- Atropine
  - 1 to 2 mg parenterally, doubled every 5 minutes until secretions are controlled
- Pralidoxime (2-Pam)
  - 1 to 2 g IV in 100 to 150 mL of normal saline over 30 minutes

When to Consult, Refer, or Hospitalize

- All patients, except those with extremely mild symptoms, should be admitted to the ICU.

Follow-up

Expected Outcomes
- Resolution of symptoms
- High doses of atropine may be needed to control secretions.
- Patients with CNS anoxic effects have worse outcomes.

Complications
- Cerebral anoxia
- Seizures
- Respiratory failure
- Cardiovascular collapse

LITHIUM TOXICITY

Description

- Lithium is used for the treatment of manic depressive illness and other psychiatric disorders.
- Toxicity is usually from renal impairment or excessive overmedication.
- A single acute overdose is less likely to result in severe poisoning.

Assessment

- Symptoms may take several days to weeks to resolve.

History
- Nausea
- Vomiting
- Diarrhea
- Delirium
- Confusion

Physical Examination
- Muscle weakness
- Tremor
- Rigidity
- Ataxia
- Dementia
- ECG changes

Diagnostic Studies
- Lithium levels > 1.5 mEq/L
  - Blood levels should be drawn 8 to 12 hours after last dose for chronic use.
- Therapeutic level: 0.6 to 1.2 mEq/L
  - Chronic intoxication may occur at levels only slightly > 1.2 mEq/L.
  - Acute overdose patients may remain asymptomatic despite having higher serum levels early after drug ingestion.
- Electrocardiogram
  - Flattening of T waves
  - Presence of U waves
  - Prolongation of the QT interval

Differential Diagnosis

- Delirium
- Dementia
- Amnesia
- Depression
- Neuroleptic malignant syndrome
- Schizophrenia
- Stroke
- Heavy metal toxicity
- Mercury toxicity
- Organic phosphorus compounds and carbamate toxicity

Management

Nonpharmacologic Treatment
- Gastric lavage may be beneficial.
- Consider whole-bowel irrigation, especially with sustained-release medication.
- Hemodialysis

- Lithium level > 6.0 mEq/L
- Lithium level > 4.0 mEq/L with chronic therapy (as opposed to acute overdose)
- Lithium level 2.5 to 4.0 mEq/L in patients with chronic kidney disease (CKD), severe neurologic symptoms, hemodynamic instability

Pharmacologic Treatment
- Activated charcoal is ineffective
- Fluid therapy
  - Volume should be restored with 1 to 2 liters of normal saline.
  - Infuse at a rate to produce 100 mL/hr of urine.

When to Consult, Refer, or Hospitalize

- Admit patients with significant signs and symptoms regardless of lithium levels.
- Admit to the ICU for severe neurotoxicity requiring hemodialysis.

Follow-up

Expected Outcome
- Resolution of symptoms

Complications
- Truncal and gait ataxia
- Nystagmus
- Short-term memory deficits
- Dementia
- SILENT: syndrome of irreversible lithium-effectuated neurotoxicity
- Nephrogenic diabetes insipidous
- Neruoleptic malignant syndrome
- Serotonin syndrome

OPIOID TOXICITY

Description

- Includes synthetic and naturally occurring compounds that are used for analgesia
  - Examples
    - Morphine
    - Heroin
    - Hydrocodone
    - Codeine

- Synthetic
  - Fentanyl
  - Methadone
  - Butorphanol
- Preparations of hydrocodone and codeine are found in combination with acetaminophen

Assessment

History
- Hypothermia
- Drowsiness
- Altered mental status

Physical Examination
- Depressed respiratory effort
- Hypercapnia
- Miosis
- Noncardiogenic pulmonary edema
- Coma
- Acute renal failure
- Rhabdomyolysis

Diagnostic Studies
- Complete blood count
- Complete metabolic panel
- Creatine phosphokinase
- Urinalysis
- Proteinuria
- Myoglobinuria
- Urine sediment
- Urine toxicology screen
- Chest x-ray
  - Will reveal pulmonary edema
- Serum opiate levels do not contribute to clinical management.

Differential Diagnosis

- Alcohol, substance abuse
- Subdural hematoma
- Syncope
- Toxicity
  - Barbituate
  - Benzodiazepine
  - Carbon monoxide
  - Clonidine

Management

Nonpharmacologic Treatment
- Establish airway
- Supplemental O_2
- Continuous ECC monitoring

Pharmacologic Treatment
- Narcan
  - Consider using low doses initially if long-term narcotic use is suspected.
    - Will decrease the severity of acute withdrawal reaction
  - 0.2 to 2 mg IV
  - Plasma half-life is about 60 minutes
    - Patients who respond should be observed for at least 3 hours after administration.
- Oral ingestion should be treated with activated charcoal 1 g/kg.
- Hypotension
  - IV fluids, vasopressors as needed

When to Consult, Refer, or Hospitalize

- Admit if a patient requires a second dose of narcan.
- Admit for a minimum of 12–24 hours any patient who exhibits respiratory depression, recurrent sedation, or any other complicating factors.
- Continued cardiac and respiratory monitoring until symptoms subside

Follow-up

Expected Outcomes
- Resolution of symptoms
- Adjustment in medication administration
- Counseling for narcotic dependence as indicated

Complications
- Acute lung injury
- IV drug abuser
- Cellulitis
- Endocarditis
- Pneumonia
- Rhabdomyolysis
- Necrotizing fasciitis
- Acute withdrawal syndrome after Narcan administration to patients with true opioid dependence

PESTICIDE POISONING

Description

- Organophosphates and carbamates are used as pesticides.
- These poisons inhibit acetylcholinersterase.
- Organophosphates may cause permanent damage to the enzyme, whereas carbamates have a transient and reversible effect.

Assessment

History
- Abdominal cramps
- Vomiting
- Headache
- Blurred vision
- Diarrhea
- Mental confusion
- Anxiety
- Drowsiness
- Urinary incontinence
- Muscle fasciculations

Physical Examination
- Sweating
- Slurred speech
- Hypersalivation
- Pinpoint pupils
- Brady or tachycardia
- Muscle weakness with respiratory depression
- Severe bronchospasm
- Intravacular volume loss

Diagnostic Studies
- Serum and red blood cell cholinesterase activity is usually depressed > 50% below baseline with severe intoxication.

Differential Diagnosis

- Gastroenteritis
- Toxicity mushroom
- Myasthenia gravis
- Gullian-Barré syndrome

Management

Nonpharmacologic Treatment
- Wash skin if exposed topically.
- GI decontamination
- Maintain airway.
- Urinary catheter to prevent retention

Pharmacologic Treatment
- Activated charcoal 1g/kg if ingested
- Atropine
  - 1 to 5 mg IV or IM initially, then double for each subsequent dose every 15 minutes until the following occurs:
    - Flushing
    - Dry mouth
    - Tachycardia
    - Dilated pupils
    - Large doses may be necessary.
      - 500 to 1,500 mg/24 hours
- Pralidoxime
  - 1 to 2 g IV over 10 to 15 minutes
  - Follow with infusion of 250 to 500 mg/hr

When to Consult, Refer, or Hospitalize

- Admit all symptomatic patients for at least 24 hours to monitor respiratory status.

Follow-up

Expected Outcomes
- Resolution of symptoms
- If occupational exposure, patient should not return to work until cholinesterase activity is > 75%

Complications
- Respiratory failure
- Seizures
- Aspiration pneumonia
- Delayed neuropathy
- Death

SALICYLATE TOXICITY

Description

- Aspirin (acetylsalicylic acid) and other salicylates are used for antipyretic and antiinflammatory effects.
- Found alone and in combination with other medications, both prescription and over-the-counter
- Salicylates interfere with the metabolism of glucose and fatty acids.
- They also uncouple oxidative phosphorylation that causes decreased production of adenosine triphosphate, accumulation of lactic acid, and heat production.
- Poisoning may result from a single ingestion (> 200 mg/kg).
- Long-term poisoning occurs in older adults, who may take large doses and increase them or develop CKD.

Assessment

History
- Nausea
- Vomiting
- Fever
- Tinnitus
- Confusion
- Lethargy

Physical Examination
- Tachypnea or hyperventilation
- Cyanosis
- Metabolic acidosis
- Respiratory alkalosis
- Dehydration
- Hyperthermia
- Coma
- Seizures
- Noncardiogenic pulmonary edema
- Circulatory collapse
  - The last four signs are typically seen with salicylate levels of > 100 mg/dl.

Diagnostic Studies
- Arterial blood gases
  - Respiratory alkalosis
  - Metabolic acidiosis
- Serum electrolytes
- Serum salicylate levels
  - Repeat every 2 hours if managing an acute ingestion
  - If levels increase, may indicate a sustained-release product
  - 6-hour post-ingestion levels
    - < 50 mg/dL: asymptomatic
    - 51 to 110 mg/dL: mild to moderate toxicity
    - 111 to 120 mg/dL: severe toxicity

- Urinalysis
  - Maintain an urine pH of 7.5 to 8 with treatment
- Liver function studies
- Coagulation studies
  - Prothombin time may be prolonged
- Salicylate-induced thrombocytopenia
- Chest x-ray if pulmonary edema is present, or there is hypoxia, or severe intoxication
- Electrocardiogram

Differential Diagnosis

- Adult respiratory distress syndrome (ARDS)
- Alcoholic ketoacidosis
- Anxiety
- Asthma
- Diabetic ketoacidosis
- Lactic acidosis
- Metabolic acidosis
- Pulmonary embolism
- Septic shock
- Toxicity
- Chlorine gas
- Ethylene glycol
- Hydrocarbons
- Iron
- Organophosphate and carbamate
- Theophylline
- Withdrawal syndrome

Management

Nonpharmacologic Treatment
- GI decontamination with gastric lavage for large ingestion (> 10 to 15 g)
- Hemodialysis
  - For patients who cannot tolerate fluid challenges
  - Worsening renal function
  - Severe metabolic acidosis
  - Serum salicylate level > 100 mg/dL
  - Patients with chronic accidental overmedication may have serious toxicity at lower drug concentrations.
    - In these cases, hemodialysis may be performed for levels > 50 to 60 mg/dL.
- Hyperventilate patient if endotracheal intubation is required.

Pharmacologic Treatment
- Activated charcoal 1 g/kg, may repeat as necessary
  - Massive ingestions may lead to prolonged or delayed absorption.
- Alkalinization of the urine
  - Infuse 100 mEq of sodium bicarbonate in 1 liter of D5W ¼ NS at a rate of 200 mL/hr.
    - Monitor urine pH.
  - May have to replace volume losses and address electrolyte imbalances first

When to Consult, Refer, or Hospitalize

- Admit patients with major signs and symptoms to the ICU.
- May need consult with nephrology for hemodialysis
- Admit patients with minor signs and symptoms to an extended observation unit or medical floor.

Follow-up

Expected Outcomes
- Resolution of symptoms
- Mortality of 1% and morbidity of 16% is associated with an acute overdose.
- Advise patients regarding the use of over-the-counter medications.

Complications
- Metabolic acidosis
- Cardiovascular collapse
- Death

SEDATIVE-HYPNOTIC DRUG TOXICITY

Description

- Sedative-hypnotic agents include barbiturates (phenobarbital, pentobarbital, butalbital, amobarbital), and benzodiazepines (alprazolam, diazepam, lorazepam, and triazolam).
- Other medications include meprobamate, glutethimide, ethchlorvynol, chloral hydrate, zolpidem, zaleplon, and buspirone.
- Used to treat anxiety or insomnia

Assessment

History
- Confusion
- Altered mental status

Physical Examination
- Slurred speech
- Lethargy
- Ataxia
- Stupor
- Hypothermia
- Respiratory depression
- Respiratory acidosis
- Absent gag, deep-tendon, and corneal reflexes
- Miosis
- Hypotension
- Bradycardia

Diagnostic Studies
- Complete blood count
- Arterial blood gases
- Complete metabolic panel
- Toxicology screen
  - Barbiturates
    - For short-acting agents: lethal dose is 3 g or a serum concentration > 3.5 mg/dl
    - For long-acting agents: lethal dose is 5 to 10 g or a serum concentration > 8 mg/dl
  - Meprobromate
    - Coma occurs at 6 to 20 mg/dl
    - Fatal at concentrations higher than 20 mg/dl
  - Glutethimide
    - Consider hemodialyis at concentrations > 3 mg/dl.
  - Ethchlorvynol
    - Charcoal hemoperfusion for ingestions > 100 mcg/ml or serum concentration of > 10 mg/dl
  - Chloral hydrate
    - Lethal dose is 10 g; a concentration of > 100 mcg/ml is toxic.
- Abdominal x-ray
  - Chloral hydrate is radiographic
- Electrocardiogram
  - May detect co-ingestion of tricyclic agents
- Urinalysis
  - Blue-green urine has been detected with zaleplon

Differential Diagnosis

- Alcohol abuse
- Brain abscess
- Delirium tremens
- Epidural hematoma
- Herpes simplex encephalitis
- Hyperosmolar hyperglycemic nonketotic coma
- Hypoglycemia
- Plant poisoning
- Isoquinoline
- Quinoline
- Cardiac glycosides
- Herbs
- Glycoside—coumarin
- Alcohol toxicity

Management

Nonpharmacologic Treatment
- Maintain airway—may require assisted ventilation
- Gradual rewarming for hypothermia
- Gastric lavage for large ingestions

Pharmacolgical Treatment
- Ipecac not recommended
- Multidose activated charcoal 1 g/kg for barbiturates, glutethimide, and meprobromate
- IV crystalloids and vasopressors for hypotension if needed
- Treat ventricular dysrhythmias caused by chloral hydrate with propranolol, 1 to 5 mg IV, or esmolol 25 to 100 μcg/kg/min
- Flumazenil is a specific benzodiazepine antagonist
  - IV administration 0.5 to 3.0 mg
  - Effects last only 2 to 3 hours; resedation may occur
  - Contraindicated if patient has ingested tricyclics or been given benzodiazepines for control of status epilepticus

When to Consult, Refer, or Hospitalize

- Observe patients with barbiturate toxicity for at least 6 hours; admit if they remain symptomatic.
- Observe patients with benzodiazepine toxicity for at least 2 hours after recovery from flumazenil—admit for recurrent symptoms.
- Patients with glutethimide toxicity must be observed for 24 hours in the hospital.

Follow-up

Expected Outcomes
- Resolution of symptoms
- Must consider co-ingestions and adjustment of medications

Complications
- Respiratory depression
- Coma
- Death
- Teratogenic or mutagenic effects

STIMULANT TOXICITY

Description

- Cocaine and the amphetamines stimulate the CNS and the sympathetic nervous system.
- Cocaine has local anesthetic properties and may cause sodium channel blockade in high doses.
- The half-life of cocaine is significantly less than that of amphetamine or methamphetamine.
- These drugs can be taken orally, snorted, smoked, or injected.
- Speedball—soluble form of cocaine injected with heroin.
- MDMA (methylenedioxymethamphetamine), or ecstasy—popular among teens and young adults
- Prescription stimulants—methylphenidate

Assessment

History
- Insomnia
- Irritability
- Dry mouth
- Anorexia
- Anginal chest pain
- MDMA
  - Euphoria
  - Sexual arousal
  - Enhanced sensory perception
  - Increased endurance
  - Increased sociability
- Diaphoresis

Physical Examination
- Dysrhythmias
- Dilated pupils
- Seizures
- Hyperthermia
- Metabolic acidosis
- Rhabodmyolysis
- MDMA
  - Hyperthermia
  - Hyponatremia
  - Seizures
  - Hepatitis
  - CVA
  - Cardiac dysrhythmias
  - Acute myocardial infarction

Diagnostic Studies
- Serum chemistry panel
- Cardiac enzymes
- Liver function studies
- Urine and serum creatine kinase
- Urine and serum toxicology screen
- Patients with prolonged seizures or altered mental status will need glucose and electrolyte evaluation.

Differential Diagnosis

- Angina pectoris
- Dilated cardiomyopathy
- Delirium tremens
- Hypertensive emergencies
- Pneumothorax
- Rhabdomyolysis
- Schizophrenia
- Septic shock
- Status epilepticus
- Meningitis
- CVA
- Subarachnoid hemorrhage
- Syncope
- Toxicity
- Amphetamine
- Anticholinergic
- Antidepressant
- Hallucinogen
- MOA inhibitor
- Neuroleptic agents

- Phencyclidine
- Ventricular dysrthythmias
- Withdrawal syndrome
- Acute myocardial infarction
- Heat stroke

Management

Nonpharmacologic Treatment
- Place patient in a quiet room.
- Treat severe hyperthermia with aggressive cooling measures.
- Myocardial infarction
  - Primary reperfusion with percutaneous intervention

Pharmacologic Treatment
- Mild or moderate intoxication can be managed with a sedative agent.
  - Diazepam
  - Lorazepam
- Severe hypertension that does not improve with sedation
  - Phentolamine 2 to 5 mg IV at 5 to 10 minute intervals or nitroprusside 0.5 to 10 µg/kg/min
- Tachycardia or ventricular dysrhythmias
  - Benzodiazepines for supraventriciular tachycardia
  - Lidocaine for ventricular dysrhythmias
  - Beta blocker may worsen hypertension because of the unopposed effects of the stimulant drug
    - Labetalol has been used safely
- Wide complex dysrhythmias should be treated with sodium bicarbonate or lidocaine
- Seizures
  - Benzodiazepines
- In patients with myocardial ischemia
  - Nitroglycerin
  - Calcium channel blockers
    - Dihydropyridine class
  - Amlodipine
  - Nifedipine

When to Consult, Refer, or Hospitalize

- Admit to a critical care unit for hemodynamic instability, myocardial ischemia or chest pain, tachycardia, dysrhythmias, respiratory distress, pulmonary edema, seizures, cerebral hemorrhage, or coma.

Follow-up

Expected Outcomes
- Resolution of symptoms
- Patients without signs or symptoms of end-organ damage do well with sedation and calm reassurance.
- Neuropsychiatric problems occur in about in about 40% of cocaine users.
- Some of the central effects of cocaine—euphoria, anorexia, hyperthermia—show tolerance and a higher dose of the drug is required to attain the same CNS effect as previously.
- A moderate number of addicts develop panic attacks.

Complications
- Seizures
- Cerebrovascular disorders
    - Hemorrhagic
    - Ischemic
- Cocaine-induced arterial thrombosis
- Infarction of the spinal cord

THEOPHYLLINE TOXICITY

Description
- Theophylline is still occasionally used for asthma and other bronchospastic disorders.
- It is available in regular and sustained-release forms.
- Aminophylline is the ethylenediamine salt of theophylline and is used for IV infusions.
- Theophylline toxicity may occur after an acute single overdose or long-term therapy.

Assessment

History
- Nausea
- Vomiting
    - Hematemesis
- Restlessness
- Agitation
- Irritability

Physical Examination
- Tachycardia
- Premature ventricular contractions
- Atrial dysrhythmias
- Seizures in severe overdoses
- Tremors

Diagnostic Studies
- Serum chemistry
  - Hypokalemia
  - Hypophosphatemia
  - Hyperglycemia
- Complete blood count
  - Leukocytosis
- Therapeutic level: 8 to 20 µg/mL
  - Levels > 100 mg/L
    - Seizures
    - Hypotension
    - Ventricular dysrhythmias
    - Serum drug levels may not peak for 16 to 24 hours after ingestion.
    - Chronic intoxication
  - Symptoms may develop at levels of 14 to 35 mg/L.
- Electrocardiogram

Differential Diagnosis

- Alcoholic ketoacidosis
- Anxiety
- Asystole
- Atrial fibrillation flutter
- Diabetic ketoacidosis
- Epidural hematoma
- Gastroenteritis
- Hypercalcemia
- Multifocal atrial tachycardia
- Septic shock
- Status epilepticus
- Subarachnoid hemorrhage
- Toxicity
- Carbon monoxide
- Cyanide
- Disulfiram
- Iron
- MOA inhibitor
- Ventricular fibrillation
- Ventricular tachycardia

Management

Nonpharmacologic Treatment
- Gastric lavage for large ingestions
- Whole-bowel irrigation for massive ingestion of sustained-release medication
- Hemodialysis or hemoperfusion for levels > 100 mg/L and recurrent seizures

Pharmacologic Treatment
- Activated charcoal 1 g/kg in repeated doses every 6 to 12 hours
- Hypotension and tachycardia are mediated through excessive β-adrenergic stimulation.
- Beta-blocker therapy: esmolol 25 to 100 µg/kg/min

When to Consult, Refer, or Hospitalize

- Admit all patients with signs and symptoms of toxicity and theophylline levels > 30 µg/ml.
- Patients with cardiovascular or neurological symptoms should be admitted to the ICU.

Follow-up

Expected Outcomes
- Resolution of symptoms
- Prognosis is dose-dependent.
- Large ingestions increase the risk of death from dysrhythmias, refractory hypotension, or status epilepticus

Complications
- Anoxic brain injury
- Status epilepticus
- Death

REFERENCES

Cooper, D., Kraink, A., Lubner, S., & Reno, H. (Eds.). (2007). *The Washington manual of medical therapeutics* (32nd ed.). Philadelphia: Wolters Kluwer/Lippincott Williams & Wilkins.

Fauci, A., Braunwald, E., Kasper, D., Hauser, S., Longo, D., Jameson, J., & Loscalzo, J. (Eds.). (2009). *Harrison's principles of internal medicine.* New York: McGraw Hill.

Irwin, R., & Rippe, J. (2008). *Intensive care medicine.* Philadelphia: Wolters Kluwer/Lippincott Williams & Wilkins.

McPhee, S., & Papadakis, M. (Eds.). (2011). *2011 current medical diagnosis and treatment.* New York: McGraw Hill.

O'Malley, G. F. (2007). Emergency department management of the salicylate poisoned patient. *Emergency Medicine Clinics of North America, 25*(2), 333–346.

Wells, B., DiPiro, J., Schwinghammer, T., & DiPiro, C. (Eds.). (2009). *Pharmacotherapy handbook.* New York: McGraw Hill.

22

Infections
Pamela Smith, MSN, RN, ACNP-BC, CCRN

NOSOCOMIAL INFECTIONS

URINARY TRACT INFECTION (UTI)

- See Chapter 8, Renal and Urologic Disorders

NOSOCOMIAL AND VENTILATOR-ASSOCIATED PNEUMONIA

Description

- Nosocomial infections of the lower respiratory tract are often associated with mechanical ventilation and are defined as a pneumonia with an onset of 48 hours after admission.

Etiology

- Aspiration of endogenous or hospital-acquired oropharyngeal (and at times gastric) flora
- Most often caused by *Streptococcus pneumoniae* and *Haemophilus* species in early onset (with the first 4 days of admission) pneumonia
- Late onset are most commonly the result of *S. aureus, P. aeruginosa, Enterbacter* species, *Klebsiella penumoniae*, or *Acinetobacter*
- Other organisms
  - *E. coli*
  - *Serratia marcescens*
- Infection is polymicrobial in 20% to 40% of cases

Incidence and Demographics

- Pneumonia is responsible for 15% to 20% of nosocomial infections.
- Responsible for 24% of extra hospital days and 39% of extra costs
- The most common and lethal form of nosocomial pneumonia is ventilator-associated pneumonia.

Risk Factors

- Administration of antimicrobial therapy
- Contaminated ventilator circuits or equipment
- Decreased gastric acidity
- Endotracheal intubation
- Decreased level of consciousness
- Presence of a nasogastric tube
- COPD
- Advanced age
- Upper abdominal surgery
- Immunosuppression

Prevention and Screening

- Handwashing by healthcare workers
  - Most effective means of prevention
- Elevate head of bed 30°–45°
- Allow sedation holiday for patients mechanically ventilated and assess readiness for extubation on a daily basis
- Use of peptic ulcer disease prophylaxis
- Use of deep-vein thrombosis prophylaxis unless contraindicated
- Meticulous care of the respiratory equipment
- Selective decontamination of the oropharynx and gut

Assessment

History
- Recent hospitalization
- Fever
- Shortness of breath
- Cough
- Changes in ventilator requirements

Physical Examination
- Purulent secretions
- Hypoxemia
- Crackles or dullness to percussion
- Tachypnea

Diagnostic Studies
- Complete blood count
  - Leukocytosis
  - Left shift
- Chest x-ray
- New or changing radiographic infiltrates
- Isolation of pathogen from
  - Sputum
  - Transbronchial aspirate
  - Bronchial brush
  - Bronchoalveolar lavage
- Biopsy
- Blood cultures
- Thoracentesis
  - To determine if pleural space is infected

Differential Diagnosis

- Atelectasis
- Congestive heart failure
- Pulmonary embolism
- Community-acquired pneumonia
- Viral pneumonia
- *Pneumocystis carinii* pneumonia

Management

Nonpharmacologic Treatment
- Handwashing
- Promote sputum clearance with incentive spirometer, chest physical therapy, and frequent suctioning.

Pharmacologic Treatment
- The susceptibilities of the hospital unit must be known.
- Antibiotic coverage is targeted broadly to include resistant gram-negative organisms.
- Early onset and no risk of multidrug-resistant pathogens
- Ceftriaxone
- Quinolones
- Ampicillin-sulbactam
- Ertapenem
- Combination antipseudomonal coverage
- Antipseudomonal beta-lactam
- Aminoglycoside
- Quinolone
- Aspiration pneumonia
- Clindamycin
- Beta-lactam or beta-lactamase inhibitor
- For the critically ill and those at risk for methacillin-resistant staphylococci
  - Vancomycin
    - Duration of therapy: 14 to 21 days
    - May be shortened to 7 days if the organism is not *Pseudomonas aeruginosa*

Special Considerations

- Nosocomial pneumonia is responsible for 24% of extra hospital days and 39% of extra costs.
- Accurate diagnosis is difficult in the hospital setting because many of the patients, especially those in the ICU, have an abnormal chest x-ray, fever, and leukocytosis, which may be attributable to multiple causes.

When to Consult, Refer, or Hospitalize

- Pulmonology consult when pneumonia is diagnosed or when patient is mechanically ventilated

Follow-up

Expected Outcomes
- Resolution of pneumonia
- Mortality is 6% to 14%.
- Risk of death is affected by comorbidities, inadequate antibiotic treatment, and the type of organisms involved, such as
  - *Pseudomonas aeruginosa*
  - *Acinetobacter*
- Creactive protein measurements may be useful in the identification of patients with poor outcome as early as day 4 and may detect patients with inappropriate antibiotic therapy.

Complications
- Acute respiratory distress syndrome
- Empyema
- Lung abscess
- Death

SURGICAL WOUND INFECTIONS

Description

- The average wound infection has an incubation period of 5 to 7 days.
- The incidence of wound infections has become difficult to assess because many procedures are now done on an outpatient basis; therefore, the incubation period is longer than the postoperative stay.

Etiology

- Wound infections are usually caused by the patient's endogenous or hospital-acquired skin and mucosal flora.
- Occasionally, because of airborne spread of flakes of skin that may be shed into the wound from members of the operating room team
- True airborne spread of infection in the operating room is rare unless there is a disseminator (group A streptococci or staphylococci) among the team members.

Incidence and Demographics

- Wound infections account for up to 20% to 30% of nosocomial infections and contribute up to 57% of extra hospital days and 42% of extra costs.

Risk Factors

- Surgeon's level of skill
- Underlying diseases
- Diabetes
- Obesity
- Advanced age
- Inappropriate timing of antibiotic phrophylaxis
- Presence of drains
- Prolonged hospital stays
- Shaving of the operative site with a razor the day before surgery
- Long duration of surgery
- Immunosuppression
- Infection at remote sites
    - For example, untreated UTI

Prevention and Screening

- National prevention efforts
    - Surgical Care Improvement Project (SCIP)
    - Surgical Infection Prevention Project (SIP)
    - Institute for Healthcare Improvement Project (IHI) 100,000 Lives Campaign
- Attention to surgical issues and operating room asepsis
- Administer antibiotics within 1 hour of surgery and discontinue within 24 hours.
- Limit any hair removal to the time of surgery.
- Use of clippers or no hair removal at all
- Maintain normal perioperative glucose levels (cardiac patients).
- Maintain perioperative normothermia.

Assessment

History
- Fever
- Pain
- Altered mental status

Physical Examination
- Purulence in the surgical wound site
- Sepsis
- See Shock section
- Cholecystectomy
- Cardiothoracic or vascular surgery
- Orthopedic surgery
- Cesarean section
- Clean-contaminated
- Colon surgery

- Penetrating abdominal or pelvic trauma
- Bowel peforation

Diagnostic Studies
- Complete blood count
- Leukocytosis
- Elevated platelet count
- Elevated sedimentation rate
- CT or MRI of affected area

Management

Nonpharmacologic Treatment
- Drainage or surgical excision of infected or necrotic material

Pharmacologic Treatment
- Common pathogens
- S. *aureus*
- Coagulase-negative staphylococci
- Enteric and anaerobic bacteria
- In rapidly progressing postoperative infections (within 1 to 2 days of a surgical procedure), suspect group A streptococcal or clostridial infection.
- Antibiotic therapy should target the most likely offending agent initially then be adjusted according to culture results.

Special Considerations

- Extensive review of infection rates by regulatory agencies and third-party payers has emphasized the importance of developing meaningful systems for wound surveillance after the patient's discharge (when 50% of infections first become apparent), the use of markers for wound infection (prolonged postoperative antibiotics), or both.

When to Consult, Refer, or Hospitalize

- Infectious disease consult for antibiotic management

Follow-up

Expected Outcomes
- Resolution of infection
- Inspect wounds at the time of discharge.
- Outpatient follow-up in 7 days
- Any discharge noted should be sent for culture and sensitivity.
- Continued surveillance until wound healed

Complications
- Dehiscence
- Necrosis or gangrene of tissue surrounding infected area
- Sepsis
- Death

INFECTIONS RELATED TO VASCULAR ACCESS AND MONITORING

Description

- Intravascular devices are common causes of local site infection and cause up to 50% of nosocomial bacteremias.

Etiology

- The infections are caused by the cutaneous microflora of the insertion site with the pathogens migrating extraluminally to the catheter tip.
- Occurs during the first week of insertion
- Contamination of the hubs on central venous catheters (CVC) or the ports of needleless systems, such as surgically implanted or cuffed catheters
- Extrinsic contamination
- Contaminated infusate
- Contaminated arterial infusions for hemodynamic monitoring

Incidence and Demographics

- Central venous catheters account for 80% to 90% of vascular access site infections.
- As many as 200,000 infections associated with central venous catheters occur each year in the United States.
- One-third to one-half of these infections occur in the ICU.
- Mortality 12% to 25%

Risk Factors

- Femoral catheterization site
- Long duration of catheter insertion
- Older patient age
- Severe underlying illness
- Parenteral nutrition
- Loss of skin integrity
- Use of nonpermeable dressings
- Bacterial colonization at insertion site

Prevention and Screening

- Education of healthcare team regarding catheter insertion and care
- Use of chlorhexidine to prepare the insertion site
- Use maximum barrier precautions during insertion
- Chlorhexidine-impregnanted patch at insertion site
- Aseptic technique for accessing transducers and other ports
- Rotation of CVC sites

Assessment

History
- Patient may be asymptomatic
- Fever
- Chills
- Pain at the catheter site

Physical Examination
- Infection is suspected because of the appearance of the catheter site or presence of fever or bacteremia without another source.
- Local erythema
- Edema
- Tenderness at the catheter site
- Warmth at the catheter site
- Tachycardia
- Hypotension
- Bacteremia

Diagnostic Studies
- Complete blood count
- Blood cultures
- Two cultures from peripheral veins by separate venipunctures
- Differential time to positivity (> 2 hours) for blood drawn through the vascular access device compared with a sample from a peripheral vein
- For infusion-related sepsis, a sample of the infusate should be taken for culture.
- Culture of the catheter tip
- Echocardiogram
  - To evaluate for endocarditis

Differential Diagnosis

- Noninfectious phlebitis
- Thrombophlebitis

Management

Nonpharmacologic Treatment
- Catheter removal
- Exchange of catheter over a guidewire
- The decision to remove a tunneled catheter or implanted device should be based on the severity of the patient's illness, the strength of evidence that the device is infected, an assessment of the specific pathogens, and the presence of local or systemic complications.

Pharmacologic Treatment
- Common organisms
- Coagulase-negative staphylococci
- *S. aureus*
- Enterococci
- *Enterobacter* spp
- *P. aeruginosa*
- *Candida* spp
- Therapy is directed at the isolated organism.
- Gram stain results can guide initial therapy.

Special Considerations

- In patients who have a track-site infection, successful therapy is unusual unless the catheter is removed.
- For suppurative venous thrombophlebitis, excision of the affected vein is required.

When to Consult, Refer, or Hospitalize

- Infectious disease consult for antibiotic management
- Cardiology consult if endocarditis is present
- Interventional radiology for tunneled catheter removal

Follow-up

Expected Outcomes
- Resolution of infection
- Blood cultures after therapy to determine effectiveness of therapy
- Serial echocardiograms if endocarditis is present

Complications
- Cellulitis or abscess at the site of catheter insertion
- Septic phlebitis
- Endocarditis
- Sepsis

MISCELLANEOUS NOSOCOMIAL INFECTIONS

DIARRHEA

Description

- *Clostridium dificile* colitis (pseudomembranous colitis) is a common cause of nosocomial diarrhea.
- Carried in the stool of symptomatic and asymptomatic individuals

Etiology

- Acquired almost exclusively in association with antimicrobial use
- Disruption of the normal colonic flora
- Spores of *C. difficile* vegetate, multiply, and secrete toxins, causing diarrhea and pseudomembranous colitis.

Incidence and Demographics

- The rate of colonization is > 20% among adult patients hospitalized for more than 1 week.
- The risk of acquiring C. *difficile* correlates with increased length of stay in the hospital.

Risk Factors

- Use of antibiotics
- Advanced patient age
- Severe underlying illness
- GI surgery
- Use of rectal thermometers
- Enteral tube feeding
- Immunosuppresion
- Antacid treatment
- Proton pump inhibitors

Prevention and Screening

- Judicious use of antibiotics
- Contact isolation to prevent spread between patients

Assessment

History
- Abdominal pain
- Fever

Physical Examination
- Heme-positive stool
- Diarrhea

Diagnostic Studies
- Positive stool culture for C. *difficile*

Differential Diagnosis

- Infectious enteritis or colitis
- Bacterial gastroenteritis
- Dysentery
- Inflammatory bowel disease
- Ischemic colitis
- Ulcerative colitis

Management

Nonpharmacologic Treatment
- Discontinue offending antibiotic
- Contact isolation

Pharmacologic Treatment
- Metronidazole p.o.
- Vancomycin p.o.

Special Considerations

- A more virulent strain of C. *difficile* has emerged in the United States and rates of infection have increased during the past few years.

When to Consult, Refer, or Hospitalize

- Infectious disease consultation to manage antibiotics

Follow-up

Expected Outcomes
- Resolution of infection
- Relapses occur in 5% to 50% of cases

Complications
- Toxic megacolon
- Sepsis
- Dehydration
- Bowel perforation
- Renal failure
- Death

TUBERCULOSIS

- See Pulmonary Disorders (Chapter 5)

MENINGITIS

- See Neurological Disorders (Chapter 7)

OPPORTUNISTIC INFECTIONS

- See Immunology and HIV section (Chapter 11)
- See Transplants section (Chapter 18)

ANTIBIOTIC-RESISTANT BACTERIA

Description

- A type of drug resistance in which a microorganism is able to survive despite exposure to an antibiotic

Etiology

- Genetic mutation of the bacteria
- The greater the duration of exposure, the greater the risk of resistance developing, even if antibiotic therapy is warranted.
- Inappropriate prescribing of antibiotics
- Poor hand hygiene by healthcare workers

Incidence and Demographics

- Approximately 440,000 new cases annually worldwide with 150,000 deaths

Risk Factors

- Prolonged hospitalization
- Prolonged or inappropriate antibiotic use
- Poor handwashing technique and infection control practices
- Emergence of multidrug-resistant microorganisms
- Unreliable specimens

Prevention and Screening

- Aggressive reinforcement of routine handwashing and infection control
- Barrier precautions for all colonized and infected patients
- Colonized personnel who are implicated in transmission and patients who pose a threat may be decontaminated.
- Daily bathing of patients with chlorhexidine
- Aggressive antibiotic control policies

Assessment

History
- Fever
- Leukocytosis
- Pain
- Altered mental status

Physical Examination
- Tachycardia
- Tachypnea
- Abscess formation

Diagnostic Studies
- Complete blood count
- Blood cultures
- Wound culture if applicable
- Urine culture
- Sensitivity testing on cultures

Management

Nonpharmacologic Treatment
- Handwashing
- Aggressive infection control measures
- Culture surveillance

Pharmacologic Treatment
- Antibiotic therapy driven by culture and sensitivity of infected site
- Pathogens that have shown antibiotic resistance
  - *Staphylococcus aureus*
  - *Streptococcus*
  - *Enterococcus*
  - *Pseudomonas aeruginosa*
  - *Clositridum difficile*
  - *Salmonella*
  - *E. coli*
  - *Acinetobacter baumannii*

Special Considerations

- Community-acquired methcillin-resistant *S. aureus* has become more prevalent.
- As much as 50% of community-acquired *S.aureus* infections in some U.S. cities are now resistant to B-lactam antibiotics.
- If these strains enter the hospital, this will cause difficulty controlling nosocomial infections.
- Many drug-resistant strains are susceptible only to colistin, which has prompted renewed use of this medication.

When to Consult, Refer, or Hospitalize

- Consult infectious disease specialist

Follow-up

Expected Outcomes
- Containment of nosocomial infections
- Resolution of infectious process
- Surveillance cultures to monitor resistance and response to therapy

Complications
- Sepsis
- Death

OPPORTUNISTC INFECTIONS

Description

- Immunocompromised patients have defects in their defense mechanisms, which puts them at a higher risk of infection from organisms that usually do not pose a threat.

Etiology

- Impaired humoral immunity
- Congenital
- Multiple myeloma
- Chronic lymphocytic leukemia (CLL)
- Splenectomy
- Neutropenia
- Impaired cellular immunity
- HIV infection

- Lymphoma
- Immunosuppresive medications
  - Solid organ transplant
  - Prolonged high-dose corticosteroid treatment
  - Asthma
  - Temporal arteritis
  - Systemic lupus erythematosus (SLE)
  - Tumor necrosis factor inhibitors
  - Etanercept
  - Infliximab
- Hematopoietic cell transplant recipients
- Immunocompromised states
- Severe burns or trauma
- Invasive procedures
  - Prolonged CVC use
  - Indwelling catheters
  - Dialysis catheters
- Central nervous system dysfunction
- Obstructing lesions
  - Pneumonia from obstructed bronchus
  - Pyelonephritis due to nephrolithiasis
  - Cholangitis due to cholelithiasis
- Use of broad spectrum antibiotics
- Diabetes mellitus

Incidence and Demographics

- Opportunistic infections rates declined and stabilized during 2003–2007 in HIV patients with the introduction of ART therapy.
- Incidence has increased in other subpopulations because of better survival of the immunocompromised patients, and increasing use of invasive devices, implants, and organ transplantation.

Risk Factors

- See Etiology

Prevention and Screening

- Effective handwashing and infection control practices
- Timely removal of foley catheters, CVC catheters
- Rotation of IV and CVC sites
- Laminar airflow isolation and high-efficiency particulate air (HEPA) filtering with hematopoietic cell transplant patients
- Use of colony-stimulating factor use during chemotherapy and stem cell transplantation
- Prevention of pneumocystis and herpes simplex infections
  - Trimethoprim-sulfamethoxazole (TMP-SMZ)
  - Dapsone for sulfa allergy
    - Check glucose-6-phosphate dehydrogenase (G6PD) levels before starting therapy.
  - Acyclovir
- Prevention of cytomegalovirus (CMV)
  - No uniformly accepted approach
  - In solid organ transplant patients
    - Valganciclovir
- Hematopoietic cell transplant recipient
  - Universal prophylaxis
    - Valganciclovir
    - Monitor without specific prophylaxis—blood sampling weekly and if positive, then begin valganciclovir
  - Preemptive therapy
    - Valganciclovir 900 mg b.i.d. for 2 to 3 weeks, then 900 mg daily until day 100
  - Use of CMV-negative or leukocyte-depleted blood products for CMV-negative patients
- Prophylatic use of antifungal agents to prevent invasive mold is routine.
  - Optimal dose or medication not yet established
  - Amphotericin B
  - Fluconzaole
  - Voriconazole
- Vaccinations for prophylaxis in the HIV patient
  - Hepatitis B
  - Influenza
  - Hepatitis A
  - Pneumococcal
  - Tdap vaccine once instead of Td

Assessment

History
- Fever, but may be blunted
- Pain
- Headache
- Night sweats
- Weight loss

Physical Examination
- Abscess formation
- Creamy white, raised lesions in the mouth (yeast infection)
- Rash
- Generalized lymphadenopathy

Diagnostic Studies
- Complete blood count with differential
- Chest x-ray
- Blood cultures
- Urine and sputum cultures if clinically indicated
- Wound culture if applicable
- Screen for latent TB

Differential Diagnosis

- Transplant rejection
- Organ ischemia or necrosis
- Thrombophlebitis
- Lymphoma

Management

Nonpharmacologic Treatment
- Reduction or discontinuation of immunosuppressive medication

Pharmacologic Treatment
- Use of hematopoietic growth factors stimulate bone marrow stem cells and produce an increase in peripheral leukocytes.
- Granulocyte and granulocyte-macrophage colony-stimulating factors
- Empiric antibody therapy—depends on the type of immunocompromise and the site of infection
- Febrile neutropenic patient
  - Broad-spectrum coverage against gram-positive and gram-negative bacilli organisms
  - Cefepime
  - Vancomycin if MRSA is suspected
  - Continued fever
    - Consider imipenem
    - Antifungal agents
    - Voriconazole
- Failure to continue antibiotics through the period of neutropenia is associated with increased morbidity and mortality.
- Low-risk neutropenic patients (neutropenia expected to last < 10 days, no comorbid complications, adequately treated cancer)
  - Ciprofloxacin orally plus amoxicillin-clavulanic acid
- Organ transplant patient

- Interstitial infiltrates
  - Main concern is *Pneumocystis* or *Legionella* species
  - Macrolide
  - Fluoroquinolone
  - TMP-SMZ
- If the patient does not respond to empiric treatment, consider adding more antimicrobial agents or perform invasive procedures to make a specific diagnosis.

Special Considerations

- The interval between transplantation and the degree of immunosuppression can narrow the differential diagnosis.
- Empiric broad-spectrum antibiotics may be used in high-risk patients.
- Culture results must be carefully evaluated and cultures not discarded as contaminated.
- Any pathogen can cause infection in the immunocompromised patient.

When to Consult, Refer, or Hospitalize

- Refer any immunocompromised patient with an opportunistic infection to an infectious disease specialist and appropriate subspecialist (transplant service, HIV specialist).
- Refer patients with potential drug toxicities and drug interactions.
- Admit for fever, suspected infection in the following groups:
  - Solid organ or hematopoietic stem cell transplant patients—especially in the first 6 months
  - Transplant recipients with recent rejection episode

Follow-up

Expected Outcomes
- Resolution of infection
- Assess for early relapse after therapy and drug toxicity.
- Maintain prophylaxis therapy.

Complications
- Sepsis
- Death

COMMUNITY-ACQUIRED INFECTIONS

PHARYNGITIS

Description

- Inflammation, infection, or both of the pharynx
- Patients develop lifelong immunity to one subtype but can be reinfected with a different subtype.

Etiology

- Group A β-hemolytic streptococcal infection (GABHS)
- *S. pyogenes*
    - 5%–15% of cases in adults
- Streptococci of groups C and G account for a minority of cases
    - < 1% of cases
- *Neisseriagonorrhoeae*
- *Corynebacterium diphtheria*
- *Corynebacterium ulcerans*
- *Yersinia enterocolitica*
- *Treponema pallidum*—secondary syphilis
- Anaerobic bacteria
- Atypical organisms
    - *M. pneumoniae*
    - *C. pneumoniae*
- Virus—most common identifiable cause
- Respiratory virus
    - Rhinovirus
    - Coronavirus
- Influenza virus
- Parainfluenza virus
- Less common
    - Herpes simplex virus 1 and 2
    - Coxsackievirus A
    - Cytomegalovirus (CMV)
    - Epstein-Barr virus

Incidence and Demographics

- Over 7 million visits to primary care physicians each year are for sore throats.
- More prevalent in the winter months and early spring

Risk Factors

- Crowded conditions
- Schools
- Household contacts
- Swimming pools implicated in Group C and D β-hemolytic streptococcus
- Industry work
- Very dry environments
- Heavy voice usage
- Smoking and alcohol use
- Chronic sinusitis
- Allergies

Prevention and Screening

- Transmitted by droplets
- Minimize droplet spread
- See Risk Factors
- A multivalent vaccine that targets streptococcus M proteins that cause pharyngitis, invasive disease, and rheumatic fever has completed Phase I trials.
- Smoking cessation
- Limit alcohol

Assessment

History
- Bacterial infection
- Pain with swallowing
- Sore throat
- Fever
- Nausea
- Viral infection
- Coryza
- Hoarseness
- Cough
- Diarrhea
- Fever
  - Adenovirus—fever for 7 days
- Scarlet fever
- History of GABHS infection
- Clinical symptoms same

Physical Examination
- Bacterial infection
  - Tonsillar erythema with or without exudate
  - Anterior cervical lymphadenitis
  - Soft palate petechiae
  - Red, swollen, uvula
  - Scarlatiniform rash
  - Posttonsillectomy patients may have less severe symptoms
  - Severe symptoms with GABHS
    - Neck swelling
    - Drooling
    - "Hot potato" voice
  - Peritonsillar abscess, infections in the parapharyngeal and submandibular spaces
    - Ludwig's angina (neck space infection)
  - Viral infection
  - Viral exanthema
  - Anterior stomatitis
- Conjunctivitis
  - Can last up to 14 days
- Scarlet fever
  - Rash
    - Develops within 24 to 48 hours of symptom onset
    - Fine, papular, bright red rash that blanches
    - Begins on the neck and spreads to extremities and trunk
    - More pronounced in skin creases; rough texture, goose-pimple appearance
    - Fades in 3 to 4 days, followed by desquamation
    - After desquamation, tongue has strawberry appearance because of edematous papillae
- Poststreptococcal glomerulonephritis
  - Occurs 1 to 3 weeks after infection
    - Hypertension
    - Edema
    - Hematuria

Diagnostic Studies
- Throat culture
  - Gold standard
- Rapid Antigen Detection Test (RADT)
  - High specificity, but low sensitivity

Differential Diagnosis

- Infectious mononucleosis
- Acute retroviral syndrome
- *Neisseria gonorrheae*
- Lemierre's syndrome

Management

Nonpharmacologic Treatment
- Rest
- Adequate fluid intake
- Warm saline gargles
- Meticulous mouth care
- Elevate the head on 3 to 4 pillows

Pharmacologic Treatment
- Viral
  - Symptom relief
    - Acetaminophen
- Bacterial
  - Delay of antibiotics 24 to 48 hours to wait for culture results does not increase the risk of rheumatic fever
  - Penicillin the antibiotic of choice
    - Penicillin VK
    - Amoxicillin
    - Penicillin G benzathine
    - For penicillin allergy
      - Kelfex
      - Macrolides

Special Considerations

- All patients should be considered infectious until 24 hours of antibiotic therapy has been completed.
- In adults, throat culture is not needed if RADT is negative.
- Stop antibiotic therapy if throat culture is negative for GABHS.
- Treatment is necessary for 10 days.

When to Consult, Refer, or Hospitalize

- ENT consult for severe neck edema
- Infectious disease consult for antibiotic management as indicated for lack of response to therapy
- Nephrology consult if glomerulonephritis is present
- Pulmonary consult for airway compromise
- Admit for IV hydration if patient unable to swallow
- Admit for management of complications

Follow-up

Expected Outcome
- Uncomplicated pharyngitis subsides in 3 to 10 days

Complications
- Suppurative
  - Spread of infection
    - Lateral pharyngeal abscess
    - Cervial lymphandenitis
    - Sinusitis
    - Otitis media
    - Retropharyngeal abscess
    - Lemierre's syndrome
    - Mastoiditis
- Nonsuppurative
  - Acute rheumatic fever
    - Occurs 2 to 3 weeks after GABHS infection
    - Starting antibiotics within 9 days of symptom onset can help prevent rheumatic fever.
  - Acute poststreptococcal glomerulonephritis
    - May occur 10 days after onset of infection
  - Poststreptococcal reactive arthritis
  - Complications from treatment
  - Antibiotic reaction
  - Drug resistance

SINUSITIS

Description

- Inflammation of the mucosa of the paranasal sinuses
- Acute sinusitis lasts < 30 days.
- Subacute sinusitis lasts 1 to 3 months.
- Chronic sinusitis lasts > 3 months.
- Most cases involve more than one of the paranasal sinuses.

Etiology

- Viral upper respiratory infections
- Allergic rhinitis
- Dysfunctional mucociliary system
- Anatomic malformations
- Polyps
- Septal deviation
- Foreign bodies
- Tumors
- Upper tooth infections
- Viral infections
- Serous sinusitis
- Bacterial infection
- Secondary infection from sinus ostia obstruction or impaired mucous clearance
- Most common pathogens
  - *Streptococcus pneumoniae*
  - *Haemophilus influenzae*
  - *Maraxella catarrhalis*
  - GABHS

Incidence and Demographics

- Affects 1 in 7 adults each year
- Women are more often affected than men.
- Whites and Blacks have a higher incidence than Hispanics.
- Older adults and the young have a higher incidence of sinusitis.

Risk Factors

- See Etiology
- COPD
- Immunocompromised patient
- Cystic fibrosis
- Use of decongestant nasal sprays
- Diabetes
- Flying
- Diving
- High altitude

Prevention and Screening

- Avoid environmental irritants
- Regular dental examinations
- Repair of septal deviation—septoplasty
- Reduction in size of the turbinates
- Limit use of nasal sprays
- Saline irrigation of sinuses
- Control allergies
- Adequate hydration

Assessment

History
- Bacterial
- Fever
- Tooth pain
- Symptom worsening following initial improvement
- Hospital-acquired
  - Rhinosinusitis that not be symptomatic
  - Source of fever in the critically ill
  - Associated with nasogastric tube (NGT)
- Maxillary sinus
- Unilateral facial fullness
- Tenderness over the cheek
- Tooth pain
- Malaise
- Headache
- Ethmoid sinusitis
- Pain or pressure over the high lateral wall of the nose between the eyes that may radiate to the orbit
- Sphenoid sinusitis
- Pansinusitis
- Headache "in the middle of the head" and may point towards the vertex
- Acute frontal sinusitis
- Pain or tenderness of the forehead

Physical Examination
- Maxillary sinus
- Purulent nasal drainage
- Nasal airway obstruction
- Dental caries
- Halitosis
- Cough

Diagnostic Studies
- Elevated erythrocyte sedimentation rate
- > 10 in men, > 20 in women
- Routine radiographs not recommended
- Noncontrast, coronal CT
- Assesses all of the paranasal sinuses
- CT scan may be used to rule out rhinosinusitis
- If malignancy is suspected: MRI

Differential Diagnosis

- Common cold
- Atypical migraine
- Tension headache
- Trigeminal neuralgia
- Temporomandibular joint dysfunction

Management

Nonpharmacologic Treatment
- Nasal irrigation with salt water
- Sinus puncture
  - Indication
    - Empyema when antibiotics have not cleared the infection
    - Used in only 1% to 2% of patients

Pharmacologic Treatment
- Mild to moderate symptoms of < 7 days duration
- Decongestants
- Proteolytic enzymes
- Mucolytic agents
- Antihistamines
- Topical corticosteroids—conflicting evidence
- Moderate symptoms > 7 days duration
- Antibiotics
  - Amoxicillin
  - Erythromycin
  - Trimethoprim-sulfamethoxazole for penicillin allergy
- Common pathogens
  - S. pneumoniae
  - H. Influenzae

Special Considerations

- A fluid level or opacification of a sinus on a CT scan is 90% specific for acute bacterial sinusitis.
- Patients with recurrent sinusitis make up 7% to 9% of all patients with sinusitis.
- Diagnosis of bacterial sinus infection is limited with plan sinus x-rays; however, a negative x-ray is an indication that a bacterial infection is not present.
- More than one-half of patients with acute bacterial sinus infection recover without antibiotics.

When to Consult, Refer, or Hospitalize

- Refer to otolaryngologist for lack of response to therapy in patients with acute bacterial rhinosinusitis.
- Any patient with extension of disease outside the sinuses should evaluated by an otolaryngologist
- Admit for:
    - Facial swelling or erythema that may be due to facial cellulitis
    - Proptosis
    - Visual changes or gaze abnormalities that are indicative of orbital cellulitis
    - Abscess or cavernous sinus involvement
    - Mental status changes
    - Immunocompromised status

Follow-up

Expected Outcome
- Resolution of symptoms in 7 to 14 days

Complications
- Chronic sinusitis
- Brain abscess
- Orbital cellulitis
- Subdural empyema
- Meningitis

CELLULITIS

Description

- A diffuse spreading infection of the dermis and subcutaneous tissue
- Usually occurs on the lower extremity
- Starts as a hot, red, edematous eruption with sharply defined edges
- No vesicles or bullae

- May progress to lymphangitis, lymphadenitis, and in severe cases, necrotizing fasciitis and gangrene
- In otherwise healthy individuals, a common entry point for lower extremity cellulitis is toe web intertrigo with fissuring.

Etiology

- Local skin trauma
- Insect bites
- Abrasions
- Surgical wounds
- Contusions
- Lacerations
- Saphenous donor site
- Common organisms
  - Gram-positive cocci
  - GABHS
  - *S. aureus*
  - In people with diabetes
    - Group B *Streptococcus*
    - Rarely gram-negative rods
    - Fungi

Incidence and Demographics

- Occurs equally in men and women and affects all racial and ethnic groups
- Exact prevalence is unknown because it is not a reportable disease.
- Slightly higher incidence in individuals over 45 years of age

Risk Factors

- See Etiology
- 20-fold more common in patients with chronic venous stasis or lymphedema
- Injection drug use
- Diabetes
- Open ulcerations
- Coronary artery bypass surgery with saphenous vein graft harvest
- Immunosuppression
- Presence of malignancy

Prevention and Screening

- If a wound is present, wash daily with soap and water.
- Apply antibiotic cream or ointment.
- Monitor for signs of infection.
- People with diabetes should inspect feet daily and wear appropriate footwear and gloves.
- Moisturize skin daily.
- Carefully trim fingernails and toenails.

Assessment

History
- Pain at injury site
- Fever
- Malaise

Physical Examination
- Tender, erythematous, indurated area of skin
- May be rapidly expanding
- Ascending lymphangitis may be present.
- Regional lymphadenopathy
- Central ulceration, pustule, or abscess may be present.
- Cellulitis caused by *S. aureus*
- Localized abscesses
- Furuncles
- Carbuncles
- Hypotension or septic shock with septicemia

Diagnostic Studies
- Complete blood count
  - Leukocytosis
  - Left shift
- Blood cultures
- Wound culture if purulent drainage present
- Full-thickness skin biopsy for culture
- MRI to rule out underlying osteomyelitis if suspected
- Ultrasound to rule out deep vein thrombosis

Differential Diagnosis

- Deep vein thrombosis
- Necrotizing fasciitis
- Sclerosing panniculitis
- Acute, severe contact dermatitis

Management

Nonpharmacologic Treatment
- Decrease physical activity and elevate area if applicable.
- If the infection does not respond promptly to antibiotic therapy, surgical exploration of the area may be warranted to establish a diagnosis and rule out the presence of necrotic or gangrenous tissue.
- Revasularization of an extremity may be warranted if delayed healing is the result of impaired circulation.
- Hyperbaric oxygenation therapy (HBO)

Pharmacologic Treatment
- Antibiotic coverage for *Streptococcus* and *Staphylococcus*
- Localized infection are treated with oral antibiotics
- IV or parenteral antibiotics may be needed in the first 2 to 5 days.
- Immunosuppressed patient and those with recurrent cellulitis should be examined for chronic sources of infection.
- Treatment in these patients should be with IV antibiotics until the cellulitis resolves, and then oral antibiotics for 5 to 7 days.

Special Considerations

- Patients with diabetes, cancer, or immunosuppression should be instructed that localized cellulitis may become a serious condition.
- If septicemia develops, hypotension followed by septic shock may follow.

When to Consult, Refer, or Hospitalize

- Infectious disease consult may be necessary to manage antibiotics
- Hospitalize for parenteral antibiotic therapy.
- Intensive care consult for systemic signs and symptoms of septicemia, septic shock

Follow-up

Expected Outcomes
- Resolution of infection
- Most cases of cellulitis are treated on an outpatient basis and respond well to standard oral antibiotics without longlasting sequelae.

Complications
- Lymphangitis
- Abscess formation
- Gangrenous cellulitis
- Necrotizing fasciitis
- Septicemia—septic shock
- Death

INFECTIOUS DIARRHEA

Description

- A production of at least 200 g of stool per day
- An increased in stool frequency and liquidity as compared to the individual's usual bowel movements
- Acute if it lasts < 14 days and chronic if it lasts > 30 days
- Two major types
  - Secretory
    - Watery
    - Large volume
    - Little or no blood or leukocytes
  - Inflammatory
    - Bloody
    - Has leukocytes
    - Small volumes

Etiology

- Infection—leading cause
- Inflammatory response to toxins
- Autoimmune disorders
- Secretory
- Bacterial
  - *E. coli*
  - *Vibrio cholera*
- Viral
  - Adenovirus (types 40 and 41)
  - Astrovirus
  - Caliciviruses
  - Rotavirus
- Protozoal
  - *Cyptosporidium*
  - *Cyclospora*
  - *Dientamoeba fragilis*
  - *Giardia lambia*
  - *Isospora belli*
  - *Microspora* species
- Bacterial
  - *Aeromonas* spp
  - *Bacteroides fragilis*
  - *Campylobacter* spp
  - *Clostridum difficile*
  - *E. coli*

- *Pleisomonas* spp
- *Shigella* spp
- *Salmonella*
- Nontyphoid *Salmonella* species
- Noncholera *Vibrio* species
- *Yersinia*
- Protozoal
  - *Entamoeba histolytica*

Incidence and Demographics

- There are between 211 and 375 million cases of infectious diarrhea with 900,000 hospitalizations and 6,000 deaths annually in the United States
- May cause severe illness in the very young, immunucompromised patients, and malnourished persons

Risk Factors

- See Etiology
- Immunosuppression
- Travel

Prevention and Screening

- Avoidance
- Limit exposure for high-risk patients
- Proper handwashing by healthcare workers
- Infection control measures when patient is hospitalized
- Probiotics
- Vaccines
- Rotavirus
  - RotaTeq
- *Vibrio cholera*
  - Dukoral
- *Salmonella typhi*
  - Vivotiv berna

Assessment

History
- Duration and frequency of diarrhea
- Inflammatory
  - Abdominal pain
  - Tenesmus
  - Fever
  - Presence of blood in stool
  - Recent travel
  - Recent ingestion of raw or undercooked poultry or seafood
  - Immunocompromised state
- Noninflammatory
  - Bloating
  - Nausea

Physical Examination
- Evaluate volume status for dehydration
- Evaluate for altered mental status
- Abdominal tenderness
- Peritonitis
- Noninflammatory
  - Watery, nonbloody diarrhea
  - Vomiting

Diagnostic Studies
- Complete blood count
- Compete chemistry panel
- Fecal leukocytes in inflammatory diarrhea
- Stool for lactoferrin, ovam and parasites, culture
- For bloody diarrhea
  - Serotyping for Shiga-producing *E. coli* O157:H7
  - Special culture requirement for *Yersinia*, *Vibrio*, and *Aeromonas*
  - Stool antigen detection tests
    - *Giardia*
    - *Entamoeba histolytica*
  - Fecal acid fast staining
    - *Cyclospora*
    - *Cryptosporidium*

Differential Diagnosis

- Inflammatory bowel disease
- Irritable bowel syndrome
- Antibiotic-associated diarrhea
- Medications other than antibiotics

Management

Nonpharmacologic Treatment
- Adequate hydration, intravenous if necessary
- Frequent feedings of tea; "flat" carbonated beverages; soft, easily digested foods—soups, crackers, bananas, applesauce, rice, toast
- Bowel rest
- Avoid high-fiber foods, fats, milk products, caffeine, alcohol

Pharmacologic Treatment
- Antidiarrheals
- Bismuth subsalicylate
- Loperamide
- Antibiotics
  - Ciprofloxacin
  - Levofloxacin
  - Targeted antibiotic therapy is based on results of stool culture
- Probiotics

Special Considerations

- Per the Centers for Disease Control and Prevention, 20% to 50% of international travelers develop diarrhea related to traveling.
- Prophylactic antimicrobial medications are not usually recommended for the prevention of traveler's diarrhea, except in the presence of immunosuppression or comorbidities that put travelers at risk for GI infection.
- The definitive etiology of diarrhea is difficult to determine because diarrhea is a nonspecific reaction by the intestine to various conditions such as infection, toxins, and autoimmune disease.

When to Consult, Refer, or Hospitalize

- Gastroenterology consult if diagnosis is unclear
- Admit for
  - IV hydration if patient unable to adequately hydrate orally
  - Bloody diarrhea that is severe or worsening to determine infectious vs. noninfectious etiology
  - Severe abdominal pain
    - Toxic colitis
    - Inflammatory bowel disease
    - Intestinal ischemia
    - Surgical abdomen
- Signs of severe infection or sepsis
- Severe or worsening diarrhea in patients > 70 years of age

Follow-up

Expected Outcomes
- Resolution of infection and diarrhea
- Usually lasts 7 days when not treated with antibiotics
- Diarrhea may persist.
- Reportable microorganisms
  - Cholera
  - *Salmonella*
  - *Shigella*
  - *E. coli*

Complications
- Dehydration
- Skin irritiation
- Electrolyte imbalance
- Orthostatic hypotension
- Confusion
- Acute kidney injury
- Metabolic acidosis
- Coma

REFERENCES

Barkley, T., & Myers, C. (2008). *Practice guidelines for acute care nurse practitioners.* St. Louis, MO: Saunders.

Beers, M., Porter, R., Jones, T., Kaplan, J., & Berkwits, M. (Eds.). (2006). *The Merck manual of diagnosis and therapy.* Whitehouse Station, NJ: Merck Research Laboratories.

Bope, E., Kellerman, R., & Rakel, R. (2011). *Conn's current therapy 2011.* Philadelphia: Elsevier/Saunders.

Cooper, D., Kraink, A., Lubner, S., & Reno, H. (Eds.). (2007). *The Washington manual of medical therapeutics* (32nd ed.). Philadelphia: Wolters Kluwer/Lippincott Williams & Wilkins.

Fauci, A., Braunwald, E., Kasper, D., Hauser, S., Longo, D., Jameson, J., & Loscalzo, J. (Eds.). (2009). *Harrison's principles of internal medicine.* New York: McGraw Hill.

Irwin, R., & Rippe, J. (2008). *Intensive care medicine.* Philadelphia: Wolters Kluwer/Lippincott Williams & Wilkins.

Marini, J., & Wheeler, A. (2010). *Critical care medicine, the essentials.* Philadelphia: Wolters Kluwer/Lippincott Williams & Wilkins.

McKean, S., Bennett, A. & Halasyamani, L. (Eds.). (2008). *Hospital medicine.* Philadelphia: Wolters Kluwer/Lippincott Williams & Wilkins.

McPhee, S., & Papadakis, M. (2011). (Eds.). *2011 current medical diagnosis and treatment.* New York: McGraw Hill.

Moreno, M., Nietman, H., Matias, C., & Lobo, S. (2010). C-reactive protein: A tool in the follow-up of nosocomial pneumonia. *Journal of Infection. 61*(3), 205–211.

Rowe, S., & Cheadle, W. (2000). Complications of nosocomial pneumonia. *American Journal of Surgery, 179*(2), 63–68.

Wells, B., DiPiro, J., Schwinghammer, T., & DiPiro, C. (Eds.). (2009). *Pharmacotherapy handbook.* New York: McGraw Hill.

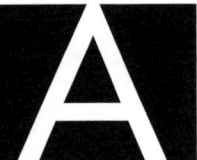

Immobility
Pamela Smith, MSN, RN, ACNP-BC, CCRN

Description

- Most disease and rehabilitative states involve some degree of immobility.
- Immobility is also related to loss of muscle mass, reduction in muscle strength and function, less mobile joints, and gait changes.
- Bed rest during hospitalization is common during acute illness, trauma, and after procedures.

Etiology

- Major trauma
- Disease states
- Stroke
- Morbid obesity
- Multiple sclerosis
- Paralysis
- Deconditioning
- Functional decline in older adults

Incidence and Demographics

- Affects all ages across the life span and is related to etiology.

Risk Factors

- Advanced age
- Major trauma or critical illness
- Neuromuscular disorders
- Paralysis
- Medical restrictions
- Deconditioning
- Altered mental status

Prevention and Screening

- Encourage early ambulation when possible.
- Mobilization with the use of appropriate assist devices
- Physical therapy
- Occupational therapy

Assessment

History
- Altered mental status
- Deconditioning
- Trauma
- Neuromuscular disorders

Physical Examination
- Inability to ambulate due to critical illness, physical limitations
- Inability to perform activities of daily living
  - Reduced exercise capacity
  - Visual impairment
- Bone demineralization
- Loss of muscle tone, decreased muscle strength
- Immobile joints
- Code for Functional Level of Classification
  - 0 – Completely independent
  - 1 – Requires use of equipment or device
  - 2 – Requires help from another person for assistance, supervision, or teaching
  - 3 – Requires help from another person and equipment or device
  - 4 – Is dependent, does not participate in activity

Management

Nonpharmacologic and Pharmacologic Treatment
- Early ambulation when possible
- Assistance is warranted for
  - Advanced age
  - Prolonged bedrest
  - Deconditioning
- Turn and reposition every 2 hours.
- Maintain limbs in functional alignment.
- Perform passive or active range-of-motion exercises, or both
- Use of antipressure devices, mattresses, beds
- Keep skin clean, dry, and moisturized.
- Encourage coughing and deep breathing.
- Use incentive spirometer.
- Volume expansion protocols
- Adequate hydration to prevent constipation
- Indwelling catheter if needed to monitor I&O, prevent skin breakdown if patient is incontinent
- Conduct ongoing evaluations to formulate individualized strategies for improved mobility.
- Assessment of nutritional needs
- Skin breakdown more likely in the setting of malnutrition
- Assess skin integrity regularly.
- Assess emotional response to immobility.
- Assess for the development of deep vein thrombosis.
  - Prophylaxis
    - Low molecular weight heparin
    - Heparin
    - Sequential compression device and TED hose
- Evaluate need for home assistive devices

Special Considerations

- Maintaining function is central to promoting health and independence in the hospitalized patient.
- Hospitalized older adults are at increased risk for decreased mobility and functional disability.

When to Consult, Refer, or Hospitalize

- Physical or occupational therapy, or both
- Dietary consult as needed
- Wound care if skin breakdown occurs

Follow-up

Expected Outcomes
- Return to highest level of mobility, independence
- Outcome is determined by underlying reason for immobility.

Complications
- Cardiovascular
  - Decreased stroke volume
  - Decreased cardiac output
  - Orthostatic hypotension
- Respiratory
  - Decreased respiratory excursion
  - Decreased oxygen uptake
  - Increased potential for atelectasis
- Muscles
  - Decreased muscle strength
  - Decreased muscle blood flow
- Bone
  - Increased bone loss
  - Decreased bone density
- GI
  - Malnutrition
  - Anorexia
  - Constipation
- GU
  - Incontinence
- Skin
  - Increase sheer force
  - Potential for skin breakdown
- Psychological
  - Social isolation
  - Anxiety
  - Depression
  - Disorientation

REFERENCES

Beers, M., Porter, R., Jones, T., Kaplan, J., & Berkwits, M. (Eds.). (2006). *The Merck manual of diagnosis and therapy.* Whitehouse Station, NJ: Merck Research Laboratories.
Gulanick, M., & Myers, J. (2010). *Nursing care plans.* St. Louis, MO: Mosby.
Hughes, R. (Ed.). (2008). *Patient safety and quality: An evidence-based handbook for nurses.* Publication 08-0043. Rockville, MD: Agency for Healthcare Research and Quality.

Intravenous Fluid Management
Pamela Smith, MSN, RN, ACNP-BC, CCRN

GENERAL PRINCIPLES

- Total body water (TBW)
- Water is approximately 60% of lean body weight in men and 50% in women.
- One liter of water weighs 1 kilogram; therefore, a 70 kg man consists of 42 liters of water as calculated by the following equation:
  60 x 70 kg
  - One kilogram weighs 2.2 pounds.
  - The distribution of water is a consistent percentage of total body water.
- It is diluted in two major compartments:
  - Intracelluar fluid (ICF)
    - Composition
      - Primarily potassium and phosphate ions
      - Low concentration of sodium and bicarbonate
    - Two-thirds of TBW is located in the intracellular compartment.
- Extracellular fluid (ECF)
  - Therapeutic fluids are administered here.
  - Composition
    - Primarily sodium salts
    - Low concentration of potassium and phosphate
    - One-third of TBW is in the extracellular compartment.

- Intravascular space (plasma compartment)
  - One-fourth of the extracellular compartment
  - Contains cells and plasma
  - Plasma is the noncellular portion of blood.
  - About 60% of blood is plasma.
  - Hematocrit is the percentage of blood volume that is red blood cells, normally about 40%.
  - The majority of cells in the blood are red blood cells.
  - Changes in plasma volume can change the hematocrit without a change in red blood cells.
    - In dehydration, the hematocrit is elevated as plasma volume is lost.
    - With IVF administration, the hematocrit may decrease by the dilution of a constant red blood cell volume.
    - Interstitial space
      - Three-fourths of the extracellular compartment
- In a 70 kg man, the total water distribution would be the following:
  - TBW: 42 liters
  - Intracellular: approximately 28L (0.66 x TBW)
  - Extracellular: approximately 14L (0.33 x TBW)
  - Intravascular: approximately 3.5L (0.25 x ECF)
  - Interstitial: approximately 10.5 L (0.75 x ECF)
- Osmolality
- Plasma osmolality is the collective concentration of all the plasma solutes.
- Calculated from the concentrations of the three plasma solutes:
  - Electrolytes
    - Any substance with a positive or negative charge
  - Non-electrolytes
    - Do not carry a charge
  - Glucose
    - $2 \times [Na^+] + [BUN]/2.8 + [glucose]/18$
    - Range is 285 to 295 mmol/L

INTRAVENOUS FLUID ADMINISTRATION

Purpose

- Repletion of volume loss and maintenance of ECF
- Volume depletion
  - Hypotension
  - Positive orthostatic vital signs
  - Tachycardia
  - Flat neck veins
  - Decreased skin turgor
  - Concentrated urine
  - Decreased central venous pressure
  - Decreased capillary wedge pressure
- Volume excess

- Hypertension
- Jugular vein distention
- Increased central venous pressure
- Increased capillary wedge pressure
- Peripheral edema
- Pulmonary crackles
- Ascites
- Weight gain
- Signs of water deficit
    - Hypernatremia
    - Serum hyperosmolality
- Signs of water excess
    - Hyponatremia
    - Serum hypo-osmolality
- Electrolyte replacement
- Administer per diagnosed deficiency
- May be IVPB or included in maintenance IVF
- Nutritional support
- TPN
    - Calories
    - Glucose
    - Lipids
    - Amino acids
    - Water-soluble vitamins
    - Trace elements
- Medication administration in water-soluble agents

Calculation of IVF Administration

- Daily weight is the best way to assess net gain or loss of total body fluid.
- The minimum requirement to maintain homeostasis in an afebrile patient with normal renal function is about 800 mL/day, which would produce about 500 mL of urine.
- In a 70 kg adult: 35 mL/kg/24 hr
- If not a 70 kg adult:
    - For the first 10 kg of body weight: 100 mL/kg/day plus
    - For the second 10 kg of body weight: 50 mL/kg/day plus
    - For weight above 20 kg: 20 ml/kg/day
- Example for an 80 kg adult:
    - 10 x 100 = 1000 mL
    - 10 x 50 = 500 mL
    - 60 x 20 = 1200 mL
    - Total = 2,700 mL/24 hours; divide by 24 to get hourly rate
- Electrolyte requirements
    - Sodium: 80 to 120 mEq/day
    - Chloride: 80 to 120 mEq/day as NaCl
    - Potassium: 50 to 100 mEq/day

- Potassium is easily interchanged between intracellular and extracellular compartments in academia or alkalemia.
- Potassium demands increase with diuresis and anabolic states.
- Calcium: 1 to 3 g/day
- Magnesium: 20 mEq/day
- Glucose requirements
  - 100 to 200 g/day
- The protein-sparing effect is one of the basic goals of IV therapy.
- At least 100 g/d of glucose decreases protein loss by more than one-half.
- Choosing appropriate IV therapy is difficult and is driven by the patient's underlying illness, vital signs, and serum electrolytes.
- For a 70 kg man:
  - D_5 0.22% NaCl with 20 mEq/L of KCL at 125 ml/hr
    - Delivers 3 L/day of free water
- Other adult patients
  - Use the preceding kg formula

Special Fluid Requirements

- Gastric loss
  - D_5 ½ NS with 20 mEq/L KCL
- Diarrhea
  - D_5LR with 15 mEq/L
  - Use body weight as a replacement guide
  - Approximately 1L for 1 kg lost
- Bile loss
  - D_5LR with 25 mEq/L (1/2 ampule) of bicarbonate mL for mL
- Pancreatic loss
  - D_5LR with 50 mEq/L (1 amp) of bicarbonate) mL for mL
- Burn patients
  - Parkland formula
    - Total fluid required during the first 24 hours = (% body burn) × (body weight in kg) × 4 mL
    - Replace with LR over 24 hours.
    - One-half of the total over the first 8 hours from time of the burn
    - One-fourth of the total over the second 8 hours
    - One-fourth of the total over the third 8 hours

Type of Fluids

- Crystalloids
- Dextrose solutions
  - D_5W
    - 50 g/L of glucose
    - Kcal/L: 170
    - Osmolality: 278 mmol/L
  - $D_{10}W$
    - 100 g/L of glucose
    - Kcal/L 340
    - Osmolality: 556 mmol/L
  - $D_{20}W$
    - 200 g/L of glucose
    - Kcal/L: 680
    - Osmolality: 1111 mmol/L
  - $D_{50}W$
    - 500 g/L of glucose
    - Kcal/L: 1700
    - Osmolality: 2 778 mmol/L
- Saline solution
  - 0.225%
    - Sodium: 38.5 mEq/L
    - Chloride: 38.5 mEq/L
    - Osmolality: 77.0 mmol/L
    - Tonicity: hypotonic
  - 0.45%
    - Sodium: 77.0 mEq/L
    - Chloride: 77.0 mEq/L
    - Osmolality: 154 mmol/L
    - Tonicity: hypotonic
  - 0.9%
    - Sodium: 154 mEq/L
    - Chloride: 154 mEq/L
    - Osmolality: 308 mmol/L
    - Tonicity: isotonic
  - 3%
    - Sodium: 513 mEq/L
    - Chloride: 513 mEq/L
    - Osmolality: 1026 mmol/L
    - Tonicity: hypertonic
- Colloids
  - Albumin
    - 25% concentration
    - 5% concentration
  - Dextran
  - Hetastarch
  - Fresh-frozen plasma
  - Blood

Composition of Body Fluids

Table B-1. Composition of Body Fluids

Fluid (mL)	Na+	Cl-	K+	HCO$_3$-	Average Daily Production
Sweat	50	40	5	0	Varies
Saliva	60	15	26	50	1500
Gastric juice	60-100	100	10	0	1500 – 2500
Duodenal fluid	130	90	5	0-10	300 - 2000
Bile	145	100	5	15	100 – 800
Pancreatic juice	140	75	5	115	100 – 800
Ileal fluid	140	100	2 – 8	30	100 – 9000
Diarrhea	120	90	25	45	

Adapted from *Clinician's Pocket Reference* (p.118), by L. Gomella & S. Haist, 2007, New York: McGraw Hill.

REFERENCES

Barkley, T., & Myers, C. (2008). *Practice guidelines for acute care nurse practitioners*. St. Louis, MO: Saunders.

Gomella, L., & Haist, S. (2007). *Clinician's pocket reference*. New York: McGraw Hill.

Marini, J., & Wheeler, A. (2010). *Critical care medicine, the essentials*. Philadelphia: Wolters Kluwer/Lippincott Williams & Wilkins.

McKean, S., Bennett, A., & Halasyamani, L. (Eds.). (2008). *Hospital medicine*. Philadelphia: Wolters Kluwer/Lippincott Williams & Wilkins.

McPhee, S., & Papadakis, M. (Eds.). (2011). *2011 current medical diagnosis and treatment*. New York: McGraw Hill.

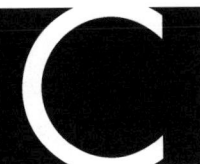

Bites and Stings
Pamela Smith, MSN, RN, ACNP-BC, CCRN

SNAKE BITES

PIT VIPER

Description
- The venom of the pit viper is cytolytic.
- Cytolytic venom causes tissue destruction by digestion and hemorrhage as a result of hemolysis and destruction of the endothelial lining of blood vessels.
- Signs and symptoms include:
  - Local pain
  - Swelling
  - Redness
  - Bleeding
  - Perioral tingling
  - Metallic taste

- Nausea and vomiting
- Hypotension
- Coagulopathy

Management

- For local symptoms
- 4 to 6 vials of crotalid antivenin by slow IV infusion in 250 to 500 mL of NS
  - Repeated doses of two vials every 6 hours for up to 18 hours
  - More serious envenomation—additional vials may be required
- Monitor vital signs
- Draw coagulation panel
- Type and cross-match
- Prophylactic antibiotics not indicated

CORAL SNAKE

Description

- The venom of the coral snake is neurotoxic.
- Neurotoxins cause respiratory paralysis.
- Signs and symptoms include:
  - Ptosis
  - Dysphagia
  - Diplopia
  - Respiratory arrest

Management

- Administer 1 to 2 vials of specific antivenom.
- Call regional poison control center.

SPIDER BITES AND SCORPION STINGS

BLACK WIDOW SPIDER (*LACTRODECTUS MACTANS*)

Description

- The venom of the black widow spider causes muscular pains, spasms, and rigidity.

Management

- Pain may be relieved with opioids or muscle relaxants.
- Calcium gluconate 10%, 0.1 to 0.2 mL/kg IV to relieve muscle rigidity
- *Lactrodectus* antivenom is effective, but is reserved for the very young or old because of hypersensitivity concerns.

BROWN RECLUSE SPIDER (*LOXOSCELE RECLUSA*)

Description

The venom of the brown recluse causes progressive local necrosis, as well as hemolytic reactions (rare).

Management

- Early excision of the bite site
- May have some success with dapsone and colchicines—unproven

SCORPION STING

Description

- Stings by most scorpions in the United States cause only local pain.
- More toxic scorpions found in the southwestern United States may cause muscle cramps, twitching, and jerking; occasionally hypertension, convulsions, and pulmonary edema.

MANAGEMENT

- No specific treatment
- Apply cool compress.
- Elevate limb to heart level.

BEES, HORNETS, WASPS, YELLOW JACKETS, AND ANTS

Description

- Target organs are the skin, vascular, and respiratory system.
- Immunoglobulin E (IgE)-mediated allergic reaction
- Anaphylaxis may occur because of sudden systemic release of mast cells and basophil mediators.
- Local reactions
    - Pain immediately after the sting
    - Edema—may extend 10 cm from site of sting
    - Bleeding at site of sting
    - Pruritus
    - Vasodilation with a warm sensation
    - Stinger may be seen in the wound
    - Nausea or vomiting
    - Visceral pain (GI tract)
- Urticaria with or without local reaction symptoms
- General reactions
    - Urticaria
    - Confluent red rash
    - Shortness of breath (SOB), wheezing
    - Edema in airway, tongue, uvula
    - Weakness

- Syncope
- Anxiety
- Confusion
- Chest pain

Management

- Remove the stinger with pinching and traction.
- Apply ice or cool packs.
- Use diphenhydramine to limit the size of the local reaction.
- Use corticosteroids in severe cases to prevent recurrent or prolonged anaphylaxis.
- H2 blockers may be given by IV.
- Use crystalloid IV infusion for hypotension.
- For respiratory compromise, inject epinephrine 0.1 to 0.5 mg of 1:1000 solution SQ or IM every 5 to 15 minutes as needed.
  - For severe anaphylactic shock, use 1 to 4 µg/min IV.

REFERENCES

Beers, M., Porter, R., Jones, T., Kaplan, J., & Berkwits, M. (Eds.). (2006). *The Merck manual of diagnosis and therapy.* Whitehouse Station, NJ: Merck Research Laboratories.

Bope, E., Kellerman, R., & Rakel, R. (2011). *Conn's Current Therapy 2011.* Philadelphia: Elsevier/Saunders.

Cooper, D., Kraink, A., Lubner, S., & Reno, H. (Eds.). (2007). *The Washington manual of medical therapeutics* (32nd ed.). Philadelphia: Wolters Kluwer/Lippincott Williams & Wilkins.

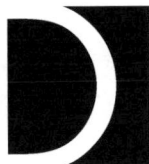

Wound Care
Pamela Smith, MSN, RN, ACNP-BC, CCRN

Description

Acute
- A wound that proceeds through the normal healing process and results in sustained restoration of anatomical and functional integrity
  - Surgical wound—clean or contaminated after surgery
  - Traumatic wound—clean or contaminated

Chronic
- A wound that fails to heal through the normal healing process or produce a restoration of anatomical and functional integrity
- Ulcers
  - Arterial
  - Diabetic
  - Venous
  - Mixed
  - Pressure
- Healing process
- Primary intention: wound that is closed
  - Surgical—wound that is sutured or stapled

- Secondary intention—wound edges are not approximated
  - Pressure ulcers, surgical wounds with tissue loss
- Tertiary intention—wound left open for several days, then wound edges approximated
- Contaminated wounds that require observation for signs of infection or inflammation

Etiology

- Surgery
- Trauma
- Arterial insufficiency
- Venous insufficiency
- Constant skin pressure—pressure ulcer
- Hyperglycemia, neuropathy, infection—diabetic ulcer

Incidence and Demographics

- Leg ulcers affect nearly 2 million people, mostly older adults.
- In 2007, 3.5 million people in Europe and North America developed pressure ulcers.

Risk Factors

- Advanced age
- Diabetes mellitus
- Immobility—constant skin pressure
- Peripheral vascular disease
- Malnutrition
- Decreased tissue perfusion
- Infection
- Immunosuppresion
- Steroid therapy

Prevention and Screening

- Tight control of diabetes mellitus
- Meticulous diabetic foot care
- Appropriate shoes
- Skin care
- Early detection of peripheral vascular disease
- Revascularization for arterial disease
- If immobilized: frequent turning, specialty beds, skin barriers
- If hospitalized: Braden score on admission and daily
- Well-balanced diet
- Anti-platelet or anticoagulation agents to prevent arterial thrombosis

Assessment

- General wound assessment
  - Many wound classification systems exist—no one system is used universally.
  - Examples:
    - Wagner Classification System—most widely recognized
    - The SAD classification—reported in *Diabetic Medicine Journal*
    - Red Yellow Black System—prominent in nursing literature
- Full medical history
- Current medications
- Lifestyle—tobacco and alcohol habits
- Location of wound
- Wound size—length and width in centimeters
- Superficial
- Partial thickness
  - Extension through epidermis, partially into dermis
- Full thickness
- Extension through epidermis, dermis, and subcutaneous layer
- Muscle and bone may be involved
- Undermining and tunneling
  - Depth and direction
- Sinus tracts
- Characteristics of wound bed
  - Necrosis
  - Granulation
  - Infection
  - Exudate
    - None
    - Low
    - Moderate
    - High
- Color of wound
  - Red
    - Healthy granulation tissue
  - Yellow
    - Exudate present
    - Debridement required
  - Beige
    - Creamy or whitish yellow
    - Yellow-green
  - Black
    - Eschar—necrotic tissue
    - Debridement required
  - Mixed
    - Identify predominant color
  - Odor
    - Present
    - Absent

- Clinical signs of local infection
  - Delayed healing
  - Odor
  - Absent or abnormal granulation tissue
  - New or increased pain at wound site
  - Excessive or increased exudates
- Condition of surrounding skin
  - Normal
  - Edematous
  - White
  - Shiny
  - Warm
  - Red
    - Dry
    - Scaling
    - Thin
    - Chronic wound pain
    - Location
    - Duration
      - Persistent/intermittent
    - Intensity
    - Quality

Ulcer-Specific Examination

- Arterial or diabetic ulcers
  - Location
  - Arterial disease
    - Below ankles, toes
  - Diabetic ulcers
    - Plantar surface of foot
    - Diminished lower extremity pulses
    - Shiny, cool skin in lower extremities
    - Sparse or absent leg hair
    - Thickened toenails
  - Abnormal Ankle Brachial Pressure Index (ABPI)
    - > 1.2 = abnormal—vessel hardening
    - $1.0 - 1.2$ = normal range—venous ulcers
    - $0.9 - 1.0$ = low—venous ulcers
    - $0.7 - 0.9$ = mild arterial disease—venous ulcers
    - $0.4 - 0.8$ = moderate arterial disease—claudication, mixed ulcers
    - > 0.4 = severe arterial disease—arterial or diabetic ulcers
  - Smooth wound margins; deep, minimal drainage
  - Atrophic, pale peri-ulcer skin
  - Cellulitis may be present with necrosis

- Diabetic ulcer—localized thickening of skin around the ulcer
- Neuropathy
- Infection
- Venous ulcers
  - Usually located above the ankle on the lower leg
  - Warm lower extremities/feet
  - Normal peripheral pulses
  - Varicosities present
  - Presence of edema in legs, feet, or both
  - Granulating superficial ulcer with irregular margins
  - Brown pigmentation in the peri-ulcer skin area (eczema may be present)
  - Moderate to large amount of drainage
- Mixed ulcers
  - Caused by both venous and arterial disease
  - Usually signs or symptoms of venous ulcers first; arterial ischemia develop over time
- Pressure ulcers
  - Classified according to stages by National Pressure Ulcer Advisory Panel
  - Localized injury to skin and tissues, usually over a bony prominence because of constant pressure alone or in combination with shear/friction force
    - Deep tissue injury
    - Purple or maroon localized area of discolored skin or blood-filled blister from damage to underlying soft tissue
      - May first express as tissue that is painful, firm, mushy, boggy, and warmer or cooler than surrounding tissue
    - May be difficult to detect in darker skin tones
    - Evolution may be rapid, exposing deeper layers of tissue even with treatment
    - Stage I
      - Intact skin with nonblanchable redness of localized area over bony prominence
      - Darker skin tones may not have visible blanching, and color may differ from that of surrounding area.
    - Stage II
      - Partial-thickness loss of dermis presenting as shallow open ulcer with a red-pink wound bed, no slough
      - May also be intact or open/ruptured, serum-filled blister
      - Shiny shallow or dry shallow ulcer
    - Stage III
      - Full-thickness tissue loss
      - Subcutaneous fat may be visible but bone, muscle, or tendon are not exposed.
      - Slough may be present but does not cover depth of tissue loss
      - Depth varies by location
      - Bridge of nose, ear, occiput, and malleolus do not have subcutaneous tissue and wound may be shallow
      - Large amount of adipose tissue can lead to developing very deep stage III ulcers.
    - Stage IV
      - Full-thickness tissue loss with exposed bone, tendon, or muscle
      - Slough or eschar may be present.
      - Often undermining or tunneling
      - Varies by location

- Can extend into muscle and supporting structures—fascia, tendon, joint capsule
- Osteomyelitis is possible.
- Exposed bone, tendon, or both are visible or directly palpable.
• Unstageable
- Full-thickness tissue loss with base of ulcer covered by slough (yellow, tan, gray, green, brown), eschar (tan, brown or black) in the wound bed, or both

Diagnostic Studies

- Lower extremity arterial duplex ultrasound
- Used to evaluate anatomy and flow of arterial system
- Ankle-Brachial Pressure Index—see earlier information
- Transcutaneous oxygen pressure ($tcPO_2$)
- Measures delivery of oxygen to the tissues
- Values > 30 mm Hg are usually needed for wound healing.
- Digital plethysomography
  - Measures toe pressure and quality of pressure wave form
  - Ratio of toe pressure to brachial systolic pressure normally 0.80 to 0.90
- Venous Doppler ultrasound
  - Evaluates for clots and incompetent valves
- Complete blood count
- Coagulation studies
- Complete metabolic panel
- Take wound culture and check sensitivity if warranted

Management

- Surgical and traumatic wounds—depends on location and type of wound—determined by surgical subspeciality involved
- Treat pain in all types of ulcers.
- Prescribe antibiotics as warranted for osteomyelitis, cellulitis, sepsis.
- Arterial ulcers
  - Wet to moist dressings
  - Enzymatic agents
  - Collagenase
  - Papain-urea
  - No occlusive dressings
  - Calcium alginate wound dressing
- Venous ulcers
  - Wet to moist dressings
  - Whirlpool
  - Surgical debridement
  - Enzymatic debridement
  - Compression therapy if normal peripheral pulses

- Diabetic ulcers
  - Wet to moist dressings
  - Incision and drainage if needed
  - Nonocclusive, nonadherent dressings
  - Enzymatic debridement
- Presssure ulcers
  - Repositioning every 2 hours minimum
  - Decrease capillary pressure
  - Specialty beds and mattresses
  - Skin barriers
  - Debridement
  - Cleansing
  - Normal saline
  - Avoid cytotoxic skin cleansers
    - Povidone-iodine
    - Iodophor
    - Hydrogen peroxide
    - Sodium hypochlorite solution
  - Dressing to keep ulcer bed moist and surrounding skin dry
  - Maintain adequate nutrition

When to Consult, Refer, or Hospitalize

- Refer for urgent evaluation and hospitalization by vascular surgeon, interventional cardiologist, or radiologist when gangrene is present, tendon or bone is visible, cellulitis, severe infection, Ankle-Brachial Index < 0.5
- Surgical consult for wet gangrene

Follow-up

Expected Outcomes
- When vascular disease is diagnosed, patient must be followed on outpatient basis to prevent the formation of ulcers.
- Patient should be followed and seen regularly for the following:
  - $tcPO_2$ > 30 mm Hg and ABPI > 1.0
  - Weak or absent pulses with ABPI < 1.0
  - ABPI > 0.5 and < 0.8
  - Poor wound healing of existing ulcer

Complications
- Osteomyelitis
- Chronic infections
- Sepsis
- Amputation

REFERENCES

Barkley, T., & Myers, C. (2008). *Practice guidelines for acute care nurse practitioners.* St. Louis, MO: Saunders.

Beers, M., Porter, R., Jones, T., Kaplan, J., & Berkwits, M. (Eds.). (2006). *The Merck manual of diagnosis and therapy.* Whitehouse Station, NJ: Merck Research Laboratories.

Bryant, R., & Nix, D. (2012). *Acute and chronic wounds: Current management concepts.* St. Louis, MO: Elsevier.

Carana, M., Bradbury, A.W., & Adam, D. J. (2005). The validity, reliability, reproducibility and extended utility of ankle to brachial pressure index in current vascular surgical practice. *European Journal of Vascular and Endovascular Surgery, 29*(5), 443–451.

Gillespie, D. L., Kistner, B., Glass, C., Bailey, B., Chopra, A., Ennis, B., ... Falanga, V. (2010). Venous ulcer diagnosis, treatment, and prevention of recurrences. *Journal of Vascular Surgery, 52*(5S), 8S–14S.

National Pressure Ulcer Advisory Panel. (2007). *Pressure ulcer stages revised by NPUAP.* Retrieved from http://www.npuap.org/pr2.htm

Rooke, T., Sullivan, T., & Jaff, M. (2007). *Vascular medicine and endovascular interventions.* Hoboken, NJ: Wiley Blackwell.

Satterfield, K. (2006). A guide to understanding the various wound classification systems. *Podiatry Today, 19*(6), 20–27.

Stein, R., Hriljack, I., Halperin, J. L., Gustavson, S. M., Teodorescu, V., & Olin, J. W. (2006). Limitation of the resting ankle-brachial index in symptomatic patients with peripheral arterial disease. *Vascular Medicine, 11,* 29–33.

Review Questions

1. A 55-year old male is admitted to the medical intensive care unit with a diagnosis of cirrhosis secondary to hepatitis B. He is confused and disoriented, with jaundiced skin, a musty sweet odor to his breath, spider telangiectasis, and asterixis. His laboratory values are as follows:

    SGOT/AST: 100 units/L; SGPT/ALT: 88 units/L; LDH: 200 units/L; alkaline phosphatase: 165 units/L; BUN: 27 mg/dl; creatinine: 1.3 mg/dl; ammonia level: 95 mcg/dl.

    Based on the above information, what is the probable etiology of his altered mental status?
    a. Loss of cerebral glucose from hepatic failure
    b. Hepatorenal syndrome
    c. Seizure activity
    d. Hepatic encephalopathy

2. A 42-year-old White female presents with acute biliary pain, fever, leukocytosis, and a positive Murphy's sign. Cholecystitis is suspected. Initial diagnostic testing to help confirm the diagnosis would be a(n):
    a. cholescintigraphy.
    b. abdominal ultrasound.
    c. serum aminotransferases and amylase.
    d. CT scan of the abdomen.

3. You are called to assess a 75-year-old male who is 5 days postoperative from a ruptured abdominal aortic aneurysm repair. His pre- and postoperative course was complicated by hypotension. His complaint is abdominal pain. On physical examination, you find he is distended and guarding. His WBC is 16K. You put mesenteric ischemia at the top of your differential diagnosis list because you know it
   a. is characterized by sudden intestinal hyperperfusion.
   b. can be caused by occlusive or nonocclusive obstruction of arterial or venous flow.
   c. presents as left-sided back pain or flank pain.
   d. typically may be seen on a plain film abdominal radiograph.

4. A 72-year-old female has been a patient in the ICU for 6 days following an abdominal aortic aneurysm repair. She was extubated 2 days ago, but has required high-flow oxygen therapy. The ICU calls you because her 0700 temperature is 101.5° F. Your initial workup would include:
   a. abdominal x-ray, blood cultures, urine culture.
   b. blood, urine, sputum cultures.
   c. chest x-ray, blood, urine, and sputum cultures.
   d. No workup is required.

5. Your answer to question 4 is based on your knowledge that the most common cause of fever in the ICU is:
   a. atelectasis.
   b. infection.
   c. drug-induced fever.
   d. dehydration.

6. Fever of unknown origin is defined as:
   a. remains febrile (> 38.3° C) with negative blood cultures after 48 hours.
   b. fever remains after suspected medications are stopped, with negative blood cultures for 48 hours.
   c. a patient who remains febrile after 7 days of antibiotic therapy.
   d. temperature > 38.3° C rectally for 3 weeks or longer without an apparent cause after extensive investigation in three outpatient visits or 3 days of hospitalization (without neutropenia or immunosuppresion being present).

7. The indications for starting total parenteral nutrition alone are:
   a. if the patient must remain NPO for several procedures.
   b. when the patient has his or her jaw stabilized with wires posttrauma.
   c. severe gut dysfunction from prolonged ileus, obstruction, or severe hemorrhagic pancreatitis.
   d. when the patient has a high risk of aspiration.

The next five questions relate to the scenario in question 8.

8. A 78-year-old female is admitted from an assisted living facility to the intermediate intensive care unit. She had not been seen in the facility's dining room for 3 days. The residence's attendant found her in room lying on the couch lethargic and weak, which is a distinct change from her baseline status. She was taken to the emergency department via ambulance. You are performing her history and physical after she arrives to the ward. Her initial vital signs and laboratory values from the emergency room are as follows:

   Blood pressure: 94/62; heart rate: 118; respiratory rate: 24; temperature: 99° F
   Na^+: 154; K^+: 4.2; creatinine: 2.5; BUN: 46; urine osmolality: > 400 mosm/kg

   Her medical records indicate her baseline creatinine is 1.0.

   Her altered mental status can be attributed to:
   a. a urinary tract infection.
   b. hypernatremia and dehydration.
   c. dementia.
   d. hypotension.

9. The etiology of her hypernatremia is most likely the result of:
   a. decreased water intake.
   b. intensive exercise.
   c. chronic kidney disease.
   d. excessive salt intake.

10. The replacement you will choose to initially correct the problem is:
    a. normal saline.
    b. packed red blood cells.
    c. D_5W.
    d. lactated ringers.

11. Once the patient's hypovolemic state is stabilized, further correction of the hypernatremia should be performed with what solution over what time frame?
    a. Lactated ringers, over 24 hours
    b. Normal saline, over 48 hours
    c. D_5W, over 48 hours
    d. D_5W, over 24 hours

12. Signs and symptoms of severe hypernatremia (Na^+ > 158 mEq/L) are:
    a. seizure, vomiting, and coma.
    b. hyperactivity and sweating.
    c. increased urinary output and hypertension.
    d. bradycardia, edema, and fever.

The next four questions relate to the scenario in question 13.

13. A 30-year-old female is brought to the emergency department by her friend. She states the patient has been depressed in recent months and took a "handful" of acetaminophen in a suicide attempt about 5 hours ago. Initial vital signs:

    Blood pressure: 104/60; heart rate: 90; respiratory rate: 24

    As the ACNP evaluating the patient, you know that with severe acetaminophen poisoning the patient could suffer:
    a. acute myocardial infarction.
    b. fulminant hepatic failure.
    c. acute renal failure.
    d. respiratory failure.

14. The antidote for acetaminophen poisoning is:
    a. nothing—there isn't one.
    b. Narcan.
    c. hemodialysis.
    d. N-acetylcysteine.

15. N-acetylcysteine may be given in what form?
    a. p.o. and IV
    b. p.o., IV, and rectally
    c. p.o. or NGT only
    d. IV only

16. N-acetylcysteine is most effective if given:
    a. within 2 hours of ingestion.
    b. orally.
    c. within 8–10 hours of ingestion.
    d. rectally.

The next two questions relate to the scenario in question 17.

17. A 49-year-old male has been admitted to your unit for complaints of fatigue, fever, night sweats, and progressive weight loss for the past 6 months. When taking the history, you discover the patient is a gay male with multiple sexual contacts. He uses sexual barriers inconsistently. When developing the differential diagnoses and workup for this patient, you discuss with him the importance of performing a test to rule out infection with HIV because:
    a. federal law requires routine testing of all inpatients.
    b. his history reveals high risk behavior for potential exposure to HIV.
    c. it is likely to be negative.
    d. he is withholding that he is aware that he is seropositive for HIV.

18. Your facility uses the rapid test Ora Quick Advance for HIV as a screening study. His test is positive; your next step is:
    a. tell the patient he is HIV positive.
    b. confirm the positive result with the Western blot test.
    c. confirm with second rapid HIV test.
    d. confirm with ELISA only.

19. A newly diagnosed AIDS patient has the following lab values:

    CD4 cell count < 300, Vial load >100,000, and is asymptomatic.

    This information indicates that:
    a. the disease is in the early stages and does not require therapy.
    b. the patient has a low risk for opportunistic infections.
    c. the disease is progressing rapidly.
    d. antiretroviral therapy should be initiated.

20. The mainstay of HIV treatment to obtain maximum efficacy is:
    a. have the patient report to a clinic in person each day to obtain the antiretroviral medication.
    b. to use combination therapy with at least three drugs simultaneously from at least two different classes.
    c. rotate the drug regimen every 6 months.
    d. reduce the number of medications used after 6 months to prevent drug resistance.

21. A 65-year-old female has been admitted from the emergency department with complaints of left lower quadrant abdominal pain and diarrhea. Her history includes coronary artery disease, hypertension, gastroesophageal reflux disease, and diverticulosis. She has a leukocytosis of 14,000 cells/mm^3 and temperature of 100° F. You suspect the etiology of her abdominal pain is:
    a. cholecystitis.
    b. appendicitis.
    c. diverticulitis.
    d. renal calculi.

The next two questions refer to the scenario in question 22.

22. A 50-year-old female is admitted to the coronary intermediate care unit with a diagnosis of acute on chronic systolic heart failure. On day 2 of her hospital admission, she complains of lower abdominal pain and has pink-tinged urine in her foley catheter. Her WBC is 12,000 cell/mm^3. You obtain a urinalysis that is positive for leukocyte esterase, nitrite, moderate blood, and numerous bacteria. The culture is still pending. You decide to treat empirically with ciprofloxacin 400 mg IV every 12 hours until the culture results come back. The patient receives the first dose, and 30 minutes later the nurse taking care of the patient calls you for unstable vital signs. The patient's vital signs and physical examination findings are as follows:

    Blood pressure: 88/60; heart rate: 120; respiratory rate: 26; O$_2$ saturation: 86% on 4L nasal cannula.

    Patient is in obvious distress, using accessory muscles and bilateral wheezing. She feels like her throat is tightening, making it difficult to breathe. You suspect the etiology of her symptoms is:
    a. hypersensitivity reaction to the ciprofloxacin.
    b. hypovolemia.
    c. exacerbation of her heart failure.
    d. asthma.

23. Anaphylaxis is mediated by:
    a. Type I: IgE-mediated hypersensitivity.
    b. Type II: antibody-mediated hypersensitivity.
    c. Type III: immune complex-mediated hypersensitivity.
    d. Type IV: cell-mediated hypersensitivity.

24. Calcinosis cutis, Raynaud's phenomenon, esophageal motility disorder, sclerodactyly, and telangiectasia compose a syndrome known as CREST. They are the defining signs of:
    a. diffuse scleroderma.
    b. limited scleroderma.
    c. systemic lupus erythematosus.
    d. anti-phospholipid syndrome.

25. The number one cause of death in patients with scleroderma is:
    a. liver failure from cirrhosis.
    b. stroke.
    c. lung disease because of pulmonary hypertension and fibrosis.
    d. sepsis.

The next three questions relate to the scenario in question 26.

26. A 42-year-old male is admitted with an exacerbation of his ulcerative colitis. He has had several episodes of bloody diarrhea with abdominal pain and tenderness.

    Vital signs are blood pressure: 100/60; heart rate: 110; respiratory rate: 24; temperature: 100° F; CBC: Hgb 8.5 g/dL; erythrocyte sedimentation rate: 30 mm/hr.

    Your initial management will include:
    a. NPO, IV fluids, electrolyte replacement, consider blood transfusion.
    b. clear liquid diet, advance as tolerated, bed rest.
    c. chest x-ray, NPO.
    d. regular diet, but limit caffeine and gas-producing vegetables.

27. The treatment for ulcerative colitis is determined by:
    a. what medications the patient is currently taking.
    b. the age of the patient.
    c. the extent of colonic involvement and severity of the illness.
    d. how long the patient has had ulcerative colitis.

28. Medications use for maintenance therapy to prevent relapse are:
    a. opiates and anticholinergics.
    b. derivatives of 5-ASA and corticosteroids.
    c. antibiotics.
    d. prednisone and opiates.

29. If needed, an appropriate choice of inotropic agent for a heart transplant patient is:
    a. norepinephrine.
    b. isoproterenol.
    c. milrinone.
    d. digoxin.

30. Immunosuppresive medications:
    a. may be weaned off after the first year if no signs or symptoms of rejection occur.
    b. prevent postoperative complications.
    c. prevent graft rejection.
    d. exaggerate the immune response.

31. One of the most common medical complications seen after solid organ transplant is:
    a. COPD.
    b. HIT (heparin-induced thrombocytopenia).
    c. arthritis.
    d. HLD (hyperlipidemia).

32. A common symptom of graft failure (rejection) of a transplanted kidney is:
    a. polyuria.
    b. hypertension.
    c. enuresis.
    d. hypotension.

33. Cardiac output after heart-lung transplantation is dependent on:
    a. blood pressure.
    b. PAOP (pulmonary artery occlusive pressure).
    c. heart rate.
    d. hematocrit > 28.

34. Pancreas transplant is indicated for:
    a. Type I diabetics.
    b. Type II diabetics with multi-organ end-stage disease.
    c. Brittle type II diabetics with CAD amenable to bypass grafting.
    d. Brittle type II diabetics with end-stage renal disease.

35. The ACNP is managing an acute hypertensive crisis secondary to pheochromocytoma. The initial agent of choice for blood pressure control should be chosen from which category?
    a. Thiazide diuretics
    b. Beta blockers
    c. Alpha blockers
    d. Calcium channel blockers

36. You are caring for a 42-year-old female in the NICU, postoperative day 2 after a transphenoidal removal of a large pituitary adenoma. She has been hemodynamically stable overnight and is being considered for transfer to the floor. After performing your exam and reviewing her chart and morning lab work, you correctly conclude that her thirst, hypernatremia, high serum osmolality, low specific gravity, and six liter urine output overnight is due to:
    a. SIADH.
    b. diabetes insipidus.
    c. cerebral salt-wasting syndrome.
    d. diabetes mellitus.

37. A 25-year-old male is admitted to the hospital with a diagnosis of acute myeloid leukemia. Six years ago, he had treatment for early-stage non-Hodgkin's lymphoma with cyclophosphamide, doxorubicin, vincristine, and prednisone and mediastinal radiation. He as a 10-pack/year smoking history and is a welder. There is no family history of cancer. His examination is significant for pallor and some petechiae on his chest, back, and lower extremities. Complete blood count reveals decreased white blood cell count, red blood cell count, and thrombocytopenia. What is the most like cause of his acute myeloid leukemia?
    a. Chemotherapy
    b. Radiation
    c. Combined modality treatment
    d. Tobacco use

38. A 68-year-old male is with bacteremia and pyelonephritis has been admitted to your service. He has no other significant medial history. After 2 weeks of treatment with antibiotics, he continues to have a fever. Repeat blood cultures reveal *Candida albicans*. His white blood cell count is normal. His central venous catheter was removed and systemic antifungal therapy was initiated. What further evaluation is recommended?
    a. Abdominal CT scan to evaluate for abscesses
    b. Chest x-ray
    c. Fundoscopic examination
    d. Transthoracic echocardiogram.

39. Which of the following regarding the insertion and maintenance of central venous catheters is correct?
    a. A guidewire exchange may be used to replace a malfunctioning catheter
    b. Full barrier technique is not needed when performing a guidewire exchange
    c. Povidone iodine is the most effective when access occurs while the solution is still wet
    d. Scheduled guidewire exchanges of central venous catheters has been shown to decrease catheter related infections in the ICU

40. When establishing a new therapeutic relationship, the ACNP must avoid making assumptions about patients and their families based on physical appearance or the type of dress because many families have blended traditional beliefs. This is an example of:
    a. cultural respect.
    b. mutual trust.
    c. professional boundaries.
    d. confidentiality.

41. In order to maintain an effective professional therapeutic patient relationship, the ACNP must practice within certain ethical guidelines. The ethical principle of beneficence is:
    a. duty not to inflict harm or evil.
    b. duty to respect others' personal liberty, individual values, beliefs and choices.
    c. duty to do good and prevent or remove harm.
    d. duty to tell the truth and not to deceive others.

Answers to the Review Questions

1. **Correct Answer: D.** Symptoms of hepatic encephalopathy are decreased brain function, especially confusion, and reduced alertness. In the earliest stages, subtle changes appear in logical thinking, personality, and behavior. The person's mood may change and his or her judgment may be impaired. At any stage of encephalopathy, the patient may have a musty, sweet odor. As the disorder progresses, the patient's hand cannot be held steady when the person stretches out his or her arms, resulting in a crude flapping motion of the hands (asterixis). In addition, the patient becomes drowsy and confused, and movements and speech become sluggish. Disorientation is common. Coma may ensue.

2. **Correct Answer: B.** In addition to the clinical findings associated with cholecystitis, an abdominal ultrasound is the first imaging study obtained and often can establish the diagnosis. Nuclear cholescintigraphy may be useful in cases in which the diagnosis remains uncertain after ultrasound.

3. **Correct Answer: B.** The hallmark of mesenteric ischemia is abdominal pain. It can be the result of an occlusive or nonocclusive obstruction of arterial or venous blood flow. Arterial occlusion is the most common type, resulting from thrombosis or segmental strangulation. Nonocclusive arterial hypoperfusion is the result of splanchnic vasoconstriction.

4. **Correct Answer: C.** Infection is the most common cause of fever in the ICU patient and should be sought early because source control is the definitive therapy. With initial fever and/or leukocytosis not attributed to medication, patient should be pan cultured (urine, blood, sputum) with a chest x-ray if one was not done on the day of fever.

5. **Correct Answer: B.** Infection is the most common cause of fever in the ICU patient and should be sought early because source control is the definitive therapy.

6. **Correct Answer: D.** This is the correct description of fever of unknown origin.

7. **Correct Answer: C.** Enteral feedings are the first choice for supplemental feedings in the critically ill patient; however, the above conditions warrant TPN only.

8. **Correct Answer: B.** When a patient is dehydrated, water shifts to the intravascular space to protect volume status and results in neurological changes. Lethargy, irritability, weakness are early signs. With serum Na > 158 mEq/L, the patient may exhibit hyperthermia, delirium, seizures, and coma.

9. **Correct Answer: A.** The hypernatremic patient is usually hypovolemic because of free water loss. It may also be seen in hypervolemia as an iatrogenic complication in hospitalized patients with impaired access to free water.

10. **Correct Answer: A.** Initially, volume needs to be restored using normal saline, which may be hypotonic relative to the serum osmolality in the severely dehydrated patient. After volume is stabilized, the hypernatremia can continue to be corrected using D_5W over the next 48 hours. Free water deficit is calculated as:

    FWD = body weight (kg) x percentage of total body weight (0.6 for men and 0.4 for women) x [(serum As/140) – 1].

11. **Correct Answer: C.** After volume is stabilized, the hypernatremia can continue to be corrected using D_5W over the next 48 hours.

12. **Correct Answer: A.** As hypernatremia becomes more severe, water shifts to the intravascular space, resulting in the neurological manifestations.

13. **Correct Answer: B.** Acetaminophen is metabolized in the liver; the normal process of metabolism and degradation is interrupted, resulting in reactive intermediate complexes attacking cell proteins in the liver, causing necrosis.

14. **Correct Answer: D.** N-acetylcysteine is the approved antidote for acetaminophen toxicity and, if given within the first 8–10 hours of ingestion, is almost 100% effective in protecting the liver.

15. **Correct Answer: A.** The antidote may be given orally and by IV infusion. The most widely used protocol indicates a 72-hour treatment time frame for oral use and 16-hour infusion IV.

16. **Correct Answer: C.** Efficacy is reduced after this time frame. If given within this window, it is highly hepatoprotecive.

17. **Correct Answer: B.** HIV is more common in males and is more common in men who have sex with men, with or without IV drug use.

18. **Correct Answer: B.** To rule out a false positive, the definitive test to confirm the diagnosis of HIV is the Western blot.

19. **Correct Answer: D.** These levels are an indication to treat in asymptomatic patients. All symptomatic patients are treated.

20. **Correct Answer: B.** This has proven to be the most effective method to suppress viral loads and help reduce drug resistance, which is a challenge in the HIV patient.

21. **Correct Answer: C.** She is exhibiting the signs and symptoms associated with diverticulitis. Cholecystitis pain is characterized by steady pain in the epigastrium or right hypochondrium. Appendicitis is characterized by colicky pain that begins in the epigastrium and then shifts to the right lower quadrant. Renal calculi presents with flank pain.

22. **Correct Answer: A.** Patient is exhibiting signs and symptoms of anaphylaxis. The signs and symptoms are similar to an exacerbation of heart failure, but the sudden onset and timing with the ciprofloxacin administration point to an allergic reaction.

23. **Correct Answer: A.** Allergy is an immunologically mediated hypersensitivity reaction to an antigen that is characterized by tissue inflammation and organ dysfunction. There are four classifications of hypersensitivity reactions:

    Type I: occurs within minutes of exposure to the antigen and includes atopy and anaphylaxis

    Type II: involves the specific reaction of IgG or IgM antibodies to cell-bound antigens, for example, immune hemolytic anemia

    Type III: occurs when antigen and IgG or IgM antibodies form a circulating immune complex and deposit it in tissues or vascular epithelium; an example is serum sickness

    Type IV: is delayed hypersensitivity mediated by T cells; an example is allergic dermatitis

24. **Correct Answer: B.** Limited scleroderma is characterized by the described syndrome.

25. **Correct Answer: C.** In diffuse scleroderma, fibrosis occurs in the skin and internal organs. Currently, lung disease is the number cause of mortality, with renal and heart failure also being common.

26. **Correct Answer: A.** Patient is demonstrating signs and symptoms of sever colitis, which requires bowel rest, hydration, electrolyte replacement, and possible transfusion.

27. **Correct Answer: C.** Patients with mild disease have a gradual onset of infrequent diarrhea (< 5 bowel movements per day) with intermittent rectal bleeding and may be treated as outpatients initially, with diet management and antidiarrheals. Those with severe disease must be hospitalized because they may progress to fulminant colitis or toxic megacolon.

28. **Correct Answer: B.** Without long-term therapy, 75% of patients who go into remission will have a relapse within 1 year. ASA derivatives alone often will be effective, but corticosteroid therapy may be added for recurrent relapses.

29. **Correct Answer: B.** Because of denervation (the result of severing the vagus nerve), medications such as atropine and digoxin have minimal effect on the transplanted heart. The inotropic agent used most commonly is isoproterenol.

30. **Correct Answer: C.** Immunosuppression manipulates the immune system, preventing or suppressing organ rejection.

31. **Correct Answer: D.** HLD, felt to be associated with the use of immunosuppressive agents, has been found to occur in 80% of transplant patients.

32. **Correct Answer: B.** There is a high correlation between hypertension and graft failure in kidney transplant recipients.

33. **Correct Answer: C.** Cardiac output is primarily rate-dependent after heart-lung transplantation. The heart rate should be maintained between 90 and 110 bpm during the first few postoperative days using temporary pacing or isoproterenol (0.005 to 0.01 µg/kg per minute) as needed.

34. **Correct Answer: A.** Type I diabetes is the only indication for pancreas transplantation.

35. **Correct Answer: C.** Beta blockers given prior to blocking alpha receptors can cause paradoxical worsening of hypertension. Calcium channels blockers may also be used with or without administration of beta blockade first. Thiazide diuretics and nitrates are not used for the treatment/management of pheochromocytoma.

36. **Correct Answer: B.** Diabetes insipidus is a common complication following removal of a pituitary tumor. This can be differentiated from SIADH because a patient with SIADH has decreased urine output, hyponatremia, and low serum osmolality.

37. **Correct Answer: C.** Long-term complications of cancer treatment happen frequently. Patients treated with radiation therapy and alkylating agents may develop malignant leukemic cells. The peak incidence is 4 to 6 years after treatment.

38. **Correct Answer: C.** Candidemia may lead to seeding of other organs. In nonneutropenic patients, the incidence is about 10%; for that reason, a fundoscopic examination is important. Seeding may occur within 2 weeks of onset of the candidemia even without fever or if the infection has cleared. The lesions may be uni- or bilateral, and are small with white retinal exudates. Patients may report blurring, ocular pain, or alteration in the field of vision.

39. **Correct Answer: A.** Guidewire exchange may be used when a catheter is malfunctioning, but if an infection is suspected, then the insertion must be changed. Scheduled guidewire exchanges have not shown to decrease infections rates. The preferable antiseptic solution to use is chlorhexidine; however, if in the rare instance povidone iodine is used, it must be dry. Full barrier technique should be used for all central line insertions, including guidewire exchanges.

40. **Correct Answer: A.** It is important to avoid making assumptions based solely on physical appearance or dress—many families have blended traditional beliefs and practices from multiple cultures. Recognizing and respecting the cultural identification of patients is viewed as being essential to establishing a therapeutic relationship. Mutual trust is a shared belief between the patient and nurse practitioner that they can depend on each other to achieve a common purpose or goal. A professional boundary is established so that the appropriate use of patient information and intimacy to meet the patient's needs while providing care is acknowledged. The rule of confidentiality is the duty to not disclose information shared in an intimate and trusted manner.

41. **Correct Answer: C.** Beneficience is the duty to do good and prevent or remove harm. Nonmalfecience is the duty not to inflict harm or evil. Respect for autonomy is the duty to respect others' personal liberty, individual values, beliefs, and choices. Veracity is the duty to tell the truth and not to deceive others.

Index

Page numbers followed by t indicate tables.

A

Abdominal aneurysm, 40, 104–106
Absence seizure, 226t. *See also* Seizures
Accreditation, healthcare institutions, 36
Acetaminophen overdose/toxicity, 349, 352, 810–813
Acid-fast bacilli (AFB), 130
Acid–base disorders, 786–788. *See also* specific disorders
Acquired immunodeficiency syndrome (AIDS). *See* HIV/AIDS
Acute adrenal insufficiency, 148, 181
Acute allergic reactions. *See* Allergic reactions, acute
Acute care nurse practitioner (ACNP)
    as advocate for nurse practitioner role, 17–18
    certification examination. *See* Certification examination
    collaboration with other healthcare providers, 18
    core competencies, 20–21
    educational requirements, 25–26
    ethical and legal issues
        informed consent, 23
        liability/malpractice, 26–27, 46–47
        medical futility, 23
        prescriptive authority, 19–20, 29
        principles, 19
        resolution of conflicts, 21–22
        risk management, 23
        state licensure or regulation, 19
    evidence-based practice, 24
    as patient advocate, 14
    patient relationships. *See* Therapeutic relationships
    practice standards, 15–16
    reimbursement/billing for services, 31–33
    scope of practice
        assessment, 27
        consultation and referral, 27
        credentialing and privileging, 17, 20
        follow-up, 28–29
        goals, 15
        management of patient care, 28
        prevention/screening, 27
        regulations, 16–17, 20, 26, 29, 31
        special considerations, 28
        standards, 15–16, 21
    time management, 17
Acute cholecystitis, 316–321

Acute coronary syndrome (ACS), 53–56
Acute glomerulonephritis (AGN), 298–303
Acute hepatic failure, 348–353
Acute kidney injury/acute renal failure
    assessment, 273–276
    description, 271
    differential diagnosis, 276
    etiology, 271–272
    follow-up, 278
    incidence and demographics, 272
    management, 277
    prevention and screening, 273
    risk factors, 272–273
    special considerations, 277–278
    when to consult, refer, or hospitalize, 278
Acute knee injury, 556–558, 559t
Acute lung injury (ALI), 137. See also Acute respiratory distress syndrome
Acute lymphocytic leukemia (ALL), 477
Acute myeloid leukemia (AML), 477
Acute nonlymphocytic leukemia (ANLL), 477
Acute pancreatitis, 370–375, 373t
Acute pyelonephritis, 252, 256–259
Acute renal failure. See Acute kidney injury/acute renal failure
Acute respiratory distress syndrome (ARDS), 137–140
Acute respiratory failure, 135–137
Acute tubular necrosis (ATN), 294–298, 296t
Addisonian crisis, 148, 181
Addison's disease (adrenal insufficiency), 180–183
Adhesive capsulitis, 556
Adjustment disorder, 580
Adrenal disorders
    Addison's disease, 180–183
    Cushing's syndrome, 177–179
    diabetes insipidus, 183–185
    pheochromocytoma, 63t, 188–191
    syndrome of inappropriate diuretic hormone, 186–188
Adult learners, 44. See also Patient education
Advanced directives, 13
Advocacy
    for nurse practitioner role, 17–18
    for patient, 14
Age Discrimination Act of 1967, 31
Alcohol toxicity, 814–818
Alcoholic cirrhosis. See Cirrhosis/chronic liver disease
Alcoholism, 582–584
Allergic reactions, acute
    assessment, 516–518
    description, 514–515
    differential diagnosis, 518
    etiology, 515
    follow-up, 521
    incidence and demographics, 515–516
    management, 519–520
    prevention and screening, 516
    risk factors, 516
    special considerations, 520
    when to consult, refer, or hospitalize, 521
Allergic rhinitis, 515, 517, 519
Allergic triggers, for asthma, 116
Alpha-1 proteinase deficiency, 112
Alpha-thalassemia, 417, 419t. See also Thalassemia
Alzheimer's disease, 240–244, 597
Amanita phalloides mushroom, 352
American Diabetes Association (ADA) dietary guidelines, 151, 157
American Nurses Credentialing Center (ANCC), computerized exam characteristics, 8–9
Americans with Disabilities Act, 31
Amiodarone overdose/toxicity. See Antiarrhythmic drug overdose/toxicity
Amlodipine overdose/toxicity. See Antiarrhythmic drug overdose/toxicity
Amyloidosis, 521–527
Anaphylaxis, 515, 517, 519, 520
ANCA-associated glomerulonephritis, 298–302
Anemia of chronic disease, 399–401, 399t, 406t
Anemia(s)
    anemia of chronic disease, 399–401
    aplastic, 402–404
    definitions, 398–399
    differential diagnosis, 399t
    folic acid deficiency, 411–413
    general approach, 398
    hemolytic, 413–414
    hyperchromic, 399
    hypochromic, 398
    iron deficiency, 405–408
    macrocytic, 399
    megaloblastic, 399
    microcytic, 399
    normocytic, 399
    red flags, 398
    sickle cell, 414–416
    thalassemia. See Thalassemia
    vitamin B_{12} deficiency, 408–411
Aneurysm, abdominal, 40, 104–106
Angioedema, 517
Ankle Brachial Index (ABI), 80
Ankle Brachial Pressure Index (ABPI), 928
Ankle sprain, 556–561
Anogenital warts, 627, 628
Anorexia nervosa (AN)
    assessment, 671, 673
    complications, 688
    description, 664
    diagnostic studies, 677–678
    differential diagnosis, 680
    etiology, 665
    incidence and demographics, 668

management, 686
risk factors, 670
Ant sting, 922–923
Anterior cord syndrome, 216. *See also* Spinal cord trauma
Anterior cruciate ligament (ACL) injury, 558
Anterior drawer test, 559t
Antiarrhythmic drug overdose/toxicity
    assessment, 818–823
    description, 818
    diagnostic studies, 823–824
    differential diagnosis, 824
    follow-up, 826–827
    management, 824–826
    when to consult, refer, or hospitalize, 826
Antibiotic-resistance bacteria, 880–882
Anticholinergic agent overdose/toxicity, 827–829
Anticonvulsant agent overdose/toxicity
    assessment, 830–832
    description, 829–830
    diagnostic studies, 833–834
    differential diagnosis, 834
    follow-up, 835
    management, 834–835
    when to consult, refer, or hospitalize, 835
Antidepressant overdose/toxicity, 835–838
Antiglomerular basement membrane/Goodpasture syndrome, 298–302
Antipsychotic drug toxicity, 838–840
Anxiety, test, 1, 6
Anxiety disorders, 588–590
Aortic regurgitation (AR), 78–79
Aortic stenosis (AS), 76–77
Aplastic anemia, 399t, 402–404
Appendicitis, 312–316
Arterial ulcers, 928, 930
Aseptic meningitis, 219. *See also* Meningitis
Aspirin toxicity, 855–857
Assessment. *See also specific disorders*
    chronic illness, 40
    elderly patient, 39
    homeless patient, 39–40
    obesity/malnutrition, 40
    tobacco and substance abuse, 40
Asthma
    allergic, 116, 517
    assessment, 116–118, 119t
    classification, 117t
    description, 115
    differential diagnosis, 118
    etiology, incidence, and demographics, 115–116
    follow-up, 121
    management, 118, 120, 519–520
    prevention and screening, 116
    risk factors, 116
    when to consult, refer, or hospitalize, 120–121
Asymptomatic bacteriuria, 259–261
Asystole, 92–93
Atopic dermatitis, 515, 517–519
Atopy, 515
Atrial fibrillation, 87–89
Atrioventricular block, 3rd-degree, 93–94
Autograft, 716
Autoimmune thyroiditis, 173. *See also* Hypothyroidism
Autonomy, patient, 15
Axillary lymph node dissection, 456

B

Balloon tamponade, 348
Barbiturate toxicity, 857–860
Bariatric surgery, 685–686
Basal energy expenditure (BEE), 663
Basilar skull fracture, 215
Beck's triad, 97
Bee sting, 922–923
Benign prostatic hypertrophy (BPH), 266–270
Benzodiazepine toxicity, 857–860
Berger disease, 299
Beta blocker overdose/toxicity. *See* Antiarrhythmic drug overdose/toxicity
Beta-thalassemia, 417, 419t. *See also* Thalassemia
Biliary cast syndrome, 696
Bipolar disorders, 580
BK-type polyoma virus, 710
Black widow spider, 921
Bladder cancer, 465–469
Body fluids, 911–912, 916
Body mass index (BMI), 649
Body temperature, 720
Bouchard's nodes, 569
Bradykinesia, 206
BRCA gene mutations, 470
Breast and ovarian cancer syndrome, 470
Breast cancer
    assessment, 452–454
    bilateral, 459
    description, 448–449
    differential diagnosis, 454
    follow-up, 460
    incidence and demographics, 449
    management, 454–458
    noninvasive, 459
    prevention and screening, 40, 450–451, 655
    risk assessment models, 450
    risk factors, 449–450
    special considerations, 458–459
    staging, 451–452
    when to consult, refer, or hospitalize, 459
Breast-conserving therapy, 455
Bretylium overdose/toxicity. *See* Antiarrhythmic drug overdose/toxicity
Bronchiolitis obliterans, 701

Bronchitis, acute, 121–123
Bronchitis, chronic, 111, 112. *See also* Chronic obstructive pulmonary disease
Brown recluse spider, 921
Brown-Sequard's syndrome, 216. *See also* Spinal cord trauma
Brudzinski's sign, 221
Bulimia nervosa (BN)
    assessment, 671, 673
    complications, 688
    description, 664
    diagnostic studies, 677–678
    differential diagnosis, 680
    etiology, 665
    incidence and demographics, 668
    management, 686
    risk factors, 670

C

CAGE questionnaire, 41, 583
Cancer
    bladder, 465–469
    breast. *See* Breast cancer
    cervical, 472–476
    colorectal. *See* Colorectal cancer
    Hodgkin's lymphoma, 488–493
    incidence and demographics, 428
    leukemias, 477–481
    lung. *See* Lung cancer
    melanoma. *See* Melanoma
    most common, 429–430
    non-Hodgkin's lymphoma. *See* Non-Hodgkin's lymphoma
    ovarian, 469–472
    prostate, 460–465
    red flags, 430
    risk factors, 428
    screening recommendations, 40
    tumor grading, 429
    tumor staging, 428–429
Cancer of the Prostate Risk Assessment (CAPRA), 465
Capitated Medicare, 32
Carbamazepine overdose/toxicity. *See* Anticonvulsant agent overdose/toxicity
Carbon monoxide poisoning, 841–843
Carboxyhemoglobin, 841
Cardiac allograft vasculopathy (CAV), 704
Cardiac glycoside poisoning, 843–845
Cardiac rhythm disturbances
    asystole, 92–93
    atrial fibrillation, 87–89
    complete heart block, 93–94
    narrow complex supraventricular tachycardia, 89–90
    ventricular fibrillation, 91–92
    ventricular tachycardia, 90–91

Cardiac surgery, risk assessment, 42
Cardiac tamponade, 96–98, 731
Cardiogenic shock, 728, 729, 731t. *See also* Shock
Cardiomyopathy
    description, 98
    dilated, 99–100
    etiology, incidence, and demographics, 99
    hypertrophic, 101–102
    restrictive, 102–104
    when to consult, refer, or hospitalize, 104
Carotid endarterectomy, 196, 198
Cauda equina syndrome, 216. *See also* Spinal cord trauma
Cellulitis, 895–898
Central cord syndrome, 216. *See also* Spinal cord trauma
Central diabetes insipidus, 183
Central venous catheter infections, 874–877
Certification examination
    characteristics, 8–9
    final preparation, 5–6
    general preparation, 1–5
    study plan, 3–5
    test-taking skills, 6–8, 7t
Cervical cancer, 472–476, 655
Cervicitis
    gonococcal. *See* Gonorrhea
    nongonococcal. *See* Chlamydia
Chancre, 619. *See also* Syphilis
ChemSTEER, 41
Child-Turcotte-Pugh scoring system, liver disease, 326t
Chlamydia
    assessment, 606–607
    description, 604
    differential diagnosis, 608
    etiology, incidence, and demographics, 605
    follow-up, 609
    management, 608
    prevention and screening, 605–606, 655
    risk factors, 605
    special considerations, 608
    when to consult, refer, or hospitalize, 609
Chlamydia trachomatis. *See* Chlamydia
Chlamydophila, 604
Cholecystitis, 316–321
Cholesterol screening, 654
Cholinergic agent toxicity, 846–848
Chronic bronchitis, 111, 112. *See also* Chronic obstructive pulmonary disease
Chronic kidney disease/chronic kidney failure
    assessment, 63t, 281, 706
    description, 279
    diagnostic studies, 282
    differential diagnosis, 282
    etiology, 280
    follow-up, 285

incidence and demographics, 280, 707
management, 282–284. *See also* Kidney
    transplantation
prevention and screening, 281, 707
risk factors, 63, 280, 707
special considerations, 285
stages, 279t
when to consult, refer, or hospitalize, 285
Chronic lymphocytic leukemia (CLL), 477
Chronic myeloid leukemia (CML), 477
Chronic obstructive pulmonary disease (COPD),
    111–115, 114t, 698
Chronic venous insufficiency (CVI), 80. *See also*
    Peripheral vascular disease
Chvostek's sign, 763
Cirrhosis/chronic liver disease
    assessment, 323–324
    complications, 328
    description, 321
    diagnostic studies, 324–325
    differential diagnosis, 326
    etiology, 322, 691
    expected outcomes, 328
    incidence and demographics, 322, 692
    management, 327
    prevention and screening, 323
    risk factors, 322, 692
    special considerations, 327
    staging, 326t
    when to consult, refer, or hospitalize, 328
Clinical decision-making, steps in, 42
Clostridium difficile colitis, 877–879
Cluster headache, 231–233, 240
Coagulation disorders
    disseminated intravascular coagulation,
        425–428
    heparin-induced thrombocytopenia, 423–425
    idiopathic thrombocytopenia purpura,
        421–423
Cocaine toxicity, 860–863
Cockcroft-Gault equation, 282
Cogwheel rigidity, 206
Collaboration
    in ACNP–patient relationship, 15
    with other healthcare providers, 18
Colloids, 915
Colorectal cancer
    assessment, 443
    description, 441
    diagnostic studies, 444
    differential diagnosis, 445
    etiology, 441
    follow-up, 448
    incidence and demographics, 441–442
    management, 445–447
    prevention and screening, 40, 442–443, 656
    risk factors, 442

special considerations, 447
when to consult, refer, or hospitalize, 447
Communication, therapeutic, 15–16. *See also*
    Therapeutic relationships
Community-acquired infections
    cellulitis, 895–898
    infectious diarrhea, 899–903
    pharyngitis, 887–891
    pneumonia, 124–126
    sinusitis, 891–895
Complete heart block, 93–94
Complex partial seizure, 226t. *See also* Seizures
Condoms, 603
Condyloma acuminate, 28
Confidentiality. *See* Privacy and confidentiality
Constipation, 636t
Continuous hemofiltration and hemodialysis, 289
Continuous quality improvement (CQI), 35
Continuous veno-venous hemodialysis, 289
Coral snake, 920
Coronary artery disease (CAD), 53–56
Credentialing, 17
Crisis situations, therapeutic relationship and, 14
Crohn's disease, 328–334
Cultural respect, 12
CURB-65 scale, for pneumonia, 126
Cushing's syndrome, 177–179
Cystic fibrosis, 698
Cystine calculi, 265. *See also* Urolithiasis/
    nephrolithiasis
Cystitis, 252. *See also* Urinary tract infections

D

DASH (Dietary Approaches to Stop
    Hypertension), 64
Dawn phenomenon, 153, 160
Death, leading causes of, 634t, 659t
Deceased donor transplant, 717
Deep vein thrombosis (DVT), 83–84
Degenerative joint diseases
    gout, 570–573
    osteoarthritis, 568–570
    rheumatoid arthritis, 563–568, 566–567t
Delirium, 245–247, 594–596, 635, 636t
Dementia, 596–598. *See also* Alzheimer's disease
Depression, 578–582, 636t, 656
Dextrose solutions, 915
Diabetes insipidus, 183–185
Diabetes mellitus, 148
Diabetes mellitus type 1, 148–153, 711–715
Diabetes mellitus type 2
    assessment, 40, 155–156
    description, 154
    differential diagnosis, 156
    etiology, 154
    follow-up, 159–160
    incidence, 148, 155

management, 157–159
prevention and screening, 155, 655
risk factors, 155
special considerations, 159
when to consult, refer, or hospitalize, 159
Diabetic ketoacidosis (DKA), 160–163
Diarrhea
　C. difficile, 877–879
　infectious, 899–903
　intravenous fluids for, 914
Diet and nutrition, 647
Diet in Renal Disease equation, 282
Differential diagnoses, development of, 42–43
Digoxin toxicity, 843–845
Dilated cardiomyopathy, 99–100
Diltiazem overdose/toxicity. See Antiarrhythmic drug overdose/toxicity
Discrimination, 31
Disease prevention
　adult immunizations, 657–658
　adult screening practices, 654–656
　description, 652
　epidemiology principles, 653–654
　influences on, 660
　risk assessment, 658, 659t, 660t
Dislocation, shoulder, 555
Dissecting aneurysm, 104
Disseminated intravascular coagulation (DIC), 425–428
Distributive shock, 728, 731t. See also Shock
Diverticulitis/diverticulosis, 334–338
Dofetilide overdose/toxicity. See Antiarrhythmic drug overdose/toxicity
Drug-induced lupus, 541
Drug overdose/toxicity
　acetaminophen, 349, 352, 810–813
　antiarrhythmics. See Antiarrhythmic drug overdose/toxicity
　anticholinergics, 827–829
　anticonvulsants. See Anticonvulsant agent overdose/toxicity
　antidepressants, 835–838
　antipsychotics, 838–840
　cardiac glycosides, 843–845
　cholinergics, 846–848
　lithium, 848–850
　opioids, 850–853
　salicylates, 855–857
　sedative-hypnotics, 857–860
　stimulants, 860–863
　theophylline, 863–865
Ductal carcinoma in situ (DCIS), 459
Duke criteria, for endocarditis, 108t
Duke staging system, colorectal cancer, 444
Dunphy's sign, 313
Dyslipidemia, 40, 57–61
Dyspnea, 636t, 637t

E

Ebstein-Barr virus, Hodgkin's lymphoma and, 489
Edrophonium test, 202
Elderly. See Older adults
Embolic stroke, 195. See also Stroke
Emphysema, 111, 112. See also Chronic obstructive pulmonary disease
End-of-life care. See also Palliative care
　incidence and demographics, 634, 634t
　special considerations, 644
　symptom management, 636t, 637t, 638t. See also Pain management
　when to consult, refer, or hospitalize, 645
End-stage renal disease/dialysis, 286–290, 707
Enteral feedings, 682–683
Environmental risks, 41
Enzyme-linked immunosorbent assay (ELISA), 511
Epilepsy, 223. See also Seizures
Equal Pay Act of 1963, 31
Esophageal varices, 339–343, 348
Esophagogastroduodenoscopy, 377
Ethanol toxicity, 814–818
Ethics, 19, 21–22
Ethylene glycol toxicity, 814–818
Evidence-based practice, 24
Expiratory reserve volume (ERV), 119t

F

Fast Alcohol Screening Test (FAST), 41
Febrile seizures, 223
Ferritin, 398
Fever
　assessment, 723–725
　description, 720
　differential diagnosis, 725
　etiology, 721–722
　follow-up, 726
　general approach, 719
　incidence and demographics, 722
　management, 725–726
　prevention and screening, 723
　red flags, 720
　risk factors, 723
　special considerations, 726
　when to consult, refer, or hospitalize, 726
Fever of unknown origin (FUO), 722
Flecainide overdose/toxicity. See Antiarrhythmic drug overdose/toxicity
Folic acid deficiency, 399t, 411–413, 667
Food allergies, 516
Food Guide Pyramid, 648
Forced expiratory flow from 25%–75% of the FVC (FEV_{25-75}), 119t
Forced expiratory volume in 1 second (FEV_1), 119t
Forced vital capacity (FVC), 119t
Fractures, 555, 561–562
Functional assessment, 13

Functional residual capacity (FRC), 119t
Fusiform aneurysm, 104

G

Gabapentin overdose/toxicity. See Anticonvulsant agent overdose/toxicity
Gallbladder, malignancy of, 320
Gallstones. See Cholecystitis
Gastric banding, 686
Gastrointestinal alkalosis, 794. See also Metabolic alkalosis
Gastrointestinal bleeding
    assessment, 341–342
    complications, 347–348
    description, 338–339
    diagnostic studies, 342–343
    differential diagnosis, 343
    etiology, 339–340
    expected outcomes, 347
    incidence and demographics, 340
    management, 344–346
    prevention and screening, 341
    risk factors, 340
    special considerations, 346–347
    when to consult, refer, or hospitalize, 347
Generalized tonic-clonic seizure, 226t. See also Seizures
Genital herpes simplex virus (HSV) infection, 625–628
Geriatric patients. See Older adults
Gestational diabetes, 155
Giant cell arteritis, 233
Gleason score, prostate cancer, 460–461
Glomerular filtration rate (GFR), 282
Glomerulonephritis, acute, 298–303
Gonorrhea
    assessment, 611–612
    description, 609
    differential diagnosis, 612
    etiology, 610
    follow-up, 613
    incidence and demographics, 610
    management, 612–613
    prevention and screening, 610, 655
    risk factors, 610
    special considerations, 613
    when to consult, refer, or hospitalize, 613
Goodpasture syndrome, 298–302
Gout, 570–573
G6PD deficiency, 399t
Graves' disease. See Hyperthyroidism
Grief and bereavement, 590–592
Group A β-hemolytic streptococcal (GABHS) pharyngitis, 889–891
Guillain-Barré syndrome, 203–204
Gummas, 620. See also Syphilis

H

H. pylori infection, 375, 377–379
Hairy cell leukemia, 477
Hampton's hump, 133
Hashimoto's thyroiditis, 173. See also Hypothyroidism
Head trauma, 214–216
Headache
    assessment, 232–233
    description, 230–231
    diagnostic studies, 234
    differential diagnosis, 234
    etiology, 231
    follow-up, 240
    incidence and demographics, 232
    management, 235–236
    prevention and screening, 232, 237–239t
    risk factors, 232
    special considerations, 239
Health Insurance Portability and Accountability Act (HIPAA) of 1996, 14, 30
Health promotion, 43
Healthcare financing, 31–33
Healthcare policy, 33–34
Healthcare quality, 34–36
Heart failure (HF), 66–69, 702
Heart transplantation, 701–705
Heberden's nodes, 569
Hemodialysis, 288–289. See also End-stage renal disease/dialysis
Hemoglobin H disease, 419t
Hemolytic anemia(s), 413–416
Hemophilia A, 398
Hemophilia B, 398
Hemorrhage, 728t
Heparin-induced thrombocytopenia, 423–425
Hepatic artery thrombosis (HAT), 696
Hepatitis A, B, C, D, E, and G. See Viral hepatitis
Hepatitis vaccines, 356–357, 657
Herniated disk, 228–230
Herpes simplex virus (HSV) infection, genital, 625–628
Herpes zoster, 232
Heterotropic, 716
HIV/AIDS
    anemia of chronic disease in, 401
    assessment, 508–511
    description, 506
    differential diagnosis, 512
    etiology, 506
    follow-up, 514
    herpes simplex virus infection in, 627
    incidence and demographics, 506–507
    management, 512–513
    opportunistic infections in. See Opportunistic infections

prevention and screening, 507–508, 655
risk factors, 507
special considerations, 513
syphilis in, 624
when to consult, refer, or hospitalize, 513
HIV rapid antibody tests, 511
Hodgkin's lymphoma (disease), 488–493
Hoehn and Young Scale, Parkinson's disease staging, 207
Homeless patient, assessment, 39–40
Horner's syndrome, 433
Hornet sting, 922–923
Hospice. See End-of-life care; Palliative care
Hospital-acquired infections. See Nosocomial infections
Human immunodeficiency virus (HIV). See HIV/AIDS
Human papillomavirus (HPV) infection, 472, 628–631
Human papillomavirus (HPV) vaccines, 473, 603, 629
Hygiene hypothesis, asthma, 116
Hyperbaric oxygen therapy, 842
Hypercalcemia, 765–770
Hypercapnia, 135, 136. See also Respiratory acidosis
Hyperchromic anemia, 398
Hyperglycemia, 162
Hyperkalemia
    assessment, 758–759
    description, 756
    differential diagnosis, 759
    etiology, 756–757
    follow-up, 761
    incidence and demographics, 757
    management, 277, 283–284, 759–760
    prevention and screening, 758
    risk factors, 758
    special considerations, 760
    when to consult, refer, or hospitalize, 760
Hyperlipidemia. See Dyslipidemia
Hypermagnesemia, 774–777
Hypernatremia, 745–749
Hyperosmolar hyperglycemic nonketosis (HHNK), 163–165
Hyperphosphatemia, 782–786
Hypersensitivity reactions, 514–515. See also Allergic reactions, acute
Hypertension
    assessment, 62–63, 62t
    classification, 61t
    description, 61
    differential diagnosis, 63
    etiology, incidence, and demographics, 62
    follow-up, 65
    management, 64
    prevention and screening, 62
    risk factors, 62

screening recommendations, 40
in stroke, 199
when to consult, refer, or hospitalize, 65
Hypertensive emergency, 65
Hypertensive urgency, 65
Hyperthyroidism, 63t, 168–172
Hypertrophic cardiomyopathy, 101–102
Hypocalcemia, 761–765
Hypochromic anemia, 398. See also Iron deficiency anemia
Hypoglycemia, 148, 166–168
Hypokalemia, 750–755
Hypomagnesemia, 770–774
Hyponatremia
    assessment, 739–742
    description, 737
    differential diagnosis, 742
    etiology, 737, 738t
    follow-up, 745
    incidence and demographics, 738
    management, 742–744
    prevention and screening, 739
    risk factors, 738–739
    special considerations, 744
    when to consult, refer, or hospitalize, 745
Hypophosphatemia, 777–781
Hypothyroidism, 172–176
Hypovolemic shock, 728, 728t, 731t. See also Shock
Hypoxemia, 135, 136

I

Ibutilide overdose/toxicity. See Antiarrhythmic drug overdose/toxicity
Ideal body weight (IBW), 647, 648t
Idiopathic pulmonary fibrosis, 698
Idiopathic thrombocytopenia purpura (ITP), 421–423
IgA deficiency, 548
IgA nephropathy glomerulonephritis, 299–302
Immobility, 905–908
Immunodeficiency disorders
    acquired, 547–548
    assessment, 549
    complications, 550
    congenital, 546–547
    description, 545–546
    differential diagnosis, 549
    etiology, 546
    expected course, 550
    incidence and demographics, 548
    management, 550
    prevention and screening, 548
    risk factors, 548
    special considerations, 550
    when to consult, refer, or hospitalize, 550
Immunosuppressive agents

for heart transplantation, 705
for liver transplantation, 695
for lung transplantation, 699
opportunistic infections and. See Opportunistic infections
for pancreas transplantation, 714
for rejection prophylaxis, 716
for rejection treatment, 717
Incidence rates, 653
Increased intracranial pressure (ICP), 200, 215
Infantile spasms, 223
Infections
community-acquired. See Community-acquired infections
nosocomial. See Nosocomial infections
opportunistic. See Opportunistic infections
respiratory. See Respiratory infections
Infectious diarrhea, 899–903
Inferior vena caval filter, 134
Inflammatory breast cancer, 458–459
Influenza vaccine, 658
Informed consent, 23
Institute for Healthcare Improvement (IHI), 36
Intracerebral hemorrhage, 195. See also Stroke
Intravascular device infections, 874–877
Intravenous fluids, 911–915
Iron deficiency anemia, 399t, 405–408, 406t
Ischemic stroke, 195. See also Stroke
Isograft, 716

J
Jarisch-Herxheimer reaction, 624
The Joint Commission, 35–36

K
Kerley's lines, 67
Kernig's sign, 221
Kidney failure
acute. See Acute kidney injury/acute renal failure
chronic. See Chronic kidney disease/chronic kidney failure
Kidney transplantation, 706–710
Knee injury, acute, 556–558, 559t
Kwashiorkor, 673

L
Lachman test, 559t
Lacunar infarcts, 195. See also Stroke
Lamotrigine overdose/toxicity. See Anticonvulsant agent overdose/toxicity
Large bowel obstruction, 363–366
Lateral collateral ligament (LCL) injury, 558
Lead poisoning, 406t
Leukemias, 477–481
Levetiracetam overdose/toxicity. See Anticonvulsant agent overdose/toxicity

Lhermitte syndrome, 494
Licensed independent practitioner (LIP), 26
Lidocaine overdose/toxicity. See Antiarrhythmic drug overdose/toxicity
Lipodystrophy, 153
Lithium toxicity, 848–850
Liver disease
acute. See Acute hepatic failure
chronic. See Cirrhosis/chronic liver disease
Liver transplantation, 327, 693–697
Living donor transplant, 717
Lobular carcinoma in situ (LCIS), 459
Löfgren's syndrome, 529
Lung cancer
assessment, 432–437
description, 430–431
differential diagnosis, 437
etiology, 431
follow-up, 440–441
incidence and demographics, 431
management, 437–439
prevention and screening, 432
risk factors, 432
special considerations, 439–440
staging workup, 434–436
when to consult, refer, or hospitalize, 440
Lung transplantation, 697–701
Lung volumes, 119t
Lupus pernio, 529
Lymphogranuloma venereum. See Chlamydia
Lymphoma. See Hodgkin's lymphoma (disease); Non-Hodgkin's lymphoma
Lynch II syndrome, 470

M
Macrocytic anemia, 398
Major depressive disorder, 578–580, 581
Malnutrition. See Nutritional imbalances
Malpractice, 26–27
Mammography, 40, 450, 453, 655
Managed care organization, 32–33
Marasmus, 672
Masked facies, 206
Mastectomy, 455
Maximum voluntary ventilation (MVV), 119t
McMurray test, 559t
Mean corpuscular cell volume (MCV), 398
Measles, mumps, and rubella (MMR) immunization, 657
Medial collateral ligament (MCL) injury, 557
Medicaid, 32
Medical futility, 23
Medical staff bylaws, 26
Medicare, 32
Medication overuse headache, 231
Megaloblastic anemia(s), 398
folic acid deficiency, 411–413

vitamin B$_{12}$ deficiency. *See* Vitamin B$_{12}$ deficiency
Melanoma
    assessment, 496–499
    description, 494–495
    differential diagnosis, 499
    etiology, 495
    follow-up, 501–502
    incidence and demographics, 495
    management, 499–500
    prevention and screening, 496
    risk factors, 495
    special considerations, 500–501
    staging, 496–498
    when to consult, refer, or hospitalize, 501
Meningitis, 219–223
Meningococcal vaccination, 220
Meniscus tear, 557
Mesenteric ischemia, 366–370
Metabolic acidosis
    assessment, 790–791
    description, 787, 788
    differential diagnosis, 791
    etiology, 788–789
    follow-up, 793
    incidence and demographics, 790
    management, 791–792
    prevention and screening, 790
    risk factors, 790
    special considerations, 792
    when to consult, refer, or hospitalize, 792
Metabolic alkalosis
    assessment, 795
    description, 787, 793
    differential diagnosis, 796
    etiology, 793–794
    follow-up, 797
    management, 796
    prevention and screening, 795
    risk factors, 794–795
    special considerations, 796
    when to consult, refer, or hospitalize, 796–797
Methanol toxicity, 814–818
Mexiletine overdose/toxicity. *See* Antiarrhythmic drug overdose/toxicity
Microcytic anemia(s), 398, 406t
Migraine
    assessment, 233
    description, 231
    etiology, 231
    follow-up, 240
    incidence and demographics, 232
    management, 235–236, 237–237t
    risk factors, 232
    special considerations, 239
    when to consult, refer, or hospitalize, 239

Mini-Mental State Examination (MMSE), 242
Mitral regurgitation (MR), 70–72
Mitral stenosis (MS), 72–74
Mitral valve prolapse (MVP), 74–75
Model for End-Stage Liver Disease (MELD), 326t, 692
Monoamine oxidase inhibitors (MAOIs), 581, 835–838
Monroe–Kelley doctrine, head trauma, 215
Multi-infarct dementia (MID), 240–242, 597
Multiple sclerosis (MS), 211–214
Mushroom poisoning, 352
Myasthenia gravis, 201–203
Myerson's sign, 206
Myocardial infarction. *See* Acute coronary syndrome
Myxedema coma, 176

N

Narrow complex supraventricular tachycardia, 89–90
National Cholesterol Education Program (NCEP), 654
National Patient Safety Goals, Joint Commission, 35–36
Nausea and vomiting, 638t
Negligence, 23
Neisseria gonorrhoeae. *See* Gonorrhea
Neonatal seizures, 223
Nephrogenic diabetes insipidus, 183
Nephrolithiasis, 262. *See also* Urolithiasis/nephrolithiasis
Nephrotic syndrome, 303–306
Neurosyphilis. *See* Syphilis
Niacin deficiency, 666, 668
Nifedipine overdose/toxicity. *See* Antiarrhythmic drug overdose/toxicity
Non-Hodgkin's lymphoma
    assessment, 484–485
    description, 481
    differential diagnosis, 485
    etiology, 481–482
    follow-up, 487–488
    incidence and demographics, 482
    management, 485–487
    prevention and screening, 482
    special considerations, 487
    staging, 483–484
    when to consult, refer, or hospitalize, 487
Non-ST-elevation myocardial infarction (NSTEMI). *See* Acute coronary syndrome
Non–small cell lung cancer (NSCLC). *See also* Lung cancer
    description, 430–431
    management, 438–439
    staging, 434–436

Normocytic anemia(s), 398
    anemia of chronic disease, 399–401
    aplastic anemia, 402–404
Nosocomial infections
    antibiotic-resistant, 880–882
    C. difficile, 877–879
    pneumonia, 127–129, 867–870
    vascular access and monitoring–related, 874–877
    wound infections, 871–874
Nurse practitioners. See also Acute care nurse practitioner (ACNP)
    demographics, 26
    educational requirements, 25
    prescriptive authority, 19–20
    regulation, 16–17, 19–20
    scope and standards of practice, 16, 25–26
Nutritional imbalances
    assessment, 670–677
    description, 663–664
    diagnostic studies, 677–680
    differential diagnosis, 680–681
    etiology, 665–667
    follow-up, 688
    incidence and demographics, 668–669
    management, 681–687
    prevention and screening, 670
    risk factors, 669–670
    special considerations, 687
    when to consult, refer, or hospitalize, 688
Nutritional supplements, 649

O

Obesity
    assessment, 670–671, 673
    complications, 688
    description, 40, 664
    diagnostic studies, 678
    differential diagnosis, 680
    etiology, 665
    incidence and demographics, 668
    management, 685–686
    risk factors, 669–670
Obstructive shock, 728, 731t. See also Shock
Obturator sign, 313
Ogilvie intestinal pseudo-obstruction, 440
OLDCARTS, for symptom attributes, 638
Older adults
    anticholinergic side effects in, 210
    antihistamines in, 520
    appendicitis in, 315
    assessment, 39
    asymptomatic bacteriuria in, 261
    corticosteroid side effects in, 520
    diverticulitis/diverticulosis in, 337
    headache treatment in, 239
    hypernatremia in, 747
    hyperthyroidism in, 171
    hypoglycemia in, 168
    hypothyroidism in, 175
    neurologic disorders in, 194
    Parkinson's disease treatment, 210
    urinary tract infection in, 255, 259
Opioids, 639–640, 641t, 850–852
Opportunistic infections
    assessment, 884–885
    description, 882
    differential diagnosis, 885
    etiology/risk factors, 882–883
    follow-up, 886
    incidence and demographics, 883
    management, 885–886
    prevention and screening, 884
    special considerations, 886
    when to consult, refer, or hospitalize, 886
Organ transplantation. See also specific organs
    complications, 696–697
    opportunistic infections and. See Opportunistic infections
    rejection in, 701, 704, 709
    terminology, 716
    types, 717
Organophosphate poisoning, 853–854
Orthotopic, 716
Osteoarthritis, 568–570
Osteoporosis, 40, 43, 656
Ovarian cancer, 469–472
Overdose. See Drug overdose/toxicity

P

Paget's carcinoma of the breast, 458
Pain, 638, 639t
Pain management
    analgesic groups, 641t
    ineffective, adverse outcomes of, 641
    nonpharmacologic, 640
    opioids for, 639–640, 641t
    patient-controlled analgesia, 640
    principles, 640
    WHO analgesic ladder, 642–644t, 642f
Palliative care, 633–635, 636t, 637t
Pancoast's syndrome, 433
Pancreas transplantation, 711–715
Pancreatitis, acute, 370–375, 373t
Pap smear, 40, 655
Paraneoplastic syndromes, 430, 434
Parkinson's disease
    assessment, 205–206
    description, 205
    differential diagnosis, 207
    etiology, 205
    follow-up, 210
    incidence and demographics, 205
    management, 207–210, 208–209t

prevention and screening, 205
risk factors, 205
special considerations, 210
staging, 207
when to consult, refer, or hospitalize, 210
Parkland formula, 914
Patient advocate, ACNP as, 14
Patient-controlled analgesia (PCA), 640
Patient education, 44, 49
Peak expiratory flow rate (PEFR), 119t
Pelvic inflammatory disease (PID), 609, 613
Peptic ulcer disease, 375–380, 380t
Percutaneous coronary intervention, 56
Pericarditis, 94–96
Peripheral arterial disease (PAD), 80
Peripheral vascular disease (PVD), 80–82
Peritoneal dialysis, 289
Peritonitis, 380–386
Pesticide poisoning, 853–854
Phalloides mushroom, 352
Pharyngitis, 887–891
Phenytoin overdose/toxicity. See Anticonvulsant agent overdose/toxicity
Pheochromocytoma, 63t, 188–191
Physical abuse, 575–578
Physical activity, 649–650
Pit viper, 919–920
Plan of care
consultation and referrals, 50
cost-effectiveness, 49
dynamic nature of, 47–48
follow-up, 50
nonpharmacologic treatment, 48
nursing process framework, 45
patient factors in, 46
patient teaching in, 49
pharmacologic treatment, 48
prevention and screening in, 47
Pleural effusion, 142–144
Pneumococcal vaccine, 125, 658
Pneumonia
community-acquired, 124–126
nosocomial (hospital-acquired/ventilator-associated), 127–129, 867–871
Pneumothorax, 140–142
Poisoning, 807–809. See also Drug overdose/toxicity
alcohol, 814–817
carbon monoxide, 841–843
pesticide, 853–854
Polycystic kidney disease, 306–309
Polypharmacy, 43
Posterior cruciate ligament (PCL) injury, 558
Posterior drawer test, 559t
Poststreptococcal glomerulonephritis, 889
Powerlessness, 593–594
Pregnancy

allergies in, 520
appendicitis in, 315
asymptomatic bacteriuria in, 261
breast cancer during, 459
gonorrhea in, 614
herpes simplex virus infection in, 627
misoprostol avoidance in, 380
sexually transmitted infections in, 604
syphilis in, 623, 624
ulcerative colitis in, 394
urinary tract infection in, 255, 259
Prerenal azotemia, 296t
Pressure ulcers, 929–931
Prevalence rates, 653
Primary aldosteronism, 63t
Primary prevention, 652
Primary T cell immunodeficiency, 550
Privacy and confidentiality, 12, 14, 30
Procainamide overdose/toxicity. See Antiarrhythmic drug overdose/toxicity
Propafenone overdose/toxicity. See Antiarrhythmic drug overdose/toxicity
Propionibacter acnes, 528
Prostate cancer, 460–465, 656
Prostatectomy, 269
Protein-energy malnutrition (PEM)
assessment, 670, 672–673
complications, 688
description, 664
diagnostic studies, 677–678
etiology, 665
incidence and demographics, 668
risk factors, 669
Psoas sign, 313
Psychosis, 599–600
Pulmonary embolism, 132–134
Pulmonary function tests (PFTs), 119t
Pulmonary hypertension, 85–87
Purified protein derivative (PPD), 130
Pyelonephritis, acute, 252, 256–259

Q

Quality improvement (QI) processes, 34–35
Quinidine overdose/toxicity. See Antiarrhythmic drug overdose/toxicity

R

Radiocontrast exposure, 273, 275
Ranson's criteria, for acute pancreatitis, 373, 373t
Rapport, establishing, 12
Raynaud's phenomenon, 533, 538
Red blood cell (RBC) studies, 398t
Red cell distribution width (RDW), 398
Reed-Sternberg cell, 489
Renal alkalosis, 794. See also Metabolic alkalosis
Renal artery stenosis (RAS), 290–293
Renal failure

acute. *See* Acute kidney injury/acute renal failure
chronic. *See* Chronic kidney disease/chronic kidney failure
Renal osteodystrophy, 284
Renal transplantation, 706–710
Research methods, 24
Residual volume (RV), 119t
Respiratory acidosis
    assessment, 799–800
    description, 787, 797
    differential diagnosis, 800
    etiology, 797–798
    follow-up, 802
    incidence and demographics, 798
    management, 800–801
    prevention and screening, 799
    risk factors, 798–799
    special considerations, 801
    when to consult, refer, or hospitalize, 801
Respiratory alkalosis
    assessment, 803–804
    description, 787–788, 802
    differential diagnosis, 804
    etiology, 802
    follow-up, 805
    incidence and demographics, 803
    management, 804–805
    prevention and screening, 803
    risk factors, 803
    special considerations, 805
    when to consult, refer, or hospitalize, 805
Respiratory failure, acute, 135–137
Respiratory infections
    community-acquired pneumonia, 124–126
    hospital-acquired and ventilator-associated pneumonia, 127–129, 867–870
    tuberculosis, 129–132
Resting energy expenditure (REE), 663
Restrictive cardiomyopathy, 102–104
Rheumatoid arthritis, 563–568, 566–567t
Riboflavin deficiency. *See* Vitamin deficiencies
RIFLE criteria, renal failure, 271
Risk assessment, 41–42, 45–46
Risk management, 23
Rolandic epilepsy, 223
Rotator cuff tear, 555
Rovsing sign, 313

S

Saccular aneurysm, 104
Safety, 651
Salicylate toxicity, 855–857
Saline solutions, 915
Sarcoidosis, 527–531
Scarlet fever, 889
Scleroderma (systemic sclerosis)
    assessment, 534–538
    description, 532–533
    differential diagnosis, 538
    etiology, 533
    follow-up, 539
    incidence and demographics, 534
    management, 538
    prevention and screening, 534
    risk factors, 534
    special considerations, 539
    when to consult, refer, or hospitalize, 539
Sclerotherapy, 348
Scorpion sting, 922
Secondarily generalized seizure, 226t. *See also* Seizures
Secondary headache, 231, 236
Secondary prevention, 652
Sedative-hypnotic drug toxicity, 857–860
Seizures, 223–228, 226t
Selective serotonin reuptake inhibitors (SSRIs), 581, 835–838
Sentinel lymph node dissection, 455
Serotonin-norepinephrine reuptake inhibitors (SNRIs), 581
Severe combined immunodeficiency, 550
Sexual assault, 604
Sexuality, 592
Sexually transmitted infections (STIs), 603, 655. *See also* specific infections
Shock
    assessment, 730–733, 731t
    classification, 727
    description, 726–727
    differential diagnosis, 733
    etiology, 728, 728t
    follow-up, 734
    general approach, 719
    incidence and demographics, 729
    management, 733–734
    prevention and screening, 729
    red flags, 720
    risk factors, 729
    special considerations, 734
    stages, 727
    when to consult, refer, or hospitalize, 734
Shoulder pain, 553–556
Sickle cell anemia, 141 416, 399t
Sickle cell trait, 414
Sideroblastic anemia, 399t
Simple partial seizure, 226t. *See also* Seizures
Sinusitis, 891–895
Slowed vital capacity (SVC), 119t
Small bowel obstruction, 387–390
Small cell lung cancer, 437–438. *See also* Lung cancer
Snake bites, 919–920
Somogyi effect, 153, 160

Sotalol overdose/toxicity. See Antiarrhythmic drug overdose/toxicity
Spider bites, 921
Spinal cord trauma, 216–218
Spirometry, 119t
Spontaneous pneumothorax, 140–142
ST-elevation myocardial infarction (STEMI). See Acute coronary syndrome
Status epilepticus, 228
Stimulant toxicity, 860–863
Stress management, 651–652
Stroke
    assessment, 196–197
    description, 194
    diagnostic studies, 197
    differential diagnosis, 197
    etiology, 195
    follow-up, 200–201
    incidence and demographics, 195
    management, 198–200
    prevention and screening, 196
    risk factors, 195
    special considerations, 200
    when to consult, refer, or hospitalize, 200
Struvite calculi, 265. See also Urolithiasis/nephrolithiasis
Study plan, for certification examination, 3–5
Subarachnoid hemorrhage, 195, 199. See also Stroke
Subjective Global Assessment (SGA), 41
Substance abuse, 41, 584–588. See also Alcoholism
Suicidal ideation, 582
Superior vena cava syndrome, 440
Surgical patients, risk assessment, 41–42
Surgical wound infections, 871–874
Syndrome of inappropriate diuretic hormone (SIADH), 186–188, 740, 743–744
Syphilis
    assessment, 617–620
    description, 615
    diagnostic studies, 621–622
    differential diagnosis, 622–623
    etiology, 615
    follow-up, 624–625
    incidence and demographics, 615–616
    management, 623
    prevention and screening, 616–617, 655
    risk factors, 616
    special considerations, 624
    when to consult, refer, or hospitalize, 624
Systemic inflammatory response syndrome (SIRS), 729
Systemic lupus erythematosus (SLE)
    assessment, 542–543
    description, 539–540
    differential diagnosis, 544
    etiology, 540–541
    follow-up, 545
    incidence and demographics, 541
    management, 544
    prevention and screening, 541
    risk factors, 541
    special considerations, 545
    when to consult, refer, or hospitalize, 545
Systemic sclerosis. See Scleroderma

T

Tabes dorsalis, 618, 620
Tensilon (edrophonium) test, 202
Tension headache, 231–233, 235, 240
Tension pneumothorax, 140–142, 731
Tertiary prevention, 652
Testicular cancer screening, 656
Tetanus, diphtheria, and pertussis immunization, 657
Thalassemia
    assessment, 399t, 406t, 418, 419t
    description, 417
    differential diagnosis, 406t, 418
    etiology, 417
    follow-up, 420
    incidence and demographics, 417
    management, 419–420
    prevention and screening, 418
    risk factors, 417
    special considerations, 420
    when to consult, refer, or hospitalize, 420
Theophylline toxicity, 863–865
Therapeutic diets, 685
Therapeutic relationships. See also Plan of care
    advance care planning in, 13
    collaboration in, 15
    components, 11–12
    crisis situations and, 14
    holistic perspective, 12–13
    patient autonomy and, 15
    privacy and confidentiality, 14
    rapport in, 12
    strategies for establishing, 12
Thiamine deficiency. See Vitamin deficiencies
Thyroid disorders
    hyperthyroidism. See Hyperthyroidism
    hypothyroidism. See Hypothyroidism
    myxedema coma, 176
    thyroid storm, 172
Thyroid storm, 172
Thyrotoxicosis. See Hyperthyroidism
Tiagabine overdose/toxicity. See Anticonvulsant agent overdose/toxicity
Time management, 17
Title VII of the Civil Rights Act of 1964, 31
TNM staging

bladder cancer, 467
breast cancer, 451–452
cervical cancer, 474
lung cancer, 434–436
melanoma, 496–497
overview, 428–429
prostate cancer, 462
Tobacco use, 41
Tophi, 572
Topiramate overdose/toxicity. *See* Anticonvulsant agent overdose/toxicity
Total body water (TBW), 911–912
Total iron binding capacity (TIBC), 398
Total lung capacity (TLC), 119t
Total parenteral nutrition (TPN), 683–685
Total quality management (TQM), 35
Transient ischemic attack (TIA), 194, 195, 198. *See also* Stroke
Transplantation. *See* Organ transplantation
Transtubular K⁺ gradient (TTKG), 753
Trauma
    ankle, 559–561
    fractures, 561–562
    knee, 556–558, 559t
    shoulder, 553–556
Traumatic brain injury, 214–216
Tremor, 206, 210
Treponema pallidum. *See* Syphilis
Tricyclic antidepressants (TCAs), 581, 835–838
Trousseau's sign, 763
Tuberculosis (TB), 129–132

U

Ulcerative colitis, 390–395
Ulcers
    arterial, 928, 930
    assessment, 927–930
    diabetic, 928, 930, 931
    diagnostic studies, 930
    etiology, 926
    follow-up, 931
    incidence and demographics, 926
    management, 930–931
    pressure, 929–931
    prevention and screening, 926
    risk factors, 926
    venous, 929, 930
    when to consult, refer, or hospitalize, 931
United States Preventive Services Task Force (USPSTF), 654
Unrelated donor transplant, 717
Unstable angina. *See* Acute coronary syndrome
Ureteral stones, 265. *See also* Urolithiasis/nephrolithiasis
Urethritis, 252. *See also* Urinary tract infections
    gonococcal. *See* Gonorrhea
    nongonococcal. *See* Chlamydia

Uric acid calculi, 265. *See also* Urolithiasis/nephrolithiasis
Urinary tract infections, 252–256
Urolithiasis/nephrolithiasis, 262–266
Urticaria, 517

V

Valgus stress test, 559t
Valproic acid overdose/toxicity. *See* Anticonvulsant agent overdose/toxicity
Valvular disease
    aortic regurgitation, 78–79
    aortic stenosis, 76–77
    mitral regurgitation, 70–72
    mitral stenosis, 72–74
    mitral valve prolapse, 74–75
Varicella immunization, 657
Varus stress test, 559t
Venous thromboembolism, 83
Venous ulcers, 929, 930
Ventilator-associated pneumonia (VAP), 127–129, 867–871
Ventricular fibrillation, 91–92
Ventricular tachycardia, 90–91
Verapamil overdose/toxicity. *See* Antiarrhythmic drug overdose/toxicity
Vigabatrin overdose/toxicity. *See* Anticonvulsant agent overdose/toxicity
Violence, 575–578
Viral hepatitis
    assessment, 357–358
    complications, 363
    description, 353–354
    diagnostic studies, 358–360
    differential diagnosis, 361
    etiology, 354–355
    expected outcomes, 363
    incidence and demographics, 355
    management, 361–362
    prevention and screening, 356–357, 657
    risk factors, 356, 692
    special considerations, 362
    when to consult, refer, or hospitalize, 362
Viral meningitis, 219. *See also* Meningitis
Virchow's triad, 132
Vitamin B_{12} deficiency, 399t, 408–411, 666, 679
Vitamin deficiencies
    assessment, 671–672, 673–677
    diagnostic studies, 678–680
    differential diagnosis, 680–681
    etiology, 667–668
    incidence and demographics, 668–669
    management, 686–687
    risk factors, 670

W

Wasp sting, 922–923
Water deprivation test, 184
Westermark's sign, 133
Western blot, 511
WHO analgesic ladder, 642–644t, 642f
Wound(s). *See also* Ulcers
    acute, 925
    assessment, 927–928
    chronic, 925–926
    diagnostic studies, 930
    infections, 871–874
    management, 930–931

X

Xenograft, 716

Y

Yellow jacket sting, 922–923

Z

Zollinger-Ellison syndrome, 377
Zonisamide overdose/toxicity. *See* Anticonvulsant
    agent overdose/toxicity

About the Authors

Pamela Ann Smith, MSN, RN, ACNP-BC, CCRN, received her undergraduate degree in nursing from California State University, Hayward in 1988 and a Master of Science in Nursing in the Acute Care Nurse Practitioner program from the University of Texas Medical Branch, Galveston, Texas in 2005. Her nursing experience has been primarily in adult critical care. She is currently employed as a cardiology nurse practitioner at Memorial Hermann Hospital–The Medical Center, Houston, Texas. In addition, she is the course coordinator for the Acute Care Nurse Practitioner Program at the University of Texas Health Science Center, San Antonio, Texas. She is currently enrolled at Texas Tech University in the Doctor of Nursing degree program and will graduate with the 2013 cohort.

Tiffany Boysen, MSN, APRN-BC, CCRN, received her undergraduate degree in nursing from University of Texas Medical Branch (UTMB) in Galveston, Texas. She continued her studies at UTMB and received a master's degree in nursing with an adult acute care focus. Tiffany is currently employed as an Acute Care Nurse Practitioner at the Memorial Hermann Heart and Vascular Institute located in the Texas Medical Center, Houston, Texas.

Julie A. Davey, MSN, RN, ANP-BC, ACNP-BC, is a 2001 graduate of Emory University's Adult/Acute Care Nurse Practitioner program. She has practiced as a nurse practitioner within the field of cardiovascular and internal medicine for the past 10 years. Julie is involved in the education of acute care and adult/gerontology nurse practitioner students and has been a faculty member at Emory University Nell Hodgson Woodruff School of Nursing since 2003. She also has experience as a text reviewer for books, including *Acute Care Protocols, Interpreting Diagnostics,* and *Advanced Practice Nursing for Older Adults in Acute Care*.

Additional experience includes developing newsletters for Practicing Clinicians Exchange and the development of online critical care learning modules for NICHE: Nurses Improving Care for Healthsystem Elders. Julie has spoken at national conferences and taught the acute care nurse practitioner review course for ANCC.

Hope Moser, DNP, ANP, BC, is an assistant professor in the Department of Acute and Continuing Care at the University of Texas, Houston School of Nursing. Moser earned her Doctor of Nursing Science (DNP) degree at Robert Morris University in Pittsburgh, PA. She completed dual MSNs in the Adult and the Women's Health Nurse Practitioner programs at the University of Pittsburgh in 2005, and her BSN at Pennsylvania's Waynesburg College in 2001. In 2009, she was voted on of "20 Outstanding Nurses" by the Texas Nurses Association (Dist. 9) for her work at Methodist Hospital.

Melanie Smith, MSN, ACNP-BC, received her undergraduate degree in nursing from the University of Illinois at Chicago (UIC). She gained clinical experience as a staff nurse at Carle Foundation Hospital in Champaign, Illinois, in the surgical intensive care unit of this Level One trauma center and then transitioned to the cardiovascular ICU, where she developed a deep affection for all things cardiac. She credits an environment of learning, leadership, collaboration, and critical thinking fostered by both physician and nursing colleagues in those ICUs for inspiring her to continue her formal education. After returning to UIC to earn a master's in nursing as an acute care nurse practitioner, she entered practice with a challenging cardiothoracic and vascular surgery service. She is now in practice in Houston, Texas as a unit-based nurse practitioner on a cardiovascular step down unit at The Methodist Hospital in Houston's Medical Center. A self-proclaimed CV surgery "junkie," she is involved in numerous hospital initiatives to improve the quality of patient care for CV surgery patients. She enjoys supporting the teaching and research needs of the hospital and precepting NP students and new nurse practitioners. She also still finds clinical practice incredibly fulfilling. Entering her 11th year of practice as an NP, she anticipates adding DNP to her credentials within the next 2 years, followed by formal teaching and clinical research focused on the role of the hospital-based NP.

Made in the USA
Lexington, KY
11 June 2016